WHAT PEOPLE ARE SA

THE CHI OF C

'If anyone is skeptical about the therapeutic power of hypnosis, this book will remove all doubts! It is an impressive work and I highly recommend it.'
Dr Walter E. Jacobson, M.D. Psychiatrist. Author of the #1 Best-Seller 'Forgive to Win'

'This fascinating book fuses the beauty of traditional thought with a modern, profound understanding of the mind and of the human spirit. Written in a style that is both timeless and fresh, 'The Chi of Change' *transcends cultures and speaks to the universal human experience.'*
Dr Richard Connolly, University of Birmingham

'Peter Field writes with rare insight into the human condition, yet does so in a way that will resonate with both reader and clinician. 'The Chi of Change' *is a major contribution to the field of hypnotherapy and indeed, psychotherapy as a whole. This work deserves a place in every therapist's library.'*
Antoine Matarasso, National President, Australian Hypnotherapists Association

'Full of insight and inspiration. It's rare for a book to impress me these days, but this one did it! A most extraordinary book.'
Terrence Watts, Chairman, Association for Professional Hypnosis & Psychotherapy. Author of 'Warriors, Settlers and Nomads'

'Synthesizes Eastern and Western insights to help people liberate themselves from profound challenges. 'The Chi of Change' *combines psychological understandings with compassion and supercharged*

hypnotherapy. I highly recommend this book!'
Jack Elias, Director, American Institute for Therapeutic Learning. Author of 'Finding the Magic: Transpersonal Hypnosis & Hypnotherapy/NLP'

'A valuable source of information for the experienced hypnotherapist, and highly recommended for any practitioner of hypnosis and/or NLP who wants a better success rate for clients.'
Roy Hunter, Best-Selling Author of 'The Art of Hypnotherapy'

'A fresh and provocative look at the difficulties in dealing with change.'
Dr Richard Harte, Director of Education, National Guild of Hypnotists, U.S.A.

'A wealth of knowledge that strides seamlessly through the extraordinary. This book is a treasure for anyone interested in the mind.'
Dr Marie Cheour, Neuropsychologist

'Using fascinating factual accounts of people he has treated, the author reveals the wonderful transformational potential of therapeutic hypnosis. 'The Chi of Change' *is a significant contribution to both our understanding of hypnotherapy and to the elevation of its status as a serious psychological intervention. An extraordinary book, by a gifted therapist.'*
William Broom, Chief Executive, U.K. General Hypnotherapy Standards Council

'The Chi of Change' *is a book authored by someone who has lived. It is a work full of compassion and one that reflects a love for humanity. In my opinion, it is a book that should be required reading for every therapist and for anyone contemplating therapy.'*
Dr F. S. Starr, M.D. FAACAP, BCIA, Psychiatrist

The Chi of Change

How hypnotherapy can help you rapidly heal and turn your life around – regardless of your past

The Chi of Change

How hypnotherapy can help you rapidly heal and turn your life around – regardless of your past

Peter Field, MA, CH, MBACP, FRSH

PSYCHE BOOKS

Winchester, UK
Washington, USA

First published by Psyche Books, 2014
Psyche Books is an imprint of John Hunt Publishing Ltd., Laurel House, Station Approach,
Alresford, Hants, SO24 9JH, UK
office1@jhpbooks.net
www.johnhuntpublishing.com
www.psyche-books.com

For distributor details and how to order please visit the 'Ordering' section on our website.

ISBN: 978 1 78279 351 9

A CIP catalogue record for this book is available from the British Library.

Design: Stuart Davies

The names, identifying details, and histories of the people whose stories appear in this book have been altered and condensed to preserve their privacy and protect their confidentiality.

Important Note

This book is not intended as a replacement for
medical advice or treatment.
Any person with a condition requiring medical
or psychological attention should consult a qualified
medical practitioner or suitable therapist.

Printed and bound by CPI Group (UK) Ltd, Croydon, CR0 4YY

CONTENTS

The Chi of Change

'The purpose of life is to kindle a flame of meaning in the darkness of mere existence.'

Carl Jung

In memory of my mother, Doris Field

Acknowledgements

There are so many people who have gone into the making of this book. To begin, I want to thank all of my clients, the people I have had the privilege of working with and who have taught me so much over the course of the years. Without them there would be no book, and my life would have taken a very different, and I am quite sure, a less fulfilling course.

Particular thanks are due to my editor, Jessi Hoffman, who worked so hard in ironing out incongruences and correcting my many errors—in thinking as well as in syntax. Without her valuable help this book would not have been nearly as cohesive or as readable as it is.

Though I thanked him while alive, I would again like to acknowledge and express my appreciation to the late Tom Brightmore for his helpful suggestions and comments on the early draft of this book. His logical mind and critical ability have made *The Chi of Change* more accessible and have undoubtedly improved its flow and coherence. Your flame shone brightly, Tom, and I thank you for the gift of your friendship.

Thanks are also due to my lifelong friend and companion Danielle Lalande, who has supported, encouraged, and believed in me for so many years, and who read the book through as it progressed in manuscript form, making many helpful suggestions. Her steadfast support and thoughtful feedback has added so much to my life, immeasurably enriching both it and this book.

I owe an enormous debt of gratitude to Dr F. S. Starr for reading my book and generously writing such a perceptive and helpful foreword.

Last but far from least, I want to thank Xinqi Ren, my veritable right hand, for patiently supporting me throughout the writing of this book, as well as in life, and for providing me with all the encouragement a therapist, or a person, could possibly need.

Foreword

As a psychiatrist, it is hard to ignore the abysmal failure of the mental health system in its contemporary form. In so many ways it has become a self-obsessed industry overflowing with diagnoses, labels, and medications.

Sadly, mental health has evolved into an industry that is more and more detached from people and their environment, something clinically distanced from the individual's own unique life journey. Little wonder that, so often, our standard treatments simply end in failure.

In so much of psychiatry, as it is largely practiced today, there does not seem to be any emphasis on real and lasting change—merely on the treatment of symptoms. As doctors, we are confronted with an endless barrage of advertising designed to promote the newest medication, the latest chemical solution.

In psychology, too, almost every other day there seems to be a new spin on therapy, a different method of improving a person's life. Yet still people remain stuck, firmly entrenched in the problems and difficulties that have led them to the doctor, the psychiatrist, and the therapist.

Your local bookstore is literally teeming with books about losing weight, getting the relationship you want, ending depression, and changing your brain. Yet self-help books are so often directed at your pocketbook and not really at your mind, body, or spirit.

The Chi of Change is different. Here is a book that is genuinely concerned with and directed at the human mind and spirit. It is a book about people and for people, one that addresses the multifaceted individual and his or her many planes of existence.

The author, Peter Field, writes from the perspective of a world traveler and keen observer of human psychology. In the spirit of Carl Jung and Joseph Campbell, he has studied the teachings and understandings of foreign cultures in order to broaden and deepen his understanding of the human psyche. It is this understanding that he brings to the therapy he practices, to the process of change, and to life.

According to *The Chi of Change*, healthy living can be accomplished through harmony with your chi—the 'life force' based on energy and information that is inherent in all that lives and which is manifested in those things that we human beings call 'feelings'.

This book explains how the events in our lives that affect—and to such a large extent determine—our 'reality' get encoded deep down in our memory systems where they are not usually accessible by ordinary therapeutic means. Because this encoding happens at the subconscious level of the mind, we simply cannot access this material in our normal, waking state.

In *The Chi of* Change Peter Field confronts the disturbing issues in mental health today and draws original conclusions and practical observations, both from his work and from his own life, providing an innovative and useful strategy for engaging with the forces (or chi) of change. In so doing he provides us with an important new approach to mental and emotional healing.

The best therapists I have met are able to transcend their training. These therapists are willing to constantly learn, grow, and update their craft. It is rare to find a therapist who has fine-tuned their craft to the degree that they can relate that knowledge in a clear and approachable manner. Peter Field has done this. In *The Chi of Change* you will read about how people can rebound from lives filled with such disturbing states as anxiety, panic, depression, addiction, and over-eating. You will learn how even your most difficult feelings and emotions can be used in order to move forward in a much more balanced, meaningful, and human manner.

As brain-imaging technology and developments in pharmacology continue to vie for and receive media attention and money, the blessed act of assisting an individual through his or her stages of change is becoming a lost art. Medication is predicated on the idea that you are a victim of your genes, a product of your biology; that you are the way you are and if you add this chemical to your own mixture of chemicals, then you will behave 'properly' and feel better. As more and more people are learning, psychiatric medication is essentially an endless turnstile of chemical after chemical, drugs administered in the hope that by luck or chance the right one might just do the trick. Often times, though, this is a practice and a strategy that can so easily lose sight of the individual.

One thing is clear: The author of this book never loses sight of the fact that we are all individuals, that we are all persons in the process of becoming what we were meant to be—balanced and healthy in mind, body, and spirit.

In addition to being well researched and beautifully written, *The Chi of Change* is a book authored by someone who has lived. It is a work full of compassion and one that reflects a love for humanity. In my opinion, it is a book that should be required reading for every therapist and for anyone contemplating therapy.

Dr F. S. Starr, MD. FAACAP, BCIA
Psychiatrist

Introduction

'If you do not change direction, you may end up where you are heading.'
~ Lao Tzu

This book is about change and transformation. It is also about hypnotherapy: how it can help to restore a person to their natural, balanced psychological state and a healthy routine of living.

My name is Peter Field, a qualified counselor, psychotherapist, hypnotherapist and nutritionist with experience guiding thousands of people back to their natural state of balance and inner peace. The information you'll read in this book is the product of the many years I have spent helping emotionally troubled individuals. It is also the product of my own life experience, the changes I have undergone and the discoveries I have made during my life journey.

We may set out on our voyage of discovery with a plan for the changes we'd like to see in our future and a clear idea of where we're going and how we're going to get there, but at times we can lose our way, wandering far from the roads we intended to take. There are times when we may feel we are back where we started, miles away from the easy, free-rolling highway we once expected to simply coast down. Such is the path that change often takes, curving around in surprising and unexpected ways.

As you move through this book, you will learn about the kinds of difficulties people bring to hypnotherapists. You will read case histories of people who—perhaps like you—found themselves stuck and bewildered, then through the therapeutic process, were able to change for the better. These individuals—all real people and clients of mine (but with changed names, of course)—freed themselves from the chains of the past and the problems that had haunted and held them back for so long.

Gautama Buddha said, 'Everything changes except change itself.' This book will explain how positive, meaningful change can be brought about through the right kind of therapy, and how even the most tenacious and overwhelming of problems can be left in the past, so you can move on with your life in a freer, more balanced, and fulfilling way. I hope that it will help you to do just that.

Chapter One

The Healing Value of Therapy

'The miracle is not to fly in the air, or to walk on the water,
but to walk on the earth.'
~ Chinese Proverb

You are a miracle. And so am I. We are miracles because, against all odds, we are here, and we are alive. We have been bequeathed the gift of life by those who have gone before—but, like them, we will not be here forever.

We are heirs to the past, indebted to those who toiled and played, laughed and cried, and passed on their life force before they died. We are the sum of all that has gone before and the bridge to all that will be. Because of this, each one of us is important; each one of us is valuable and worthwhile, and each one of us is unique.

Sometimes we can forget this. Weighed down by our cares and burdens, we can become trapped, fooled into thinking that perhaps this is all there is and all that we can look forward to. The awful feeling that we are somehow stuck in a rut, losing our grip, or wasting our life can rob us of the simple joy of being alive. This sense of having wasted our energies, talents, and time can leave us feeling exhausted, frustrated and unmotivated. In fact, many of the people who visit me in my role as a therapist feel just like this.

Some of us live like this for years, thinking that this is just the way things are or the way we are. We do our best to push the pain away and grit our teeth as we struggle on regardless. But in doing this, we become even more of a stranger to ourselves, out of touch with what our feelings and our symptoms are really trying to tell us.

I know this because this is the way I lived for a very long time, and I spent my early years running from those uncomfortable feelings and unsettled emotions whose only purpose seemed to be to disturb. What I did not realize then, and what I realize now, is that the difficult feelings were actually there to help me—a form of energy whose function it is to initiate change. I call this energy 'chi'.

Before I could help others to instigate change in their lives in a positive way, I needed to understand how change worked in my life. The only way I could do this was to experience it myself, to go out into the world and live. To understand change I had to change.

Much of my life has been spent outside my native England, and my journey took me far and wide, to all Earth's continents. For many years I lived, studied and worked in the Far East—in Japan, India, and China. There I learned the term chi—or *qi* to give the word its Chinese Pinyin spelling. The concept of chi is borrowed from the five-thousand-year-old Chinese philosophy of Taoism.

Chi is commonly translated as *life force* or *life process*. In China, an understanding of chi is contained in the written language—the oldest continuously used system of writing in the world. A literal translation of the Chinese character (or *hanzi*) for 'health', for example, is 'original chi', while the character for 'vitality' may be translated as 'high-quality chi'. According to tradition, chi is brought into the body primarily through the air we breathe, but also through the food we eat.

In Japan, chi is known as *ki*, and in India it is approximated by the words *shakti*, or *prana*, the agent of all change. In the Taoist tradition, chi is regarded as having two aspects: *energy* and *information*. Neither of these is static; each exists in a constant state of flux. Chi is regarded as the force that brings about all change.

The world of physics has shown us the vibratory nature of all that is, and also that the universe and everything in it is composed of these two things: *energy* and *information*. They run as warp and weft through the fabric of existence. Like it or not, each of us functions within and is influenced by their basic law, affecting our physical, mental, and emotional life.

From the Taoist perspective, our bodies are comprised of patterns of energy—or, one could say, of the flow of chi. The feelings generated by our subconscious mind are also chi—energy suffused with information—and this produces the emotions and thoughts that are the instigators of change. I like to call the messages and feelings that come from our subconscious mind 'the chi of change', because this form of chi is primarily responsible for all the significant changes we make in our lives.

In many ways, the human mind is like a massive biological computer, and the most powerful part of this computer is the largely hidden, subconscious part. Much of the information we rely on in order to respond to life is held in the vast storehouse of the subconscious mind, just as programs are held in the hard drive of a computer. In the subconscious, the experiences we undergo are processed and then transformed into beliefs (*information*) and feelings (*energy)* that influence the interpretation of subsequent experiences. The feelings and beliefs we hold—and hold onto—at a subconscious level inform us about the nature of life and of our place in it. They inform us about the nature of existence.

But when the information stored within our subconscious is the result of faulty processing, then the information is inaccurate, and this creates distorted, false beliefs discordant with reality. Our invalid beliefs and the flawed information they are based on create uncomfortable feelings that misdirect and block our energy, giving rise to difficulties in how we think and function. Faultily processed information, energetically transmitted, disturbs our 'original chi' (our natural state of balance).

In the midst of our difficulties, we tend to focus on the frustration and discomfort that the unsettling experiences are producing within us. We are so caught up in the unfairness or the confusion of the problems that are overwhelming us that we fail to see the good in their existence. When we are struggling with our problems, all we really want is to be rid of them. It is only later—and often only much later—that we are able to see the positive changes that our difficulties may have brought about within us. Some of us never arrive at this kind of understanding, so the potential positive changes never crystallize into reality. We continue to resent those uneasy experiences and to suffer because of them. Fearing the future and holding steadfastly onto the past—or perhaps more correctly, onto our interpretation of the past—we lick and nurture our wounds, not realizing that, in so doing, we are keeping those wounds open and alive. In this way we resist change, and this, in turn, makes us even more uncomfortable and more neurotic.

Change is usually made in response to uncomfortable feelings and messages sent to us by our subconscious mind when something is not right in our lives: We change to get rid of the discomfort and to get our lives on an even keel again.

For genuine, positive change to occur in the life of a troubled person, a reprocessing has to take place—the chi must be realigned or unblocked. The programs that have been running deep within the subconscious mind need to be rewritten—new beliefs must be generated—freeing the person to feel good again, to respond to life from a healthier belief perspective more congruent with reality.

As long as we draw breath, change will be in that breath. The chi of change is as constant as the air that surrounds us, as close as the breath that sustains us. When we learn to work with that chi, we learn how to live.

Yet change seldom occurs in a straight line or instantly. It usually takes place gradually and in a curve. Even when change does happen linearly, its piercing arrow hitting straight home (a birth, a marriage, a death, the end of a relationship or loss of a job), the change can take some time to sink in and manifest itself. Indeed, our most important changes—whether constructive or destructive—sometimes come long after the experiences that were their catalyst.

One thing is certain: For better or worse, change will surely come, but it will usually come in ways unanticipated, and rarely on our terms or according to our schedule. Often it will happen in subtle, mysterious ways—ways that feel so natural we hardly notice we have altered until someone points it out to us, or we find ourselves reacting in a manner different from how we previously did. Nor do we always notice the way this occurred, the chi at work behind and within the process. We just seem to find ourselves adjusted in some way.

Whether we change in affirmative, constructive ways that help us adapt and move forward with our life, or in ways that restrict and narrow our world, it really is up to us. And this is what this book is all about. *The Chi of Change* is not a self-help manual, an instruction book, or a book on Eastern philosophy. It is a book about how hypnotherapy can help people change for the better, no matter how stuck they are or how long they have been stuck. In these pages, you will learn how hypnopsychotherapy is used to reprocess the subconscious mind and end inner conflict and how it can help bring about a real transformation in the way we feel and think.

When people have lost their balance and life has become a struggle, it is not easy to independently go back to the source of the hurt and bring about the healing that is so needed. This is because many of those things that disturb us may have happened when we were very young, so we may not remember or be able to put our finger on them. The things that have wounded us can be major, traumatic experiences, but much more often they are not. In fact, they are usually small incidents now almost completely lost to conscious recall. When we are young, even little things can appear to be very big.

Sometimes, though, we hurt because, consciously or not, we are so tenaciously hanging on to the anger, guilt, or resentment caused by our past that we can't move beyond it. Burdened by a history that is only partly understood, we are unable to discern the cause of our malaise, defuse the mechanisms, and unblock the troubled chi—the disturbed emotional energy—that continues to fuel our uneasiness. On we soldier, wearing the bravest of masks, but all the while something gnaws away inside us, a feeling we do our best to deny. Small wonder then that so many of us turn to medication, substances, or compulsive and irrational behavior in an effort to distract ourselves from our inner discomfort.

In this way we remain the victim of the difficult experiences through which we have passed. We remain filled with fear, resentment, and blame, martyr to that half-buried internalized anger or guilt that continues to hurt not only ourselves but also those who care about and reach out to us.

When the discomfort of those unhealed wounds becomes too much to bear, when it impinges on our life and robs us of the simple joy of being alive, then we may arrive at that place where we truly are ready to change. By this time, we may well have developed symptoms that have taken us to doctors. Those doctors will probably have done their best to take the edge off our discomfort, attempting to lessen the inconvenience of our difficult feelings by drugging them away. Some of us will even have bought into the false belief that there is something terribly wrong with us, that the way we are feeling and responding is so abnormal that we are mentally ill.

If this rings a bell with you, I want you to know one thing: You are almost certainly not mentally ill. You are simply experiencing real difficulty in living. There is nothing fundamentally wrong with you. Just as you are reading this book for a reason, you are here in this place with these difficult feelings for a reason.

Although there is nothing fundamentally wrong with you, in

the sense of a mental illness, there may be something out of sync in the way your mind currently perceives and processes information. You are probably running on programming that is lagging behind present reality. The energy being generated by your subconscious mind and carried in your chi is transmitting information that has, in some way, been incorrectly interpreted. Your chi is disturbed, and so, therefore, is your perception. But this is not who and what you are, and this state can be altered.

In this book we will be talking a lot about feelings and emotions, and we will also talk about thinking. Always remember that these things are not you. They are things you experience and do, but you are not your thoughts, or your feelings. You will always be something more than this.

In reality, *our difficult feelings are the chi of change*, information energetically surfacing from our subconscious, urging us to respond. They are messages sent by our inner self to inform and prod us into action. Inconvenient and unwelcome though they well may be, they are there to help us.

When our chi flows freely, we seem to flow with life. We feel good. We sense we are well and on the right path. But when the chi sends us uncomfortable feelings, it causes distress. The uncomfortable feelings can only be ignored or denied for so long. Sooner or later they insist on our attention, surfacing at the most inconvenient times, leaving us in a confused and lonely place where even doctors, drugs, friends and family seem powerless to help.

Your pain and discomfort have not been wasted if they lead you to this place. It is here that positive change can start to occur. Here real learning and growth can take place. And it is here that the right kind of hypnotherapy can play an important role in bringing about the vital transformation so that you can return to your true nature, with your life force flowing unimpeded through your body and psyche, as you rejoice in the simple joy of being alive.

Sometimes a great deal of time needs to pass before we arrive at this place. Some of us spend long years trying to run from our difficult feelings rather than stopping to listen to the message they are trying to convey. For some of us, a whole catalog of discomfort, worry, frustration, anxiety, and heartbreak may have to be endured before we can come to the state where transformation can occur.

Others of us get lucky. We are able to work through these things on our own to arrive at some kind of clarity, acceptance, and a degree of inner peace. Through the practice of meditation, mindfulness, and perhaps prayer, we may arrive at this calmer place independently, but many will find this impossible to achieve without help. This is where good hypnotherapy can be of enormous value.

One of the primary goals of hypnotherapy is to bring a greater awareness into being so that we may live an authentic and ethical existence and, no matter our past, experience harmony in our feelings and with the world around us.

I will be using the word 'authentic' many times in this book, so I'd like to clarify its meaning. People are authentic only to the extent that they are connected to their true self, a self that is not a sham or false but spontaneous and largely at peace.

But what is this true self? What we call 'the self' is really a combination of several different states and different aspects of our identity, each with its own part to play. In psychology these different aspects are known as *ego states*. We each have our own different ego states, and these are developed according to our individual histories. So the self is not so much a lone agent as it is an array of selves, or ego states, each with its own particular history, its own particular role.

According to Dr Gordon Emerson, of Victoria University, Melbourne, perhaps the leading authority on the branch of psychotherapy known as Ego State Therapy, most of us have up to one hundred underlying states, but only five to fifteen surface states are commonly used. Some of our underlying states can hold trauma and because of this they will sometimes surface, triggering those uncomfortable, upset feelings.

Most of us are not consciously aware of which part is in charge at any given moment. We assume that it's our 'self'. In a manner of speaking, whichever ego state comes forward to take charge more or less has the steering wheel until some other part surfaces to take over. When an ego state does this, we say that it has 'gained the executive'. Sometimes a part of us just does not want to hand over the wheel. It wants to continue to have its way, to drive and direct things against the wishes of some other part of us. When this happens, we become 'conflicted' within, and this creates a problem.

This conflict disrupts our sense of inner harmony and peace, disturbing the chi, as we are pulled this way and that. This is the reason for the 'one part of me wants this, but another part of me wants that' kind of feeling—it quite literally is true.

Sometimes, also, a part of us may be so overcome by negative experiences that it can no longer function. When this part gains the executive it can produce very difficult feelings and the sense of being out of control or overwhelmed to the point of collapse.

The lesson here is that no one is a one-dimensional entity. If we were, we would be more like cartoon characters than people. We are all composed of a multiplicity of different parts. Inside each one of us, there is a whole team of players.

Living means changing, and in change all our ego selves are involved. But sometimes, either through learned fear or because it is working to an outdated program and faulty set of beliefs, a certain ego part may not want to change. It can resist, and in so doing, may cause problems. Such a part may insist on remaining in a role it learned in childhood, in 'retro' mode, even though this is to the detriment of the person.

The writer Anaïs Nin seems to have intuitively touched on

this when she remarked: 'Life is a process of becoming, a combination of states we have to go through. Where people go wrong is that they wish to elect a state and remain in it. This is a kind of death.'

In a very real sense, we are all works in progress, travelers on a never-ending journey, and so we will always be in the process of becoming our true, authentic self, or, more accurately, our authentic selves. Stagnation is death, movement is life, and movement means change. It is our nature to move, to dance with the chi of change.

When we are consumed by the problems and difficulties we experience on our journey, we tend to become fractured; we drift away from our natural harmony, somehow becoming our problems and difficulties. As our different parts clamor and clash, it can feel as if there is a war going on inside us. Life becomes even more of a struggle because we are continually conflicted. We seem to go around in circles, our chi becoming 'luan chi'—disordered chi—a disruptive energy that brings difficult feelings, messages from our own subconscious mind that tell us something needs fixing. Our tendency is to run from these feelings, to try to ignore and suppress the luan chi, but in so doing we become even more fractured, distanced from ourselves and what our feelings are trying so hard to tell us. In a word, we become 'inauthentic'.

Being authentic means that we are unified and centered within, all parts working largely in harmony together, flowing with the chi of change. In this natural state, we respond to life in a spontaneous and positive manner, living in the here and now because this is all there ever really is. In this state we need no scripts and have no need of contrivance or façade. The winds may blow and Earth may move, but we will remain anchored, safe and secure, balanced from within. This does not mean we will become an enlightened Master or a Buddha; it means we are an authentic person and not a sham.

It is this authenticity that the best hypnotherapy encourages and fosters, guiding the person who has been experiencing difficulties in living to at last open to the healing they so deeply need and deserve.

Let me assure you that you, too, can achieve this state. You really can be authentically you. No matter what the past has been, no matter what the present is, you can change, and when you change so does your life. You can become balanced and whole and free of whatever symptoms have caused you so much discomfort. But in order for this to happen, you will need to go on a journey of self-discovery. You will need to work with and not against your feelings, opening yourself to the chi of change. It is a process that will alter both you and the energy and information that flows through you, the chi itself. During your travels, you will come face-to-face with old feelings and emotions, with old thoughts and unhelpful ways of thinking.

This will bring up memories of the things that produced those old thoughts and feelings that pushed and pulled and bent you out of shape, forcing you to endlessly repeat the same patterns of living as if frozen in time, somehow getting older while going nowhere.

Commit to the journey of therapy. Treat it as an adventure, and you will learn how to integrate your various selves, reprocess faulty and unhelpful beliefs, and awaken your mind from the subconscious rituals and responses that your past may have programmed into you. You will learn how to come home to yourself—the person you were born to be.

Simply because people are experiencing difficulties in living does not mean that they are mentally ill. Nor does every irregular human behavior or difficulty have a mysterious underlying psychological driver that needs ferreting out and treating. Because we veer from the 'norm' does not automatically mean that there is something wrong with us. A couple of experiences spring to mind that may illustrate this point.

As a younger man living in the Caribbean, I shared a house with a psychologist who belonged to the Freudian psychodynamic school of thought. One day he noticed that I turned a can of beans over before opening it.

'Are you aware that you always turn the can over before opening it?' he commented. I answered that I was. 'I very much doubt it', he said, 'but it is very interesting.'

The shelf on which the beans were stored was quite dusty, so I thought it only sensible to turn the cans over in order to keep the dust from falling into the food. I had no particular fear of dust or of germs; it simply seemed the right thing to do. But for my friend the psychologist, my action was not reasonable. What for me was an ordinary and completely rational action was to him the symptom of an obsessive behavior. And any attempt to explain my action was simply 'a defense mechanism'.

I remember, too, the case of a young boy, many years ago when I was in India. Once an excellent student, the boy had been doing poorly in his new school. His grades had been falling, and he was obviously struggling to keep up. His mother had brought him to me, hoping I could uncover the underlying psychological reasons for this and get him back on track.

In my preliminary talk with him, I asked whether he had made many friends in his new school, and he told me that he had. I asked him if he liked the school, and he said it was okay but very traditional, with a built-in 'pecking order'. Because he was new, he was forced to sit at the very back of the class and, unlike at his previous school, he was not encouraged to ask questions of the teacher.

'In your last school, where did you sit?' I asked. He replied that he had always taken his seat at the very front. 'And can you see the chalkboard clearly from the back?' I enquired.

'Oh, no,' he said. 'It's very difficult to see what the teacher writes on the board, and the light reflects off of it, but I have to keep quiet and not ask anything.'

This was all there really was to the boy's difficulties. He needed a pair of glasses and to be seated where the reflected light wouldn't affect his view! Yet no one had thought to check anything as obvious as his eyesight or whether he could see the board. It was simply assumed that if he was having difficulty in school, there was a psychological reason for it. A standard eye test found that he was, in fact, short-sighted. With glasses fitted and seating altered, the boy soon settled down and proved, once again, to be an excellent student.

Before looking for any complex or convoluted psychological reason for our difficulties, we must first exclude the more obvious but often overlooked explanation. This is the reason why I always advise those who come to see me to take care of the basics, to make sure that they are eating right, perhaps adding some nutritional supplements in the beginning of therapy to ensure they have all they need to function and feel well.

If more obvious causes and remedies have been explored and difficulties continue to persist, we have the responsibility to do something about them. It is here that good therapy can prove useful.

Therapy is really a very big word, and it encompasses many different approaches. Just as no one type of shoe will suit every single person, no one psychological approach will suit everyone.

How are we to know which therapy is right for us, which one works, and which doesn't? These are perfectly valid questions, and in order to offer some kind of answer, I need to explain a little of how I came by my own therapeutic approach and how I came to use hypnosis in psychotherapy.

In my life, I have filled many different roles and my learning has been wide and varied. My studies began with food and nutrition, and this made me aware of the intricate connection between food and the mind, food and feelings. This led me to become even more interested in how the mind works, and so I set about learning as much as I could in these areas, too. I journeyed far and wide, residing in many different countries and absorbing as much as I could from the cultures in which I found myself. With years of psychological study, extensive reading, and life experience behind me, I went on to train in psychotherapy and counseling—what are known as 'the talking therapies'. I used the skills and insights I had acquired in an effort to help people deal with their difficulties.

My starting point was my own personal experience. Because I had been an alcoholic, in the beginning my energies were focused on helping people with alcohol problems. Later I expanded my work to include addictions, as I, too, had been an addict. I worked with these issues for a good number of years and then found myself back in the U.K. working in the field of HIV and sexual health. My only brother, Bob, had died of HIV-related illness, and that made the field matter greatly to me. I started working with people who had been diagnosed with HIV and were finding it hard to come to terms with their diagnosis, as well as those who were troubled by their sexual orientation or who firmly believed they had contracted HIV despite all evidence to the contrary. There were those, too, who had gone out of their way to acquire HIV, people who so despised themselves and their lives that they had sought infection as a means of coping.

As I progressed on my journey as therapist, I became increasingly frustrated. While I was often able to help people achieve a much clearer understanding of their problems and how their mind worked, and while I could also provide emotional support, all too frequently my assistance didn't enable them to change in any profound way. Even with insight into the nature and origin of their difficulties, people often appeared powerless to bring about the change they knew was so desperately needed.

Like so many of those working in the talking therapies, I was approaching people's problems in a purely rational—but not necessarily an intuitive—manner. There seemed to be no other way, and my training had taught me that this approach was correct. I saw myself as empathetic and non-judgmental, yet I was appealing to the conscious, logical part of the person's mind—the cognitive, thinking part. I was actively listening and questioning, challenging clients and explaining strategies to help them manage their thinking and hopefully thereby change how they were feeling and acting.

Yet all too often, people's *feelings* remained unchanged. Their chi remained unsettled and blocked. They continued to be afraid, anxious, angry, or depressed even though they knew full well that they had no logical reason to be and even though they now had strategies and knew how to examine and challenge the thoughts and habits that appeared to be fuelling their difficulties.

The best I could do was to help my clients try to cope with their symptoms, in the hope that the better they became in this, the less their symptoms would trouble them. But it was as if I were teaching them to cope with having a massive boa constrictor coiled up in their living room. With the best efforts of their intellect and powers of reasoning, these people continued to respond to life primarily through their feelings, despite the strategies they had learned.

Some of the people I worked with were able to get through life in this way, but I asked myself, was this really enough? How much better it would be if the boa constrictor simply was not there. If we could just evict it, they would not need to cope with it.

People came to me because they were *feeling* bad. Their naturally free-flowing chi had turned into disordered luan chi. Their thoughts had a lot to do with their feelings, but the strategies I taught them seemed to work only at the conscious, thinking level. We seemed to be focusing only on the symptoms, and not on the underlying *cause* of the difficulty. All too often people appeared powerless to alter the fundamental drivers of those unsettling symptoms—their *feelings*. No matter how much they tried to change their thinking through cerebral strategies, their feelings all too often remained disturbed.

Intuitively I knew that in order for real and lasting change to happen, what was needed was a way to reach deeper inside, to work not so much with the conscious, thinking mind but with the subconscious, feeling part of the person. I found myself turning to something I had studied years before while living in India, a powerful tool that I had used in my own life and also in order to help friends and family: hypnosis. I sought out experienced therapists and great teachers who could help further refine my skills and answer my questions. And in hypnosis, I found a way to evict that boa constrictor.

With hypnosis we are able to bypass the critical, conscious mind and communicate directly with the subconscious, feeling part of ourselves. In hypnosis, with the strategies it facilitates, we are able to accomplish what might otherwise be impossible: We are able to work with and alter *feelings*. In so doing, we clear the chi, changing emotions that, despite all logic, have troubled the individual and held them back for so long. Through hypnotherapy, we can actually revise the faulty information that has been programmed into the subconscious and that causes the negative attitudes and feelings.

If you change the way you feel about something, the way you think about it will very quickly follow suit. When our feelings change, then so, in a very fundamental way, do we.

Many people have the wrong idea about hypnosis. They see it as some kind of mind control or as magical entertainment and think that if they allow themselves to enter the hypnotic state, they will end up clucking like chickens. They have viewed such things on TV, have read about them, or have seen hypnosis used this way in theatres. Stage hypnosis is light years away from the kind used in therapy. Here hypnosis is used exclusively as a tool that allows you to communicate directly with the subconscious, feeling part of your mind in a beneficial way.

Used in this manner, hypnosis is the most rapid, effective, and natural way to modify behavior, thought processes, and their origin: feelings. Both the American Medical Association and British Medical Association have approved the use of hypnotherapy as a psychotherapeutic tool for more than sixty years. Despite the impression given in films and on television, a person in therapeutic hypnosis remains in control at all times. The individual simply encourages the conscious mind to change its focus and relax, thereby allowing a deeper part of the mind to open. This is an entirely natural thing for the mind to do. In fact, most of us do this automatically several times a day—we just don't call it hypnosis.

Let me explain. If you have ever found yourself drifting into a daydream, your gaze unfocused, your attention deep in thought, you were actually in a hypnotic state at the time. If you've ever driven along the road with your mind wandering, then realized you missed your turnoff, it's because you were actually in a state of hypnosis. Similarly, if you've ever sat in front of a TV or computer when an hour or two just seemed to fly by, you were in a hypnotic state. In fact, time distortion is a common phenomenon when we are in a hypnotic trance.

Hypnosis is an entirely natural state that has been around since primitive man first gazed into the fire and drifted off into thought. Of course, there is a difference between that kind of hypnosis and the kind a person experiences in a hypnotherapy session. The fire-staring, daydreaming kind of hypnosis is automatic. The person doesn't intend to go into trance; it happens spontaneously. But in the kind of hypnosis used in hypnotherapy, the person is guided systematically into the trance state in a safe, structured and controlled manner. You are aware of everything around you and remain in control throughout.

Hypnosis, though, is merely a tool. It's what happens when we are in the trance state that matters, and this is where the therapy part comes in. Hypnosis gives us the means to communicate directly with the subconscious mind, and hypno*therapy* allows us to work with the mind in a therapeutic manner—realigning, reprogramming, and rebalancing it so it functions in a more life-affirmative way. This is why I often refer to hypnotherapy as "hypno-psychotherapy". It is the single most effective means of helping people psychologically that I have found. And this is why I use it. I use it because it works.

But we cannot properly treat the mind—the psychological software that has been so influenced and shaped by past experiences—without regard for the body and the brain (the mind's hardware). In fact, the more we learn about the mind and body, the more we come to see that the two cannot be separated. Each is an extension of the other. Body, brain, and mind are all part of the same thing. Indeed, it can be difficult to know where hardware ends and software begins. Just as the mind influences the body, so the body influences the mind. And both are dependent on energy, or chi.

Our experiences influence our brain chemistry at least as much as our brain chemistry influences our experiences. Each one of us is a complex interplay of biography and biology. Because of this, any comprehensive therapeutic approach needs to consider both body and mind.

If our mind and our emotions are to function in the healthiest possible way, with our chi flowing freely, then we need to maintain the right biochemical balance in the body and brain. If we have been experiencing emotional difficulties, we must correct any possible nutritional deficits. After all, the body's chemistry is dependent on that from which it is constructed—the food we eat. Nutritional deficits can cause the brain (and therefore the mind) to fog up, become erratic, and so react and think negatively.

Because of this mind-body interconnection, our therapeutic journey will need to include an awareness of the important role nutrition plays in our mental and emotional health. Our chi, or life force, is brought into the body through the air we breathe and the food we eat. Like all living things, food is filled with chi, gaining its energy from sun and earth, and we absorb this energy by eating.

For many years, a substantial and ever-increasing body of research, conducted at the best universities and research centers around the world, has demonstrated that certain nutrients and micro-nutritional elements do indeed have a direct effect on our mental well-being. If we have been experiencing emotional or mental difficulties, then we may well benefit by eating more of those whole foods that contain these important elements and nutrients.

Sometimes we might also benefit by supplementing specific nutrients—particularly certain amino acids, essential fatty acids, and individual vitamins and minerals—in quite large quantities, at least *in the early stages* of the therapeutic process. Though *The Chi of Change* is not a book on nutrition or orthomolecular science, I will mention food and nutritional supplements as we move through its chapters.

Simply eating wisely can ease so many of our health problems, both mental and physical. After years of living and years of practicing therapy, I am more convinced than ever that without the correct nutrition we simply cannot balance and maintain our health. Without the right nutrients, our chi can never flow freely. When our eating is out of sync with nature, it affects us in a negative way—physically, mentally, and emotionally.

For many of us, learning how to eat the right foods will involve leaving our comfort zone. We will have to adopt a new and (perhaps in the beginning) a less convenient way of eating. But such effort will be more than rewarded by the positive results that come with it. All food carries energy, or chi. When we eat fresh, vital foods, then we absorb this chi and so enhance our own.

I firmly believe that we need to get away from the idea perpetrated by Big Medicine that pharmaceuticals hold the solution to our mental and emotional difficulties, that they can cure us of our troubled mind and disturbed spirit—our luan chi. We need to see that prescription drugs can never really provide us with a lasting solution to an inner turmoil that continues to provoke symptoms such as depression, anxiety and insomnia.

No matter what we eat or what therapy we engage in, the things and people that surround us and the world in which we live will continue to influence our perceptions, feelings and actions. This is inescapable. But we must always remember that though these things will continue to affect us, they are not us.

According to Plato, 'The part can never be well unless the whole is well.' The best kind of therapy treats the whole person, working with mind, body, and spirit. In the process, one realigns one's relationship with oneself, restoring balance, confidence, and self-esteem.

While good therapy can realign our belief system into something positive and productive and free us from many illusions that stopped us from living life to the fullest, no one ever completely loses every one of their illusions. Indeed, a degree of illusion seems necessary for us to function and live in this world.

Sooner or later, though, we have to face the fact that we were born into a world that is, in many ways, imperfect and unjust. We will need to come to terms with this if we are to face life with emotional and mental stability.

We may begin our journey with the highest ideals, believing we really can change the world—and, indeed, every one of us *can* change the world, though only some of us will—but we will never change the way that life is. Life will continue to be life, despite our desires and remonstrations. It does not have to be fair, it does not have to be just, and it does not have to always make sense. All it has to do is all that it can do: It has to be itself. In the sage words of Lao Tzu, founder of Taoism, what we have to do is 'let reality be reality'.

This is true, also, as it applies to each of us: We must allow ourselves to be ourselves. Finding out who that self is, or more accurately who those selves are, is a very big part of becoming authentic, of becoming real.

When we understand and accept this, when we stop demanding that life be something other than it is and that we become something other than we are, then we stop swimming against the current, and our passage through life becomes so much easier.

There are times when we have to trim our sails and steer a course that leads to the shores of compromise. We may not like this, but then again there is no 'Great Law' that says we have to like everything in existence. The trick, of course, lies in knowing when to compromise and when not to. When something cannot be changed, it is senseless to keep on banging our head against it. The fortunate ones among us find the serenity to accept the things that we cannot change, the courage to change the things that we can, and the wisdom to know the difference, to quote from Reinhold Niebuhr's Serenity Prayer, so wisely adopted by Alcoholics Anonymous and other Twelve Step groups.

As long as we do our very best, then we will have done all we can—even if, at times, the best we can do is to hold our head above the water and keep right on breathing. Our feet will always find dry land as long as we do not give up hope.

Who knows how many people we might one day help because of our own difficult experiences? Although we may not see it at the time, nothing need ever really be wasted. Everything has its value.

Our true solutions, like so many of our problems, lie within. We need to work from the inside out, not from the outside in, to bring about real change and restore an inner balance that will endure.

If you pause and glance back over your life, you will recognize that, no matter your age, you have already learned many things. The fact that you are able to understand these words means you have learned to decipher the printed word, and the fact that you can think about their meaning proves you have learned how to think. Yet these things took effort. You had to actually do some work in order to acquire such learning. You do not have to be as old as a sequoia tree to see that life's learnings rarely come gift-wrapped or with glowing candles on top. You know only too well how often your best learnings came at the cost of leaving the familiar behind and journeying past the borders of your comfort zone.

Indeed, many of life's major lessons come in the form of uncomfortable surprises. Often they arrive as unpalatable and apparently overwhelming experiences that upset, shake, and challenge. The emotions we feel at such times are the chi that leads us to change.

The truth is that real learning comes at a real price. It is a price that each one of us, in our own unique way, must pay if we are to fulfill our potential and live in harmony and peace with ourselves and with our world.

Sometimes, paying this price can prove painful, so the tendency is to try to dodge it. Reality can be hard, and our human inclination is to avoid the hard and to opt for the softer, easier way, even if that means anesthetizing ourselves to reality, denying the way things are. But the attempt to avoid paying the necessary price of growth and learning is the cause of our mental and emotional instability. When the discomfort that comes from maintaining our denials and illusions exceeds the pain of surrendering them, then we are ready for real change.

The great psychologist Carl Jung—a keen student of Chinese Taoism—believed that 'there is no coming to consciousness without pain'. He saw neurosis as an attempt to flee from this necessary pain. In his opinion, neurosis was simply some kind of 'substitute for legitimate suffering'.

My work and life have convinced me of the truth of Jung's observation. It is in attempting to deny and run away from our difficulties that we open the door to real mental and emotional malaise and imbalance.

When we have become stuck in the way we feel, mired down by our emotional difficulties, it is usually an indicator that we have been avoiding our underlying problems and the painful symptoms they can produce. Typically, we have refused to properly examine and deal with our problems.

Because our problems often emanate from the hidden, subconscious, feeling part of the mind, it can be extremely difficult to independently manage the largely unconscious mechanisms that drive these problems. The fact that they stem from the subconscious makes them all the more confusing, unsettling, and in many ways frightening. But it is in continuing to ignore our problems—and the feelings they generate—in the vague hope that they will simply go away, that we open the door to some very unsettling, even harsh consequences.

Difficulties such as depression, anxiety, panic attacks, alcoholism, addiction, overeating, insomnia, and phobias—not to mention unhealthy habits and compulsions, such as hair pulling, skin picking, teeth grinding, and nail biting—point to an unwise stoicism, an attempt to soldier blindly forward, ignoring our issues.

Sometimes this strategy is fuelled by a misplaced and false sense of pride. From our earliest years, we may have been encouraged to be self-sufficient, and this is how it should be. But we also need to recognize that we are not islands, that we are all somehow in this together, interconnected and mutually dependent: The part cannot be separated from the whole. In Buddhism the belief that everything is mutually dependent on everything else and that phenomena arise only in relation to other phenomena is known as 'dependent origination'. Just as the mind needs the body and the body needs the mind, whether we like it or not, we need each other.

Human beings are social animals, and as such we can benefit from the wisdom and guidance of our fellow travelers who have learned something of the lay of the land. The best therapists have been properly trained. They have learned how to navigate the difficult waters and the rough terrain, and they have experience helping others to do the same. But above all, they have lived.

Being human, they have resisted change and been battered in the process. They may have walked a rocky path not unlike your own. They have stumbled, fallen, and been bruised as they fought against the chi of change. They have learned something about the territory that lies beyond the confines of maps and classrooms, outside the covers of books.

One of the greatest fallacies about therapy is that seeking it is a sign of weakness. Nothing could be further from the truth. Recognizing the need for help and doing something about that need, far from being a sign of weakness, is an indication of maturity and strength. It is a manifestation of the individual's essential humanity and of their courage and determination to live a balanced and meaningful life. This surely merits respect. Indeed, there are times when most of us could use the assistance and support of an experienced professional who is equipped and trained to guide, advise and help us on our way.

Sometimes people come to the therapist already placing that person on a pedestal. Seeing the therapist as 'the expert', they imagine this individual to have always been well-balanced, wise, and completely 'sorted'. But the therapist is a human being, and human beings are not born with all the answers, nor will we ever acquire all of them.

The good therapist knows the solutions to a person's problems already exist within that person, deep within their subconscious mind. It is the therapist's job not to provide answers or impose remedies, but to help the person discover their *own* solutions.

In my life I have met and known many therapists. I have come to believe that the very best—those who excel at moving people forward and helping them grow—were once themselves forced to struggle and overcome serious difficulties. Most have known what Rudyard Kipling called 'those two imposters': triumph and disaster, success and failure. And every one of them will tell you the same thing: If you are lost, confused, or in pain, do not despair. Do your very best to see what you are going through as part of your human education, something that life is asking you to pass through so that you can become a more whole, authentic person. Though it might be difficult to accept at this moment in time, your difficulties can give you valuable insight that will lead you on to a deeper understanding and a better life.

Whether we recognize it or not, we are all somehow dancing with the chi of change, no matter how disturbed that chi may be. And this process will continue until we leave this world. Good times and bad, easy and difficult, thick and thin, confused and clear, all must go into life's mix.

Some, of course, never make it. They never awaken from the dream they have created or been led into, and everything they experience becomes processed and performed within the confines of their illusory reality. Some may become lost to such a degree that it seems impossible they could ever return to the right path, but they *can* return if they summon their courage, have the honesty to recognize their error, and possess a powerful desire to become whole.

A very few others may become completely trapped in their own confused state, the center of their own universe, devoid of any capacity for empathy, their daily reality forever processed through the filter of their illusion-filled brain. It is in this dissociated, fragmented state that the murderers, terrorists, and the criminally insane largely dwell.

We do not solve our difficulties by pretending they are not

there. Our problems flourish in the darkness of denial, so we need to shine the light of truth on denial itself and see it for what it is. It is a form of dishonesty. It is our way of attempting to fool ourselves or others into believing this is just not happening, or if it is, then we don't want to know about it, so we'll pretend that it's not.

In the state of denial, it is easy to look to external remedies and panaceas—medication, drink, drugs and behaviors intended to distract us from the difficult feelings carried so forcefully in our chi. However, our attempt to run from these unwelcome feelings distances us further from ourselves and from any real solution to our difficulties. It is this same denial that is perpetuated by the vested interests of a multibillion-dollar and pound pharmaceutical industry and by the medications so casually prescribed by well-meaning physicians.

Antidepressants, anxiolytics, tranquilizers, and sedatives are nothing more than attempts to use chemicals to gloss over people's fundamental problems. These drugs further restrict the chi—the energy and information our subconscious mind is using to tell us something within is out of sync, conflicted, and in need of resolution. Instead of encouraging an individual to open up their poorly processed experiences—uncovering their own damaging beliefs and subconscious programs and then repairing them—this chemical warfare (for that is what it amounts to) attempts to shut people down and pretend the problems are not there. (We will talk more about drugs such as antidepressants, and how they are supposed to work in a later chapter.)

Only when we end our attempts to avoid the messages coming from our powerful subconscious can we begin to acknowledge things as they truly are and actually do something about them. When we accomplish this, we are no longer compelled to squeeze ourselves—or anyone else—into some preconceived image or learned blueprint of what is 'normal'. There is no longer a need to doggedly follow that old and circular trail we have stumbled down for so long, the one we mistook for life's highway.

For Sigmund Freud, 'the goal of life is death'. But in this he seems sadly to have missed the point. What he failed to recognize is that the true goal of life lies in the journey itself and not in its terminus. Freud's contemporary Carl Jung had a different vision. For him, 'The purpose of life is to kindle a flame of meaning in the darkness of mere existence'.

The flame of meaning is fuelled by chi, illuminating the darkness with energy and information, lighting our way towards clarity. What do our feelings mean? What are they really trying to tell us? To live by this light requires courage and honesty, yet it is this that guides a person back home.

'The way to do is to be,' said Lao Tzu, and each one of us is in the process of becoming. As we begin to become, we change. We no longer need to run away from, deny, or attempt to distract ourselves from our difficult emotions. We learn to face them and deal with them. In doing this, we move nearer to the creative person we truly are within and closer to the profound understanding that there is nothing fundamentally wrong with us.

The great majority of us have no organic dysfunction. We are not mentally ill. With our chi disturbed, we have simply been running in the wrong direction, looking in the wrong places, buying into the wrong stories and the wrong beliefs, feeding our mind and brain with the wrong things. We have been 'normal' all along. Not average, but normal. We just didn't know it.

This is the understanding—forged in the fires of experience and honed by learning, shaped by tumult and joy and by the simple humility gained from having lived—that the best therapists bring to each new client and to each human being they meet. It is an understanding that is at the heart of all good therapy.

In the therapeutic setting, people are given a safe place where they can reveal themselves without fear of judgment, criticism or rejection. Indeed, nothing is more essential than a person feeling safe and completely accepted as they enter into and move through any form of psychotherapy. This is what good hypnotherapy is— psychotherapy conducted in hypnosis. Without the feeling of safety and acceptance, it is doubtful any therapeutic movement would be possible.

With hypnotherapy we are able to systematically work our way through a process that brings positive, meaningful change at the deepest psychological level. The kind of hypnotherapy I practice is called 'brief therapy' because it does not require the investment of years in soul-searching analysis—although it does require some soul-searching honesty. The process rarely exceeds half a dozen sessions, and many difficulties (such as phobias and habits) may be cleared in only a couple of sessions. Because it is a brief therapy, it does not require a bottomless pocket in order to fund.

It is a therapy that can be very demanding of both client and therapist; in it there is no room for dishonesty or deceit. Good therapy is a means of freeing oneself from such things. Intense as it is, it is the very intensity, the exacting honesty, that makes it so truly rewarding and life-changing.

At the end of their therapeutic journey, many people tell me they feel they have at last come home to themselves. Frequently they say that the struggle or war within is over and that they now are so much calmer and more at peace. Yet, as a therapist, I must admit that despite all my training, experience, and successes, I have no exact map that will lead a person back home. That is because only the client, not the therapist, knows where home truly is.

A skilled hypnotherapist can help you find your way, but it has to be *your* way. Just as no two birds ever fly along the same path in the sky to arrive at their own nest, so each one of us must move forward in our own special way, prompted and guided by the feelings and emotions that our experiences elicit, our own unique chi of change.

In therapy, as in life, the metaphor of a journey is entirely appropriate. Therapy is indeed a journey of discovery. Through it, we come to look at our life from a fresher, more balanced perspective. As the French writer Marcel Proust so aptly put it: 'The real voyage of discovery consists not in seeking new landscapes, but in having new eyes.'

With the hypnotherapy you will read about in this book, we employ a comprehensive approach to the person as a whole—an approach that has proven highly effective in helping countless people free themselves of their difficulties, flow with their chi, and move on with their life in a much more positive, balanced, and creative manner.

But at the outset of any therapeutic journey, one thing needs to be understood: No therapist is God. Like you, we are all human. Unfortunately, there are far too many poorly trained and ill-informed practitioners who ply their wares under the banner of 'hypnotherapist'. Some have done nothing more than taken correspondence courses and written a few short assignments in order to receive their diploma from a 'school' that is only too happy to award its 'qualification' in return for a fat little fee.

I have even spoken with graduates of some of the most 'prestigious' courses in the country only to learn that too much of what they have been taught is either faulty or plainly ineffective in the real-life world of therapy. Indeed, I have often found myself shaking my head in bemusement as graduates recounted some of the erroneous things they have been taught.

Yet a therapist's ability to be of real help to a client is not wholly dependent on their academic qualifications. I know some therapists who hold doctorates whom I would no sooner refer someone to than I would go to myself. Conversely, I know of others—some of whom were among the best therapists I've ever met—who had little formal training and no academic degree or advanced qualification in the work, but who knew their healing art inside-out. They accomplished wonders for the people fortunate enough to consult with them.

If you are contemplating therapy, the best way of finding an effective therapist is to ask around. Check with friends and enquire whether they know of anyone who has benefited from sessions with a hypnotherapist. Above all, speak to the therapist before booking sessions and allow your gut feeling, your intuition, to be your guide. It helps enormously if you use your common sense.

Perhaps the most important thing when it comes to success in therapy is the relationship between client and therapist—something called the 'therapeutic alliance'. Only with trust and empathy can therapy really be effective. Remember, though, that while a good therapist is friendly, they cannot be your friend. The therapist is there for one purpose only: to help a person change and move on with their life.

It is the therapist's job to shepherd, to walk a while with each person who comes for assistance, to clean metaphorical windows and to help open doors. But it is not the therapist's job to foster dependence. There comes a time when the person must accept responsibility and let go of the therapist's hand, venturing forth on their own. If the therapist has done a good job, the person will accept this transition willingly, aware that they alone can live their life.

Albert Einstein said that there are only two ways to live your life. One is as though nothing is a miracle. The other is as though everything is a miracle. Like that ancient Chinese philosopher whose words opened this chapter, I believe the true miracle of life is that you and I are here, walking the earth. And we are here to thrive—not merely to survive. My hope is that this book will help you to do that.

Chapter Two

Feelings and Emotions—Who Needs Them?

'Thoughts are the shadows of our feelings.'
~ Friedrich Nietzsche

Whenever we experience an emotion, we feel. Feelings inform us we are alive. They have been with us since we were in the womb, and they will be with us until we die. Take away our ability to feel, and we would not simply be living life flat, we would be dead.

Our very earliest experiences brought with them feelings. Before we learned to think, we felt. Through feelings, we learned to respond to the world. The baby whose nappy is wet, for example, experiences that uncomfortable sensation and responds with an emotion that produces a cry for assistance.

Feelings are the chi that provides the information and energy needed for us to respond to life's stimuli. As such, feelings are the precursors of change.

For feelings to make sense, however, we must first decipher their information and interpret their meaning. We must *perceive* them. And it is this perception—whether taking place in present time, remembered, or imagined—that gives rise to our emotions. Perception is our own personal interpretation of what our feelings mean, what they are telling us. Thus, perception is at the very heart of emotion.

Strictly speaking, feelings are the sensations that inform and trigger our emotions, while emotions are our response to those feelings and to the thoughts we have come to associate with them. For convenience sake, though, I will be using these words more or less interchangeably throughout this book.

As we mature, we acquire a whole repertoire of experiences.

Each experience is twinned with accompanying feelings, so that our perception of what is happening in the present is based on the meaning we have ascribed to our feelings—and to the situations that produced them—in the past.

The difficulty is that so much of that meaning was ascribed when we were very young and not in the best position to properly process our experiences in any objective or balanced manner. Our perception was simply the *opinion* of a child, and opinion is not fact. It was something viewed from the younger self's limited perspective and understanding and not necessarily a true reflection of what was actually taking place. In other instances, it was influenced by the perception of others, by *their* interpretation of experiences, which was passed on to us.

The way in which we perceive can have been formed at any time—but it has *always* been formed in the past. To a large extent, we are a product of the meaning we have given to past experiences, so our version of the memories we carry, especially at the subconscious level, continues to influence our interpretation of reality. Perhaps this is what the Czech writer Franz Kafka meant when he wrote in one of his letters: 'I am a memory come alive.'

Whatever reasons people may have for consulting a hypnotherapist, the one common denominator they all share is the way they are feeling. By the time they arrive in the therapist's office, practically everyone, in one way or another, is feeling unhappy. Often people will have spent a very long time trying to conceal their unhappiness from others. In the safety of the therapist's office, they soon find themselves releasing this pent-up emotion, often crying as they do so, yet feeling guilty and apologetic for it.

Whenever this happens, I swiftly reassure the person that this is indeed a safe and appropriate place to release their emotions, and I encourage them to do this without apologizing. As Benjamin Disraeli once said: 'Never apologize for showing feeling. When you do so, you apologize for the truth.'

A big part of this unhappiness and the emotion that permeates almost every difficulty a person brings with them into therapy is the emotion of *fear*. So powerful is this emotion that according to many spiritual teachers, fear and love are the only real human emotions; every other emotion is simply derived from them.

When we feel afraid, our primary human instinct is to run from the source of our fear. But fear is a powerful emotion and it is not easily shunned. When we have tried and failed to deal with our fear and yet it persists, then its energy can easily become transmuted into anger or hatred and directed towards others—sometimes even those closest to us, the ones with whom we feel most safe.

Some of us may try to hide our fear behind an arrogant attitude or by acquiring material possessions. Some live recklessly, often harming others and themselves in the process. And some simply become overwhelmed by the burden, retreating into the surety of habitual worry or the numbness of depression.

My professional experience clearly demonstrates that fear underpins and supports not only every single phobia, but that it is present in a range of issues, from anxiety to low self-esteem. But with the exception of phobias, hardly anyone comes straight out and says: 'I'm here because I'm afraid.'

But what exactly is fear? If we consider it for a moment, we'll see that fear is nothing more than the belief that something bad is going to happen. This emotion arises in an attempt by the subconscious mind to protect us, to warn us of danger, and to get us out of harm's way. Without the emotion of fear, we would not have survived as a species. The ability to discern danger and then to take steps to evade or neutralize it is hard-wired into us. As such, the emotion of fear is entirely healthy; in fact, it is essential. But when fear exists in the absence of a real threat or danger, then it is neurotic fear, and something needs to be done about it.

Many people who visit the therapist are unaware that it is often the fear of fear that they find problematic. Because they have experienced fearful feelings in connection with certain activities, locations or objects in the past, these things have become subconsciously linked with fear in their minds. The person develops an expectation that the awful *feelings* of fear—the pounding heart, labored breathing, and panicky sensations that tell them they are afraid—are somehow lying in wait for them whenever they encounter a similar set of circumstances. This keeps the person in a constant state of vigilance, which can be exhausting. It is this state people refer to when they say, 'My nerves are bad.'

Even though emotions may surprise us, they do not really spring out of nowhere. As we have seen, they are inextricably tied to the experiences we have had in the past when we felt, perceived, and gave meaning to our feelings.

Soon emotions and thoughts became so intermingled that one easily triggered the other, and we became caught up in a cycle of constant feedback that influences the interpretation of our current reality. By themselves, thoughts may be abstract, wispy things, but when they are endowed with emotion, they become something more substantial and powerful.

If we reflect, we can see that those times when we felt emotion are more easily remembered than times that provoked little or none. Think back to a memorable time in your past, and you will almost immediately access a feeling or emotion that is linked with that time. This is because our senses are keener when we are in an emotional state, so the experience is rapidly registered in the feeling, subconscious part of the mind.

Our society is rife with anxiety and fear. It is scripted into our soap operas. It's the mainstay of our newspapers and of the ten o'clock news (a good reason not to watch the news just before sleeping). In one way or another, anxiety and fear seem to be built right into modern existence.

So ubiquitous and universally powerful are the emotions of fear and anxiety that marketing specialists regularly employ them to influence and manipulate our buying habits. With a savvy understanding of people's subconscious psychological drivers, they know that many of our daily decisions are motivated by fear. This psychological insight was first employed about half a century ago by the giant American conglomerate IBM, whose marketing department cleverly created the formula known as 'FUD', which stands for 'Fear, Uncertainty and Doubt'. With a keen eye on the bottom line, an entire advertising strategy was built around the concept that bad things would happen if someone bought a competitor's product. Fortunes were made, as the company capitalized on people's fear of making the wrong choice, the wrong decision. A strategy neatly reflected in a slogan of the day: 'Nobody ever got fired for buying IBM'. Today the FUD formula is subtly used to sell us just about everything—from cars, TVs, iPods, and items of fashion (the fear of not looking 'hip' and up to date), to concert tickets ('be there or be square'), insurance policies and mouthwash.

But anxiety and fear not only influence our consumption habits and unsettle our inner peace. They produce a harmful effect on our bodies, sending waves of powerful chemicals and hormones (such as cortisol, adrenaline, and norepinephrine) through almost every tissue, washing through the brain like a tsunami, unbalancing and leaving mayhem in their wake. Chronic anxiety leads to broad and harmful alterations in every single organ of our system, from our heart to our stomach to our brain.

While harmonious, balanced feelings—carried in our free-flowing, healthy chi—result in mental, emotional, and physical well-being, difficult feelings produce the emotions that upset and disrupt. Both kinds of feelings have a direct and powerful impact on our health and lives. Indeed, so powerful are our feelings and emotions, that they can even influence us at the genetic and immunological levels.

This understanding is at the heart of Taoism and traditional Chinese medicine, which see no separation between body and mind, both being manifestations of the energy that is chi. Quietly recently, a field of study known as epigenetics has come to the fore, focusing on the way in which factors such as stress, anxiety and even parental attachment can trigger and activate genes, turning them on and off.

And over the last forty years, another branch of medicine known as psychoimmunology has developed in the West. It studies the relationship between the immune system and emotions and is posited on the same ancient belief that body and mind are inseparable. Neuroscientists involved in the field of psychoimmunology and epigenetics have clearly shown that emotions produce biochemical reactions and activate or deactivate genes that can either harm or heal the human body.

This is why, if you are experiencing a lot of anxiety, you need to address not only the psychological reasons for it but also the foods that you eat. Eating foods that provide the macro and micronutrients that can ameliorate or repair the damage caused at a physiological level and help restore your chi is the wise thing to do. We will be talking a bit more about nutrients and health-promoting foods later in this book.

Anxiety and fear are present in practically every form of emotional disturbance and psychological imbalance that exists. They underlie virtually every symptom of profound uneasiness—from depression to phobias, low self-esteem to lack of confidence, unmanageable anger to insomnia.

Drilling down directly to the feelings that are connected with those symptoms always reveals the source of a person's problems, and this is an important strategy used in hypnotherapy. The therapist also pays close attention to the thoughts and images that drift through the mind, topics the client tries to avoid, and the language they use to express their thoughts and feelings. These are all useful indicators of the source of their discomfort, which the conscious mind may not recognize.

For most of us, our troubled luan chi—the energy and information that is the driving force of emotional discomfort—is hardest to ignore in quiet moments such as daydreaming, just before sleep, or while waking from sleep—all essentially trance-like states when we are more in touch with our subconscious. It is frequently during these times that the early, usually subtle symptoms of our problems first manifest themselves, although we often don't recognize them at the time.

Those 'four in the morning' feelings are generally the moments when our mind seems to wander in the direction of unwelcome worries and emotions. Inevitably we find that behind those worries and emotions are memories of previous times when we felt this way. Something in our present life resonates with and triggers similar feelings we experienced in our past.

In his book *The Secret Language of Feelings,* Californian therapist and renowned hypnotherapy teacher Calvin Banyan explains this mechanism very well: 'Our nervous system is made up of water, minerals, proteins, fats, and so on. When we're in a particular emotional state, there are changes in our physiology that can be measured—changes in muscle tension, heart rate, and brain wave frequencies, to name just a few. Each time this occurs, the changes are stored in the subconscious ... along with our other memories ... These stored emotions can be recalled in an instant when something occurs that we associate with them.'

It is those memories, sometimes clearly recalled but so often incorrectly processed, lodged within the subconscious and then repressed and forgotten by the conscious mind, that cause those feelings which give us so much trouble. Our difficult feelings—energy suffused with chaotic or flawed information—produce the emotions that upset and disrupt. This is what affects our mental and physical balance, producing what we know as 'symptoms'.

Yet it is these same uncomfortable feelings that are the precursors of change. Each painful emotion is a message that contains an opportunity for personal growth, an invitation to become better balanced and healthier—provided we are wise enough to listen and to act upon the message. Our troubling feelings are there to tell us that something needs attention. When attempting to escape these feelings, we stifle our ability to put things right and to fully experience the more joyful, positive emotions that life has to offer.

And so we stumble on in the darkness, as if following a badly drawn map, something roughly sketched from the memory of our past travels, our past experiences—or from hearsay gleaned from others. We depend on our map to guide us safely away from fear and discomfort, but often we find ourselves instead being led even further from the solution that we so desperately need.

But just as a map can never be the territory itself, merely a representation of that territory, so a memory can never be the actual experience. It is simply our representation or *translation* of that experience, our internalized *perception* of the experience. It is these perceptions that form our beliefs, working much as programs might work in the bio-computer of our powerful subconscious mind.

In neat symmetry, these beliefs become the filter through which we apprehend reality—or to be more accurate, our version of reality. As the American philosopher Henry David Thoreau observed, 'The question is not what you look at, but what you see.'

The British scientist Sir John Lubbock took this understanding a step further when he noted that *what we see depends mainly on what we look for*. In other words, we human beings have the tendency to see what we expect to see. When we are in a state of fear, we usually look for and expect the worst. The anxious, fearful person will almost always give a negative interpretation to an experience or situation. What's 'out there' will always be filtered through what's 'in here', and when there is fear within, that which is without will very often appear intimidating, threatening, or downright dangerous. When we are afraid, then harmless teenagers at dusk can appear to be menacing thugs, and as any child frightened of the dark can testify, 'things that go bump in the night' can be terrifying monsters up to no good.

It is through our perceptions, then, that we experience the world. It is also through our perceptions that we build our beliefs, and it is our beliefs that influence, and in so many ways determine, the life that we live.

Unfortunately, some of our beliefs may be flawed because, as we have seen, they may well be based on faulty perceptions and incorrect information acquired in the distant past. They are the product of our much younger self's distorted translation of past experiences, or of other people's translations (their value systems and interpretations). Or they may be based on information that might once have been correct, but no longer is. So many personal problems stem from this kind of faulty belief—a belief out of sync with current reality. Such beliefs will continue to disrupt our lives until they are somehow reprocessed and changed.

Because so many of our basic beliefs are formed in early childhood, our faulty representations of reality are usually the product of the limited perceptions of a child, though now embedded in the mind of an adult. Psychologists now know that each child is essentially in a state of trance until around the age of five or six. Before this age, practically everything is brand new. Young children have not had time to develop the comparative mechanism or 'critical factor' that allows the mind to separate correct from incorrect information. They have not yet developed a sufficient data bank against which new information can be compared. Incorrect information can 'slip in under the radar' because at this early, formative age there is, as yet, no radar in place. Our early interpretations of the difficult or confusing experiences through which we have passed strongly shape our adult understanding—or misunderstanding—of how the world operates and of our place in that world.

What happens 'out there' is not nearly as important as what happens 'in here', because what happens externally is usually filtered through what has happened—and continues to happen—internally. Within us lie beliefs that form the bedrock of our attitude towards self, other people, and life experiences. We see things not as they are, but as we *believe* they are. This points to an important understanding: *Life is mostly a matter of how we perceive it, and this largely determines the attitude with which we approach it.* Once we realize this, we are in an excellent position to bring real and lasting change into our life.

The inner self cries out in the form of troubling feelings and physical symptoms when old programmed beliefs create fear in the present. But it is not enough to understand this. Even if we can identify some of the incidents that created our false beliefs, that does not generate our healing. The conscious mind, the part of us that reasons and comprehends, is relatively powerless to do anything that will change the situation.

This is because uncomfortable feelings, and the luan chi that brings them to us, spring not from the conscious mind but from the deeper subconscious. And the subconscious mind does not speak the same language as the conscious. Try as we might to logically explain things to the subconscious, in our normal waking state it will usually remain stubbornly inattentive and essentially deaf to our rational reasoning. Feelings, after all, can quite easily crowd out reason.

In our evolution as a species, emotion existed in advance of rational consciousness—our very survival depended on it.

Feeling was there long before conscious thought, so it is not really surprising that even today emotion can lie beyond reason's reach. Emotion is ill at ease with the logical, conscious mind. Being primeval and instinctual, it is more at home with the unconscious and subconscious mind.

The language of the subconscious is not rationality, but imagination and metaphor. Our deeper mind speaks in symbols, often given to us during sleep, in our dreams. This is why the 'talking therapies' of psychoanalysis, traditional psychotherapy, and counseling tend to fall short and often fail to bring about the needed change. It is because we *talk* with our conscious mind, but *feel* with our subconscious. And as we have seen, feelings are what bring most clients to the therapist.

People usually know they have no 'good reason' to hold onto irrational beliefs. Those with phobias, for instance, know very well that spiders, birds, or elevators will not really harm them, but their logic is powerless to prevent the feelings of fear and anxiety these things trigger. They simply cannot will or reason that fear away with the conscious mind. While a person may be taught cognitive strategies in an attempt to manage their fear and to desensitize it, the fear will often remain at some profound level within, as the person tries to live their life around it in a logic-oriented, practiced coping strategy.

Please don't misunderstand: I am all for logic, and some people find cognitive therapy quite effective. But I don't believe it's the best way for most people to communicate with their subconscious mind, because logic can so easily be defeated by feelings—especially by the feeling of fear. Neither is it enough to simply know the origin of our fears. Few things are more disempowering than knowing the reason and the cause of our problems but feeling unable to do anything about them. This sense of powerlessness can so easily lead to or reinforce feelings of failure, futility, and despair.

Charles was a gaunt-looking man in his mid-forties who

visited me because of feelings of depression, anxiety, insomnia, low self-esteem, and lack of confidence. Though a successful businessman and CEO of his own company, he had struggled for years with strong feelings of despondency and depression. Although outwardly successful, inwardly he felt as if he were an abject failure. Nothing he could do or achieve seemed to lessen his feelings of profound self-disappointment and deep-seated unhappiness.

At the beginning of our sessions together, Charles brought in an old photograph to show me. It was of a boy, no more than five or six, sitting rather forlornly and alone on some grey concrete steps. The expression on the boy's face was one of bewilderment, as though he had not expected a camera to be there. It was a picture of a little boy who was very unhappy.

'This is me as a kid', Charles said. 'I don't look too happy, do I? Do you know why? It's because I don't believe I ever knew what happiness was. I don't think I've ever really felt happy in my whole life.'

For years Charles had invested time, money, and a good deal of energy in various forms of therapy as he attempted to free himself of his burden. For the past five years he had been in weekly therapy with an analyst who had helped him to painstakingly drill down and uncover what he now saw as the origins of his difficulties. But still he remained stuck; still those terrible feelings seemed to haunt him like dark shadows, yet something inside told him that there must be more than this. A friend of his who had been in therapy with me had passed him my number.

'I would finish my sessions each Friday, get into my car, hit my head on the steering wheel, and weep', he reported when talking of his most recent therapy. 'The work we'd done had helped me to understand why I felt so bad. We'd taken all of those things out of the box, but then I was left with them, not knowing what to do or how to put them back again in the right order. To make matters worse, my therapist didn't seem to know either. She seemed to believe this was not really her job, that I should be able to figure out the solution. It was enough for her to have helped me uncover the cause of my misery, but then she seemed to expect me to do something with all that—but what could I do? All I was left with were questions.'

Although Charles had indeed been helped to increase his knowledge of himself and of his problems, those problems still remained, only now he felt even more helpless and vulnerable. He felt incompetent as a person. This fuelled his self-criticism because now he saw himself as even more incapable, an even greater failure. All he had been offered was the opportunity to continue to talk of these things, and this he had done in the lengthy and costly procedure of analysis for the past several years.

'We just kept going around in circles', he said. 'But no matter how much we talked, no matter how much I was questioned and challenged, I still kept right on feeling bad.' An even more confused and desperate mood had arisen. For Charles, the implicit had indeed become largely explicit, but this had only made matters worse.

What needed to happen, of course, is that his subconscious needed to reprocess what his conscious mind now better understood—and it needed to find a way to do this. The sensitizing experiences through which he had passed in childhood and that shaped the way he felt and responded to life needed to be reinterpreted at a deeper level, below that of the conscious mind. To continue with our computer analogy, the subconscious programs that continued to make him feel so bad needed to be re-written.

In hypnosis, Charles was taken back to those formative experiences where his perceptions of events were uncovered. Here his younger selves were shown how to reprocess the experiences and restructure his understanding in a more helpful way—one that would create no inner conflict for him in the future. With hypnotherapy, Charles found great relief in a brief period of time. It did not take years, only weeks. When last I saw Charles, he said to me, 'When I think about the picture of that little boy now, he's smiling—and so am I.'

In addition to the primary emotion of fear, anger and guilt are two of the most powerful emotions and ones frequently present in those who come to see me. Odd as it may seem, people often are much more willing to admit to feelings of guilt than of anger. In fact, whenever I hear the words: 'I'm not an angry person' or 'I don't get angry' or some such version of these statements, I know only too well that in all probability I am talking with a person who is extremely angry at some deeper, internalized level.

Why is this? It is simply because in our modern 'civilized' society, anger is so frowned upon and disparaged that we are taught to deny and internalize it. After all, few other emotions have the power to fill us with such fear. We are afraid of anger in others as well as in ourselves.

As children we were told off, or else heard someone else being chastised for being angry. Because of this we learned to stuff it down inside, to hide and deny anger like some shameful secret to which we must never admit—but we were not taught why it is there, how to respond to its message, or how to release it in any positive way.

Most of us have little difficulty allowing pleasant, joyful feelings to be expressed when they arise. Often, as soon as we become aware we are feeling happy the feeling quickly subsides. In fact, almost all human emotions are short-lived. As with any other form of communication, once heard, our feelings need to be properly responded to, processed, and then stored at a deeper level so that our conscious awareness channels remain open for other information to be received and transmitted. In this way, our chi is free to flow in a naturally healthy manner.

But when we disrespect our feelings and emotions, attempting to dismiss or deny their existence, then what we are really doing is trying to silence our own inner voice, to block our chi. When we try to wish away troubling or inconvenient feelings, they do not simply pack up and leave town. Like tenacious resistance fighters, they go underground, driven down deep until they find some other way of grabbing our attention and being heard.

They produce the symptoms that disturb and unsettle us—the headaches and migraines, the insomnia and depression, the teeth-grinding and panic attacks, the malaise and the neuroses—and they will continue to disrupt our life until we arrive at that place where our life becomes increasingly unbearable and something just has to be done to address and deal with their demands. Until the luan chi is converted into free-flowing, vibrant chi, it will persistently apply its disturbed energy. It will continue to inform us that something is out of harmony, needing attention.

Usually the process of denying and attempting to bury troublesome, inconvenient, and scary feelings begins where our beliefs began, in the formative years of our infancy when the balance of power was so unequal. After all, in the rather primitive state of childhood, the law of the jungle appears to rule: It is the biggest and strongest—the adults we depend upon for our safety and therefore have a desperate need to please—who have almost all of the power and authority.

If we grow up in an environment, a family, or a society that devalues feelings and frowns upon emotion, then we absorb that attitude, and it informs our values. Psychologists call values we pick up from others 'introjected values'. They are not really ours but are more or less imposed on us as we subconsciously incorporate them into our own belief system and the way we respond to things.

Anger is one such devalued, yet natural human emotion. As we know, anger differs from other emotions in its ability to fill us with fear. So many people are afraid both of becoming angry and of witnessing anger in others. Because of this, anger is unique among the emotions. Few other emotions have the power to repel us to this extent or are viewed as being so 'wrong', but if anger is so very wrong, then why is it a part of every single human being's nature and an essential component of our emotional vocabulary?

If we reflect, we will recognize there are times when anger is, in fact, justified. Indeed, sometimes in life, the only really appropriate response is anger. Who has not felt angry when treated in an unjust manner or when learning of someone else being treated unfairly? What right-thinking person does not feel a sense of anger when learning of cruelty to an animal? Anger itself is not wrong; it is what we do with the anger that falls within or beyond the boundaries of morality.

When we suppress our anger, it goes down deep inside us where it ferments and foments, easily becoming repressed and lost to the conscious mind as it begins to work its own special mischief. Although it might be years later, ultimately this mischief will manifest itself. When this happens, that ancient anger erupts, as if out of all proportion to the present stimulus, taking us and others by surprise as we become ever greater strangers to ourselves, further distanced from our true nature: our real and authentic loving and loveable self.

Then why do we need to feel anger? Like all other emotions, it has its origin in our perception. Anger exists because we *perceive* that someone has been very unfair or unjust, either to us or to someone or something we care about. It is our emotional response to having been wronged or denied or learning that this has happened to others with whom we empathize.

Anger is the other side of the coin, the twin of *guilt*, which is also cut from the fabric of injustice. If anger stems from the perception that someone else has been unjust, then guilt stems from the perception that we ourselves have in some way been unfair. Guilt is the feeling we get when we believe we have violated our own internalized standards. It is a form of inner-directed anger. Both anger and guilt have their positive uses, since they can activate our ability for corrective action.

When our internalized and repressed anger or guilt becomes too great, however, we can easily find ourselves experiencing disturbed moods and engaging in all manner of self-abusive or other-abusive behaviors. Taken to their extreme, anger or guilt can manifest as murder or suicide. Anger and guilt have the ability to so disrupt our chi that our entire nervous and immune systems become compromised, making us vulnerable to illness and disease. Until we find a way to express our anger in a healthy way, to change what has caused it, or to forgive those who occasioned it, we will continue to suffer because of it.

Each one of us can and does experience both anger and guilt. The potential for both exists within us at all times. Without these emotions, there would be no conflict between people and a good deal less inner conflict to torment us. But this is simply not the way that life is put together. People can and will sometimes be unfair, intentionally or unintentionally, and both we and other people will perceive this unfairness. Anger is such a basic human emotion that as long as there are human beings, it will always be in this world, and it is futile to deny it.

Yet this is exactly what so many of us have been taught to do since early childhood. Time and again we have forced it down until we no longer recognize its existence. Then all that is left is, 'I don't do anger', 'I'm really not an angry person', or 'I don't even remember the last time I got angry.'

Of course, I am not suggesting that we go around venting our anger indiscriminately or looking for things to be angry about, but I *am* suggesting that we allow ourselves to recognize anger and other scary and difficult emotions when they arise, so we can listen to their important messages and respond to them in an appropriate way.

Interestingly, anger appears to be more acceptable in boys and sadness more acceptable in girls as gender, too, plays a role in our ability to connect with and express emotion. Though slowly changing, in our culture women are usually allowed and even encouraged to connect with their feelings, while men are encouraged not to be emotional. Little girls are granted permission to show feelings much more commonly than little boys ever are. But by and large, we see the pattern of females being allowed to feel and men not being allowed to feel. Women are believed to have a greater degree of emotional intelligence or 'EQ' than men, while men are believed to excel in the colder, more cerebral type of intelligence called 'IQ'. Both of these perceptions are culturally inherited.

So many men have grown up in an ethos that finds expression in comments like 'boys don't cry' and 'don't be a sissy'. It's as if the ability to feel is in itself a sign of some terrible weakness, an unspeakable sin. If a boy or man allows himself to show his feelings, he is in danger of being considered 'girly' or effeminate.

This learned inability to connect with or acknowledge emotion is perhaps one of the major reasons why men are, generally speaking, more reluctant to visit a doctor when feeling unwell and why women outnumber men in seeking help for their emotional difficulties. Women are less likely to continually ignore their feelings of inner discomfort than men, so they may well be in a better position to actually do something about them.

Emotions are at the very heart of our relationships. If we have absolutely no feelings for a person, we are very unlikely to have any kind of relationship other than the most cursory and essential. Imagine a relationship in which there are no emotions, and you are imagining a pretense, a hollow shell. Like or dislike, love or hate, when it comes to human relationships of any kind, emotion is a factor. Without emotion there would be no relationships. Without relationships there would be no intimacy. Without intimacy there would be no humanity—neither you nor I would exist.

But men and women can view emotions quite differently, with each gender prioritizing and valuing different ones and appearing to have different emotional needs. Women, for example, tend to prioritize caring, while men might prioritize trust; women might seek understanding, while men may want acceptance; women may look for devotion, while men may seek admiration; women may want reassurance, while men might want encouragement, and so forth.

Problems arise when each gender believes the other gender values and needs exactly the same things it does. The discrepancy between partners' values, needs, and wants is at the root of many relationship breakdowns. Conversely, a better understanding of how one's partner differs from oneself helps create more empathetic, stable, and long-lasting relationships.

There also appears to be a real difference in the way each gender stores and processes memories of emotional events and experiences. Research has shown that women consistently recall more childhood memories than men (Davis, 1999) and are generally quicker in accessing such memories. This difference can be ascribed partially to socialization and also to physiological differences in the sexes, in particular to differences in the part of the brain that is involved in processing emotional responses and emotional memory, the amygdala.

Of course, human beings of both genders always did and always will have emotions. In fact, it is impossible to imagine us without this capacity. It is one of the essential things that separate us from machines, one of the things that lend us our humanity.

An interesting and important aspect of emotion is its ability to dramatically narrow our field of focus. Emotion can easily close down our awareness of the choices we have. When we are really angry, for example, all our attention is focused on the person or thing that has provoked our angry feelings. When we feel fear, our attention is directed almost exclusively towards the source of the perceived threat.

It is this focusing of attention and the consequent inability to see our options that exacerbate so many of our problems, from depression to anxiety attacks. Interestingly, it is just such honing in, this same narrowing of focus and disregard for options, that is at the heart of our ability to fall in love or to be overwhelmed with joy.

When we deny powerful feelings, we are refusing to listen to the language of our own subconscious; we are trying to block our chi, to silence our own wise inner voice. In so doing, we inevitably begin to build a potential tidal wave of trouble for ourselves. Each denial may seem to be nothing special, a polite little compromise, a nod to civilization and past conditioning, but add the energy of all these little suppressions, repressions, and denials together, let it accumulate over the course of years, and what we are left with is an angry sea, a tempest of emotional, mental and even physical trouble.

Our troubled feelings are messages asking us to go to the source of that trouble and do something about it. They are not an invitation to foolishly attempt to drug these uncomfortable symptoms into oblivion. The luan chi is trying to tell us something important, and try as we might, we cannot dismiss and deny our uncomfortable feelings forever. As we move through this book, we will learn how hypnotherapy can help a person effectively heal the causes and greatly ease the distress that our disturbing emotions can provoke.

But anger, guilt, and fear are by no means the only emotions that disturb and guide a person into therapy. Among the other common ones are sadness, loneliness, low self-esteem, frustration, boredom, and perhaps the most devastating of them all—that thing we call depression.

Because of the prevalence of depression, I will be devoting two entire chapters to its discussion. For now, though, suffice it to say that depression is simply a cry from within that says: 'My unhappiness is too great—and I just can't cope anymore.' It is the feeling that seeps out from the inner belief that life is too overwhelmingly difficult or meaningless, and the only thing left is in some way to give up.

Stress is a common difficulty that brings people to the therapist. When we are stressed, we experience a combination of feelings that have built up to such an extent that we can no longer deny them, so the overriding feeling is that of being overwhelmed. We feel stressed when we have been trying to do too much, or when we have been trying to do it too soon or too well, juggling too many things. In some ways stress is similar to frustration because we feel it when what we've been doing has not been effective. And stress is a killer. The feelings that it produces are the subconscious mind's way of sending us urgent messages. The luan chi says to stop what we are doing and change. We would be wise to heed the message because failure to do so will almost inevitably lead to ill health and some form of system breakdown—mental, physical, or both.

While stress is a combination of emotions, there are really only half a dozen or so primary emotions to which human beings are heir. These are fear, love, joy, anger, sadness, disgust, and surprise—although, as we've seen, some believe the only primary emotions are fear and love. Practically all of the other emotions that we experience are based on one or more of the primary emotions. Guilt is a form of anger, for example. That makes guilt a secondary (or second-tier) emotion. Some emotions, such as jealousy, are tertiary (or third-tier). Jealousy is based on the feeling of insecurity (a secondary emotion), and insecurity is based on fear (a primary emotion). You get the idea.

As we have seen, each of our emotions exists for a reason; each has its own particular meaning and wisdom. Carried within each feeling are messages from our subconscious mind. They are the agents of change, the harbingers of the chi—information and energy—necessary for change.

In school we were made to study academic subjects, but we were taught nothing about what feelings are for and why we have them. So we face life ill-equipped to deal with them when they arise. The reason we were not taught about emotions, of course, is that the adults who taught us were as mystified by emotions as we children were. If you had asked your teachers *why* we have emotions, it is doubtful you would have received a clear answer. And if you had asked *how* we manage to have feelings, chances are that unless you were speaking to a really good teacher of human biology, again you would have received a vague answer.

But there is no need to go on being perplexed. Now you are in an excellent position to better understand your emotions, and in so doing, you can respond to them in a much more effective manner. In order to properly comprehend our feelings, we need to know a little bit about the mechanics that make them possible. This means understanding something of our nervous system and the divisions of our mind because without them, we would be incapable of feeling anything. This basic understanding isn't difficult to grasp, so don't worry. Just getting a general understanding of the process will be fine. It will greatly help as you advance through your own personal chi of change and will also help you to understand yourself better.

Let's start with the mind itself. The mind is a non-physical thing: We can't cut the body open and put our hands on it. Some equate the mind with *the soul*; others call it *consciousness*. We'll avoid getting into a philosophical discussion of the nature of the mind, but many psychologists agree we can talk in terms of three of its aspects: the conscious mind, the unconscious, and the subconscious.

The *conscious* mind—the part that reasons, thinks, perceives, judges, and decides—functions through the area of the brain known as the *neocortex*. This part of the brain, which forms the top layer of the brain's two hemispheres, takes time to develop, and the process isn't completed until we are in our twenties. The job of the conscious mind is to analyze, question, measure, critique, plan, organize, and doubt. The conscious mind is the part responsible for intellectual activity, reading, writing, information processing, and decision making. It is also the home of willpower. Though we rarely like to admit it, in many ways our conscious mind is quite limited. For example, it can hold only six to nine bits of information at any one time, whereas the subconscious mind appears to have no such restrictions.

The conscious mind can learn, but it learns in an 'intellectual' manner, keeping the things it has learned to a relative few that remain in its short-term working memory bank. The rest is sent down into the long-term memory bank that holds those things we know—or believe we know—but which we don't need to consciously think about anymore. The conscious mind does this so that it has room to hold new information that comes in, ensuring our working memory remains fresh and functional.

The conscious mind's job is to try to make sense of things, to rationalize. The problem is that some of the things it tries to make sense of, it doesn't really understand because those things are connected with feelings, and the conscious mind may be brilliant at *thinking* (which psychologists call 'cognitive' processing), but it's extremely poor at *feeling*. It speaks the language of logic, not of emotion. Because of this, it is so often mystified by that other, powerful part of the mind, the part of the mind that deals with feelings—the subconscious. I call the conscious mind 'the cognitive mind' or 'the thinking mind'.

Then there is the unconscious or the *reactive* mind. This part of our mind functions through the base of the *brain stem* in the oldest, most primitive part of the brain. (It is 'oldest' in terms of evolution, this being the part of the brain that developed first in the earliest prototypes of our ancient human ancestors.) This instinctual part of the brain is responsible for the operation of all of those bodily functions we usually take for granted—breathing and heartbeat, regulation of body temperature, sense of balance, and automatic reflexes. This is the part of the brain that reacts instinctively whenever we experience an abrupt, unexpected stimulus. It makes us suddenly jump when startled and automatically flinch when something is thrown near our eyes.

The unconscious mind has its very own memory system, which operates on conditioning. Stick your hand near a hot stove just once, and your unconscious will learn very quickly not to do that again; it will make sure your hand is withdrawn instinctively when near such heat in the future.

When confronted with an unexpected stimulus, the unconscious mind rapidly computes the following four questions: Do I quickly withdraw from it? Do I fight it? Do I eat it? Do I mate with it? The unconscious does not pause to think about this; it just reacts instinctively. This primitive instinct is the mechanism that has ensured the survival of the human race. I call the unconscious mind 'the instinctive mind'.

Finally, we have the subconscious, or the *emotional* mind. It functions mainly through the part of the brain known as the *limbic system,* located deep inside the brain beneath the two hemispheres. This is the mind's real powerhouse, where emotion is generated. It is also the part of the brain that houses beliefs that run just like programs in a computer. Emotional memories are regulated by a region of the brain called the *amygdala.* They also involve an area that affects mood and decision-making, known as the *orbitofrontal cortex.*

Unlike the conscious mind, the subconscious mind's storage capacity is unlimited, just as imagination is unlimited. The subconscious mind is the source of imagination and the storehouse of all memories from our past—even those no longer available to our conscious mind, our normal waking-state awareness. The subconscious always retains a wonderful childlike capacity; its job is not to weigh and analyze—that's the task of the conscious mind. The subconscious has the tendency to trust, just as a child trusts, and it trusts *feelings*.

In the subconscious, all our programs, inner maps, and

blueprints—the things that so greatly influence how we respond to life as adults—are stored. Our five senses are processed in the subconscious, along with music and visual images. Things we have perceived with our senses bypass the conscious mind and go directly to this part of the brain or to the unconscious part. Because of this, we can actually alter our chemistry on a profound neurological level by listening to music and by viewing images or looking at light frequencies and sequences.

The subconscious is the creative, imaginative part of the mind. It doesn't 'speak logic'. Its language is imagination, and its currency is feelings. One of the interesting things about the subconscious is that it cannot really distinguish between the imaginary and the real, and it does not really understand time very well either. For the subconscious, past and present simply seem to intermingle as one. It feels much more than it can think, and so I call the subconscious mind 'the feeling mind'.

When we feel an emotion like fear, the feeling can easily overpower our rational, conscious mind. The fear may be triggered by something real, of course—a rabid dog or a person with a bomb. But it can also be triggered by an image, a face, a word, a situation—or even a thought or sensation—which is not in itself inherently threatening but which does, in some way, resemble a *previous* experience that was perceived to be dangerous, threatening, or uncomfortable.

Every day we encounter new experiences, and the mind needs to make some kind of sense out of each one in order to respond. To do this, the subconscious rapidly scans its memory bank of experiences, looking for a link to a previously drawn-up 'map'. Then it connects this information—based on what it believes happened in the past—with whatever is happening in the present, to try to make sense of the moment. In doing this, it searches for the best explanation, the most appropriate response.

In other words, it looks to those programs already installed by our interpretation of previous experiences in order to respond to what is happening here and now. It is not the rabid dog or the possible bomb that enters the mind because objects cannot enter. The only thing that can enter the mind is a *perception* of things.

The problem is that what the subconscious mind is really scanning at lightning-fast speed is not the actual reality of what previously happened but our registered *interpretation* of what previously happened. Because we filter our present experiences through the data bank of past experiences—which are now programmed into us—we see and respond to things not because of how they actually are, but because of how *we* are—because of how we've *learned* to see things. In this way, our history regularly repeats itself.

How does the subconscious manage to send messages to us via our feelings? It uses the physical circuitry in the brain and of the entire body to stimulate sensations we identify as particular emotions. Let's look at how this works.

The human brain is a universe of activity. In it, electrochemical signals shoot back and forth like spaceships across a galaxy of more than thirty billion nerve cells called *neurons* that connect and form the brain itself. In fact, there are more connections in the human brain than there are stars in the sky.

These neurons release what are known as *neurotransmitters,* or chemical messengers. It is their job to stimulate the transmission of electrical signals between the neurons in the brain and throughout the nervous system. There are more than sixty different messenger molecules. Serotonin, norepinephrine, and dopamine are prime examples of such neurotransmitters, and you will be hearing more about these important substances as we move through the book.

When it comes to emotions, the neurotransmitters convey messages called *neuropeptides,* sometimes called 'molecules of emotion' (Pert, 1997). These travel through the system like chi, carrying information and energy. They go not only to the brain, but throughout the entire body because there are nerve receptor sites virtually everywhere. The neuropeptides travel to the muscles, causing them to contract or relax, creating tension or relaxation; to the digestive system, where they affect the stomach, bowel, and related organs; as well as to the blood vessels feeding the skin, heart, lungs, and other organs of the body. They also travel to the immune system.

Much like tiny rockets, the neurons fire neurotransmitters across the gaps that lie between neurons. Such gaps are called *synapses*. Having been fired across a synapse, neurotransmitters automatically lock onto receptor sites in nearby neurons, just as spaceships might lock into their own landing docks.

There can be as many as ten thousand receptor sites on each neuron. Each kind of neurotransmitter has its own unique docking site. For example, the neurotransmitter dopamine—responsible for triggering the rewarding 'feel-good' sensations that come from some foods and the ecstatic highs that can come from sex and certain drugs—has its own special receptor sites as does serotonin, the 'happiness' neurotransmitter, and so forth.

Once enough receptor sites get hit by neurotransmitters that lock into position, the neuron automatically fires off, forwarding an electrical signal to the next nearby neuron. This process is then repeated down the line, from neuron to neuron, until the information is conveyed to an area of the brain (or elsewhere in the body) where the message is felt and perceived as a physical sensation and/or emotion.

Where once we believed consciousness functioned exclusively through the brain, we now know that consciousness communicates throughout the entire body via the signal molecules—part and parcel of our chi. We also know that neural receptors are present on the vast majority of the body's cells, allowing every area of the body to receive messages of emotion—in the form of physical sensations—from the subconscious mind.

It has been said that emotions are the bridge between the

spiritual and the physical. They have a physical component (sensation), but they also convey a message that is beyond the physical—a message of happiness, sadness, anticipation, regret, anger, and so forth, that appears to have little to do with the body. The messages come from the subconscious mind, which is itself non-localized and non-physical. (Even the most skilled surgeon cannot physically open the brain or body and pull out the subconscious—or any other part of the mind for that matter.) This is one reason why our emotions should be regarded as important and even rather sacred because they come from a non-physical intelligence within us that's trying to tell us something.

But let's get back to neurons for a moment. While located throughout the entire body, they have a particularly high concentration in three places: the brain, the spinal cord, and—this may surprise you—the gut. The stomach and intestines (sometimes called the *enteric nervous system*) are actually loaded with neurons. These send and receive messages, just like the neurons in the brain. The gut contains over a hundred million neurons—even more than the spinal cord!

The enteric nervous system—the gut—has a complex circuitry that acts independently of the brain, enabling it to learn and remember and produce *feelings*. Where once we believed that it was something of a one-way street, with the brain affecting the stomach and digestive system, we now know the enteric nervous system produces and sends messages that influence the brain.

Practically every chemical that controls the brain has been identified in the gut. This includes hormones and neurotransmitters such as serotonin, dopamine, glutamine, norepinephrine and GABA. (GABA, by the way, plays a major role in regulating neuronal excitability throughout the nervous system.) So important are such neurotransmitters to the balanced, healthy functioning of the enteric nervous system that 95 per cent of all serotonin in the body is located in the gut. Because of this, neurobiologists have nicknamed the enteric nervous system 'the second brain' and 'the second nervous system'.

As research continues on the circuitry that links these 'two brains', we are beginning to understand more about human actions and feelings. While they are completely independent systems, so similar are the 'head brain' and the 'gut brain' that both share natural ninety-minute cycles during sleep, and both affect the way we function and feel when we are awake. For the brain atop the shoulders, the ninety-minute cycle involves slow brainwave sleep patterns interrupted by periods of dreaming, which are distinguished by rapid eye movements. For the brain in the gut, the ninety-minute sleep cycle entails slow waves of muscle contraction, broken by short bursts of rapid muscle movement.

In traditional Chinese medicine and in Taoist belief, the body is not a mechanistic device devoid of its own intelligence. Rather, the gut is seen as a reservoir of chi. In most psychiatry and psychology, however, the health of the gut is very rarely, if ever, taken into account. The fact is that just as the brain has the ability to disturb the digestive tract, so the gut, in turn, can disturb the brain.

The message is clear: If we wish to feel and be well, then we need to pay attention not only to the brain in our head, but to the brain in our gut. We need to give *both* brains all they need in order to function in a balanced, healthy manner. I believe there can be no comprehensive therapeutic approach to emotional and mental health that fails to take the enteric nervous system into account.

No matter their point of origin, however, neuropeptides (the signal molecules that carry messages) have the same essential purpose: to carry information and energy that the receptor sites will transmit to certain places in the body. Energy and information, you will remember, is the very definition of chi. The messages chi sends are experienced as feelings. If we listen to these instead of repressing them, we will understand what our subconscious is trying to tell us, and that is a major step in becoming a more integrated and balanced person.

For this messaging process to work efficiently, we need to get our brain/body chemistry right. If our chemistry is imbalanced, so too are our perceptions, our mood, and the way we feel about life. We need to be mindful of what we put into our bodies—namely, the foods we eat—and how they affect the body and the brain.

The nervous system is dependent on specific micronutrients in order to function. Without a constant, steady supply of these vital factors (which include amino acids, essential fatty acids, minerals, and vitamins), we could not survive. An imbalance in any of these critical micronutrients can cause real problems in the way we think and feel. In Taoist terms, such imbalance creates luan chi.

Foods contain their own chi, their own life force, because they, too, are living things. When we eat, we absorb that life force, and it becomes part of us. In traditional Chinese medicine, food is considered the most basic and essential means of correcting illness and rebalancing the body's chi.

Good nutrition is absolutely essential if we are to live a healthy life. Eating poor, lifeless food creates imbalance and can contribute to mental, emotional, and physical difficulties. But it is only one piece of the puzzle; food is not the whole picture.

Perhaps it's becoming apparent that if we want to be healthy on all levels, we can no longer afford to view ourselves in the reductionist manner that so much of Western medicine encourages. Neither Prozac nor food supplements can ever really heal a wounded spirit or calm a deeply troubled mind.

As ancient Chinese wisdom knew and modern neuroscience clearly shows, body, brain, and mind are indivisible. They are not just interconnected; they are one. If we are to live a healthy, balanced life, we need to take this into account. Most mental and emotional difficulties stem from a *combination* of faulty subconscious programming (the incorrect or unhelpful meaning given to past experiences), poor cognitive processing (humorously called 'stinking thinking'), *and* nutritional and lifestyle imbalance.

If a person is suffering because of deep-seated, unresolved issues from the past, if their problems emanate from psychological conflict, then a truckload of organic whole foods, vitamins, amino acids, and other supplements alone are not going to make much of an impact. On the other hand, if a person is suffering from a lack of folic acid or a sensitivity to wheat, if they have been living off lifeless processed foods devoid of chi, then psychological reprocessing or realignment of inner ego states will not be enough to heal them.

Let's close this chapter by looking again at our earlier question: What are emotions for? They are barometers of our mental, emotional, and physical health and guideposts for how to maintain these. Without emotions, we would stumble apathetically through life, existing more than living. As Carl Jung put it, 'There can be no transforming of darkness into light and of apathy into movement without emotion.'

Yet emotions can only help us when we respect them and listen to the messages they attempt to deliver. This process begins with understanding that there is no such thing as a right or a wrong feeling, only feelings that are comfortable or uncomfortable. There really are no unhelpful feelings. All are a form of chi and all of them have value; they help us maintain or regain inner balance and guide us towards positive and meaningful change. Attempting to consistently bury or deny our feelings is a sure way of creating emotional, mental and physical imbalance. It is only by respecting our feelings, and the feelings of others, that we can live a life in harmony with ourselves and the world.

Once we lose our fear of emotions and learn to rely and act upon their wisdom, we develop an emotional intelligence that makes us more rounded and fully human. It is an intelligence that supports us, guiding us through the peaks and valleys of life. Through feelings, we respond to our world and everything in it. Through feelings, we learn to change and to fully live. In the next chapter we will look more closely at how hypnotherapy can assist in this process of change.

Chapter Three

The Beginning of Change

'When I let go of what I am, I become what I might be.'
~ Lao Tzu

When we have had enough of the rollercoaster ride of difficult feelings, we can arrive at that state within ourselves where we are ready for the essential transformation. At last, we are ready to work with the chi of change.

When we reach this place, the crack within us has become so great that it just cannot be pasted over and concealed. All meaningful change comes at a cost, and that cost always involves some discomfort. Because of this, it's a human tendency to change only when we absolutely must. After all, very few of us like the feeling of discomfort.

In order for real, constructive change to happen, we must first make up our minds that we are going to do this. We have to end our resistance to change. We must get to the point where we are ready to do whatever it takes to reclaim our life and bring things back into balance.

The idea that individuals need to accept responsibility for their own change can come as a surprise to some people. They are accustomed to behaving as passive participants in their own well-being, almost completely handing over responsibility for their life to doctors and other 'experts'. So the idea that they now must take responsibility for their own change can be quite unsettling. But if a person wants to move forward, leaving the problems of the past behind and becoming more integrated within, this shift in perception is essential.

Usually I amplify this element of personal responsibility with the analogy of shoes. 'If your feet hurt, does it really make the slightest bit of difference if I change *my* shoes?' I enquire. 'I believe that I can help you, but *you're the one who needs to do the changing*. Are you ready to accept responsibility for that?'

The truth is that neither I nor any other therapist can force a person to change. It has to come from within them. A person will change only when they themselves are willing to accept responsibility for that change.

Today many people suffer from what is known as 'magical thinking'. Our swift-paced, microwave society—fuelled by convenience foods, liposuction and glamorous TV makeovers—has turned us into believers in the quick fix, the 'magic bullet'. So many of us have bought into the belief that there is some mystical concoction or magic spell out there that can do the work *for* us. It's as if we are constantly on the lookout for an instant solution, something external to ourselves, some easy remedy that can absolve us of the responsibility for our own life.

This belief fuels the pill-for-everything craze so prevalent in modern medicine. It's a belief that inhibits our growth, preventing us from doing what is necessary to make the changes that would allow us to truly feel better. It is a belief that blocks the chi of change.

In therapy, this attitude is reflected in people who expect a quick fix without their having to put in any work at all. They assume they can simply pay a fee, lie back, be 'put under' hypnosis the way they might be put under anesthetic, and then be awakened to a life that has been instantly and magically transformed.

Sometimes this is, in a way, possible. With simple phobias, for example, we can often bring about the required change in just two or three sessions, and the person can leave with the fear that has handicapped them for so long permanently removed. This is because something like a simple phobia usually has a single and easily identifiable cause that can be quite rapidly reprocessed at the subconscious level, and it rarely carries with it unresolved issues such as guilt or anger that need to be worked through. But even with phobias, the person has to do *some* work to bring about the needed change. They cannot simply lie back and be a passive participant in their own transformation.

But for more complex issues like depression, overeating, addictions, low self-esteem and so on, real change takes a while longer to bring about, and it comes at the cost of a good deal of emotional energy. It also usually means the person will have to work their way through uncomfortable feelings, accumulated over the years, before their personal metamorphosis takes place.

Is it really a coincidence that the rise in consumption of prescription drugs and pharmaceuticals coincides with the rise in people's inability to face their problems and accept the responsibility to actually *do* something about them? The evidence is there for all to see: The more diet pills that are produced, the fatter we continue to become; the more tranquilizers we are prescribed, the more anxious we seem to be; and the more antidepressants available, the more depressed we are. Who then can deny there is something seriously lacking in this approach?

As a therapist, I specialize in helping people to genuinely change. After years of experience, I still marvel at the changes I have come to expect but which still continue to amaze me. I never allow myself to forget that I am simply a catalyst, someone who knows something about the process of change and how to facilitate it. I have never actually 'changed' anyone. My clients change themselves.

Meaningful change is not something that can be done *to* a person; it is something a person has to work for and allow. Inner growth means an alteration in the way we perceive. And when our perceptions alter, then so do we. As the sage Thoreau put it: 'Things do not change, we change.'

Change always involves a leap into the unknown. What we know is familiar, and there is always a sense of security inherent in the familiar. Change demands that we leave the familiar behind and strike out into a new, unfamiliar direction. Such a leap can seem quite scary.

When first consulting a hypnotherapist, it is entirely natural for clients to feel a degree of apprehension, even anxiety. That's because the person is facing a brand new experience, and new experiences take us out of our comfort zone. But a client's apprehension is sometimes based on a misunderstanding about the nature of hypnosis. They may have the false belief that in hypnosis they might lose control and say or do something that could embarrass or compromise them. This, however, is not possible in responsible hypnotherapy. Hypnosis is not a truth serum. Even in hypnosis, people choose what they wish to disclose, and they retain control and awareness even while in the trance state (in the same way you remain in control and aware when you are in the trance state induced by watching an enthralling television program).

Sometimes a person contacts the therapist because someone else has insisted they change some aspect of their behavior and has more or less pushed them into going. Often the therapist receives enquiries on behalf of other people, with partners, parents, brothers, sisters and friends calling to make appointments for those they care about.

Many times such calls are entirely appropriate, especially if they are made on behalf of someone with difficulty telephoning—a person who is extremely nervous, for example, or someone with very low self-confidence. But before any therapist can ethically accept anyone into therapy, they must know the person is coming of their own accord—because they *want* to change, not because someone else wants them to.

Anyone who has been pushed into coming in order to please or pacify some other person is almost certain to fail because they will be unprepared to do the work needed to bring about change and growth. The genuine desire for change, like the readiness to accept responsibility for that change, is a prerequisite for successful therapy.

Once the desire and the decision to act on that desire—the readiness—are there, the person can work effectively with the therapist. Then real change can take place, often with surprising rapidity. This inevitably means facing up to the problem. Each of us has the capacity to do this if we allow ourselves to access just a little of our inner courage.

Andrew was a well-groomed, intelligent, heterosexual man in his late thirties who consulted me because of what he termed 'sexual difficulties'. He suffered erectile dysfunction—he simply could not obtain or maintain an erection when with a woman—a much more common difficulty in men than is generally acknowledged and one I am often called on to treat. (We will be looking more deeply at this particular issue when we come to Chapter 5, on anxiety.)

Since he was a teenager, Andrew had been involved in a life of crime that included breaking-and-entering and burglary. He had spent most of his adult years incarcerated. Having served his sentence, he inevitably went right back to his old miscreant activities, only to be caught, arrested, and sentenced once again to time behind bars.

Four times in his life he had attempted intimacy with women: the first time when just fourteen, an abysmal affair that had filled him with feelings of shame; then a year or two later; then a couple of times in his twenties. Each occasion had produced the same result—no erection, leaving him with intense feelings of humiliation and the terrible feeling that he was inadequate.

Andrew came from a home where 'being a man' was held in the utmost esteem. Born into a large family with many brothers, he had always been encouraged to be something of a 'bad boy', a 'Jack-the-Lad' (as it is referred to in the U.K.), and his brothers had constantly teased him because he had no girlfriend. His brothers had even bamboozled him, as a teen, into going to a prostitute they had paid for. Much as he tried, he did not get an erection, and so, to save face, Andrew covertly paid the woman even more money to tell his siblings he was a really virile performer in the bedroom.

In the safety of the therapy room, where confidentiality is ensured, Andrew voluntarily disclosed all of this and also explained how he had discovered a way to escape from his difficulties: He would commit 'brave and manly crimes' that would be sure to send him to prison where he would not have to face his inability to have erections with women. In his cell there would be no feelings of humiliation and shame because there would be no women there. In other words, Andrew's desire to run away from his erectile dysfunction and the feelings of shame and inadequacy it gave him had taken him time and again into a life of petty crime and imprisonment.

Perhaps you will think that a man like Andrew would never visit a hypnotherapist with such a problem, but you could not be more wrong. When people have lived long enough with their difficulty, have tried so many times to find relief and yet failed, they then become open to exploring new avenues they previously would have dismissed. So often I hear the words: 'You are my last hope.'

When Andrew came to see me, he was tired of the constant fleeing and running. He was finally ready to do whatever it took to bring about the change he wanted so desperately in his life. He had had enough of being sent to prison, enough of living in a state of ongoing isolation, shame, and confusion. At last he was ready to work with the chi of change.

Building from the ground up, we first established that Andrew was taking no medications or drugs and had no underlying medical issues that might be causing his problem. At my request he had visited his doctor for a check-up; his testosterone levels were within the normal range, and he had no sign of vascular disease or diabetes.

Next we looked at Andrew's eating habits. I recommended he

make certain dietary changes to ensure he was getting all the correct micronutrients to support healthy functioning of the reproductive system and to help rebalance his chi. I advised him to increase his intake of zinc by adding such things as wheat germ and pumpkin seeds to his breakfast cereal, and perhaps also adding a zinc supplement to his diet for the next few weeks. The wheat germ would also increase his vitamin B6 intake, and he could further add to this by eating foods such as bell peppers, spinach, and broccoli. I asked him to naturally increase his vitamin E intake by adding some sunflower seeds and almonds to his morning cereal. I also suggested that he take a supplement of red Korean ginseng.

Having taken care of this basic nutritional and orthomolecular support for the healthy functioning of his body, we began the psychological therapy. In a few sessions of brief but intense therapy, we were able to delve down and uncover the psychological cause of his difficulties and then do something about it.

In hypnosis, Andrew quickly returned to a childhood event where he had been teased by his older brothers for having a perfectly natural, spontaneous erection that showed through his short trousers. The embarrassed, guilty feeling this had produced within the boy had been reinforced later when, as an adolescent, his mother unexpectedly entered the room in which he was masturbating. Subsequently, this embarrassed, shameful feeling came to be subconsciously associated with erections—particularly when anyone else was present—and it stood in the way of a healthy sex life.

Once we had uncovered these important sensitizing events, we were then in a position to help Andrew reprocess the experiences and rewrite the programming that had prevented him from getting an erection with women—the real reason for his constantly being on the wrong side of the law. As the therapy progressed, we also worked on increasing his sense of self-esteem, helping his subconscious mind alter its preconceived ideas and perceptions so that it began to see sex not as a performance or test of his masculinity, but as a pleasurable act of intimacy and joy. His therapy completed, Andrew soon put a permanent end to his life as a criminal and within time established his own security consulting company. Soon he had created a new and much better life for himself.

About a year and a half after our final session together, I received a small package delivered by hand to my office. In it there was a piece of wedding cake and a slip of paper with the following words: 'Thank you. Andrew'.

As Andrew's story demonstrates, for change to occur, a person has to stop running. People with emotional difficulties need to allow the part of themselves causing the problem to release its hold. The compulsive overeater has to allow the overeating part to let go of its old habitual way of doing things and assume a more constructive role; the depressed person has to allow the despondent part to change its 'job description' to something more helpful, and so forth.

This process can feel a little unsettling, as if real loss is taking place. For genuine growth to occur, some misguided part of the identity that may well have been integral to our self-definition has to be altered. For the butterfly to be born, the caterpillar first has to fade.

In the therapeutic process, when the sense of loss over giving up a false or redundant part of ourselves feels overwhelming, the ego may become overly protective, and we may encounter the psychological phenomenon known as *resistance.* In fact, resistance is usually a synonym for fear, and that fear has everything to do with the conscious or subconscious perception that part of the self is being threatened with abandonment. It is in danger of being surrendered and lost, and so we resist.

As Andrew's case demonstrates, *all behavior has a positive intent.* Even our most bizarre negative reactions and actions try, at some level, to accomplish something useful for us. The same is true of our symptoms; they have a positive intent behind them. They are luan chi, there to alert us that something is seriously wrong and needs attention. The more severe our symptoms, the more urgently we need to take action.

But when we have lived with a problem for a long time, it can begin to feel almost comfortable because of its familiarity. When confusion abounds, there is something about a long-standing problem that seems somehow dependable, predictable, even reassuring.

Depressed people, for example, may become so associated with the depression that they have a subconscious reluctance to let go of it. In losing the depression, they may feel they are losing a part of themselves that makes them who they are. They may understandably be fearful of putting their trust in life and entering a new and unfamiliar world in which they have little real experience, an unpredictable world of uncertainty and perhaps even greater vulnerability. Something in them may be reluctant to get up and do what is necessary to bring about the essential change. A powerful part may wish to remain as they are, on the floor, because after all, no one can really fall off the floor. Such reluctance can show itself as resistance to change.

As we have already seen, it is the nature of the conscious mind to question, doubt, rationalize, analyze, organize, and compare. It also has a natural tendency to search for an easier way, the path of least resistance, because given the choice between the easy and the difficult, it is only logical to choose the easy. Although the conscious mind may *think* it welcomes a particular change, we can sometimes produce considerable resistance to that change. To a degree, of course, resistance is needed for rational thought; it is integral to how the conscious mind organizes the world—comparing and rejecting, filtering out many things it simply does not want to deal with, managing to function within the apparent safety of known and familiar parameters.

When I was attempting to recover from my own alcoholism and drug dependency many years ago, resistance took hold of me. Something within me fiercely fought giving up the dependent part of myself. Alcohol and drugs had, after all, once been my friends and unfailing companions.

I was a true child of the '60s, and a powerful part of me—my self-identity as a free-spirited, using, bohemian rebel—felt strangely threatened as it faced recovery. I learned that I had to surrender this part of myself, or more correctly, to give it another job to do. My former alcoholic, drug-dependent, and depressed identity—a false, inauthentic self-image—felt like it was dying and was trying everything it could in order to hang on. This experience taught me first-hand that a human being facing real and profound change can experience intense feelings of loss and anxiety and mount strong resistance to the very change they want and so desperately need.

Having lost my appetite for food, I had been reduced to a skeleton: six feet tall and only ninety-eight pounds, or forty-five kilos, in weight. The doctors had given up on me, saying that if I didn't change my behavior, I had only months to live. But they did not tell me *how* I might change my behavior, so I sunk even deeper into despondency.

So lost had I become that I had reached 'the jumping off place', that place where I knew I had to decide either to die or to live. The choice was clearly mine and mine alone, but it needed to be made—it could be delayed no longer. I knew then, as I had never known before, that I did not wish to die. I wanted to live. And the only way I *could* live was to at last accept the responsibility for doing exactly that and say goodbye to that part of myself that wanted me to continue in the self-destructive patterns even though they were killing me. In order for me to live, a part of me just had to let go.

I had to accept the responsibility of *choosing* to take an enormous leap of faith and put my trust in life, in my own natural ability to somehow come through it all, and in a power I could barely believe in. Only then could I bring an end to the resistance and ease myself forward and upward into recovery and health.

From my own personal experience, I learned that the only true antidote for resistance is trust. There is a time and a place for doubt, but in therapy, as in life, without trust, little can be accomplished. For change to happen, people have to abandon resistance, listen to the chi of change, and allow it to flow freely.

In order to be effective, a therapist needs to be aware of possible resistance, as well as of the fear and sense of loss that may drive it. With this understanding, the therapist provides a safe, non-judgmental space where the client can explore even the most uncomfortable feelings. Having established good rapport and the vital trust needed to move past resistance, the therapist guides the client through whatever rough waters they may encounter.

When resistance is too strong, a person can sabotage their own therapy, sometimes without even realizing it. Fortunately, this seldom happens, but it does occasionally. It is important to remember at such times that the therapist does not control the client's mind; therapy is not 'brain-washing'. Each of us possesses a sufficient degree of free will, and this means we each have the ability to choose. In the end, it is the individual who must choose to allow the walls of resistance to come down. If a person really wants to move on and be free of the problem that brought them to the therapist, it is that person's responsibility to *choose* to let go of resistance, to take whatever leap of faith or trust is necessary to allow the therapeutic process that will bring about the change they desire. A skilled therapist can indeed open doors, but it is the client who must choose whether or not to walk through them.

Resistance can present itself in various ways. For example, some people, even though they have passed all tests for being in the trance state, will emerge from hypnosis and say, 'I don't think I was hypnotized'. Sometimes, this is a normal reaction after one's first hypnotic experience. Even though explanations have been given to the client prior to induction into trance, the person's preconceived ideas of what hypnosis is and what it *should* feel like still persist. These notions often differ considerably from the actuality. In the very first session, I usually conduct a series of tests designed not only to check for the level of hypnosis, but also to provide objective evidence to the client that they were indeed hypnotized.

With some people, especially those who are particularly analytical or those with a powerful need to believe they are in control at all times—so called 'control freaks'—the conscious, logical mind can find it difficult to accept that it was not entirely running the show during hypnosis, so it resists any evidence to the contrary. It may be reluctant to admit that another part of the mind—the hidden, subconscious part—was more in control. No matter how strong the evidence may appear, the person's conscious mind can insist on rationalizing and denying what it does not wish to believe just happened, that they were, in fact, in hypnosis.

Of course, resistance may manifest itself for perfectly valid reasons. We must never forget that there is always a reason for our symptoms and that our symptoms may serve a useful psychological function. If, for example, a person compulsively picks at his or her skin because it is the only way to gain a degree of release for an unexpressed inner rage that has yet to be properly processed at the subconscious level, then the mind will be very reluctant to give up the skin-picking behavior (a condition known as dermotillomania) unless it has some other way to release the anger or something else to replace it with. The subconscious mind is fully capable of resisting any attempt to force it to give up what it believes to be a behavior that is serving a useful psychological function—despite the wishes of the conscious mind or the very best intentions of the therapist.

In addition, resistance is almost always present when the subconscious mind feels the need to protect itself and its beliefs—even when some of those beliefs are faulty—so it more or less forces the conscious mind to rationalize and offer some logical explanation for its resistance. When this is the case, resistance is a symptom of fear, and until that fear is assuaged, there is little that can be done in hypnosis or with hypnotherapy. Though resistance can be worked through, if the mind insists on maintaining it and the resistance remains too great, then therapy will, of course, not be effective. Indeed, it may not be possible at all.

Once any resistance has been effectively dealt with, then we may truly begin to co-operate with the process of change. We are free to uncover those old, redundant programs that have been causing such difficulty so that we can do something about them; free to realign the ego states that have been causing so much inner friction.

Many people are astonished to learn that this need not be a lengthy process. Unlike other modalities, therapies that may demand an investment of months or even years, effective hypnotherapy can usually accomplish its healing surprisingly swiftly, with the entire therapeutic process seldom taking more than half a dozen sessions for most presenting issues and far fewer for simple phobias. This often comes as a surprise to people accustomed to thinking of therapy as a protracted, lengthy, and drawn-out process.

This is not to say that the more lengthy talking therapies do not have their value. There are times when an individual is simply not yet ready to change or to respond to rapid-change therapy. In other instances, individuals who have successfully resolved their presenting issues and problems through hypnotherapy choose to benefit from an ongoing, lengthier form of continued emotional support, feedback, or life-coaching. So the talking therapies can be useful for many people.

People who have strong neurotic tendencies can also find solace in good counseling. Such individuals find it hard to maintain a balanced sense of responsibility. That great psychologist, Alfred Adler, once said that the neurotic is nailed to the cross of their own fiction. But for the subconscious mind, there is no great difference between fiction and fact, the imaginary and the real.

Neurotic people tend to extremes. At one extreme they can assume far too much responsibility for that which is really beyond their control, and they often feel guilty for things that go wrong that are not their fault and for which they have little responsibility. In so doing, they easily make themselves despondent and unhappy. I have coined the term 'intro-neurotic' for such people. At the other extreme, there are neurotics who simply shun all responsibility, placing the blame for anything that goes wrong on other people. These people I call 'extro-neurotic'. The intro-neurotics make themselves unhappy, while extro-neurotics make others unhappy. A person can swing between both states, and few people are exclusively one or the other. Neither position is balanced or healthy.

In all the above cases, counseling and the more traditional forms of psychotherapy can be useful. Although Freudian psychoanalysis is, in my opinion, a highly questionable endeavor, often verging on a religion for those heavily invested in it, there are other counseling modalities that can be beneficial.

I believe that humanistic existential counseling may be particularly helpful for people with neurotic tendencies, and I sometimes refer clients to an experienced counselor for this. Existential counseling, in common with the best hypnotherapy, seeks to continually encourage a person's self-honesty, thereby promoting a more balanced sense of responsibility and personal authenticity. Unlike the determinism of Freud and psychoanalysis where so much is considered to be pathological and 'written in stone', existential counseling helps individuals to explore the choices they make and to accept responsibility for those choices.

Of course, there are other forms of counseling available, the most common being what is known as 'person-centered'. If you are considering counseling, the most important thing is to work with a counselor with whom you feel a connection. Research has demonstrated that the therapeutic relationship is often more important than the counselor's particular school of thought—and this is true for most forms of psychological therapy.

But for rapid and truly powerful change, little can really compare with a therapy that goes directly to the root cause of an individual's issues and then changes the programming that created and continues to drive them. This capacity to rapidly bring about profound and lasting change through brief yet intensive strategies is what makes hypnotherapy such an excellent tool for healing.

As we have seen, change seldom comes in the manner people expect. It has its own special way of functioning and revealing itself. As we mature, we come to understand that genuine change rarely happens via lightning bolts or mystical winds that sweep us to the heights of the mountaintops. Rather, it usually occurs in subtle, almost inconspicuous ways and there is a reason for this.

Because our problems never really were us, once they have been cleared, it can feel entirely normal to be without them. It feels natural and organic to be authentically ourselves, and we may not even notice how profoundly we have changed. It is often only later, when we realize we have responded to a life situation in a very different manner than we previously would have, that we recognize how much real change has occurred.

For some, of course, this lighter, freer self takes a bit of getting used to. That heaviness or tightness in the chest, those butterflies or knots in the stomach are simply no longer there. The tension has been lifted. It has been replaced with an almost strange and unaccustomed lightness, which some may experience as a kind of emptiness. In the beginning this can feel a little peculiar. Some people experience it as an almost dizzy feeling, but they soon adjust to this wonderful lightness of being as they become accustomed to spontaneously approaching life with a much more affirmative, balanced attitude.

It is important to understand that once formal therapy has ended, the fresher, freer life can be maintained only by cultivating balanced, healthy interests that will fill whatever place the problems and difficulties previously occupied. Life will continue to be life, with all of its ups and downs and challenges. Having moved through therapy, the person needs to develop interests that will continue to absorb and assist in personal growth and development. Here self-hypnosis or meditation can be very helpful.

As we have now seen, many of our problems and difficulties can be traced back to our infancy, to experiences that were misinterpreted or only partially understood by our younger self. For many people going through therapy, it is sometimes hard to believe that a seemingly small and insignificant event that occurred so long ago could ever have been the cause of their difficulties. Because their problem has become so large and overwhelming, they expect it to have been caused by something equally as large, some major traumatic event that has perhaps been lost to conscious recall. While this can sometimes be the case, in reality it is very rarely so.

Generally speaking, life's major traumas tend to be remembered by the conscious mind, while the smaller ones that produce so much later difficulty and so many distressing problems down the road are very often forgotten, registered only in the subconscious.

Surprisingly, while people do visit therapists because of major traumatic events and their consequences, most of the time the difficulties that bring a person to the therapist's couch are the result of quite mundane experiences. Usually these occurred during the early years, and they often involved an interaction with a relevant other, such as a parent, sibling, teacher, friend or peer. They may also be the product of some other experience through which the younger self passed that did not involve anyone else, or the person may have subconsciously modeled their responses and reactions on those observed in someone else.

The compassionate therapist empathizes with the troubled and often upset client, aware that it is the worrying and disruptive symptoms that have guided the person to seek help. Yet the therapist must never allow those symptoms to distract from the real issue. For the experienced therapist, *symptoms are simply signals*. As troublesome as they are, they are not the real problem. They are luan chi, messages manufactured by the subconscious to direct the person's attention to an issue that needs to be addressed. The real problem is the *driver* of those symptoms—the improperly interpreted and poorly processed experiences and conflicted ego states that caused and continue to fuel the person's difficulties.

In hypnotherapy, we use symptoms to guide us towards the real issue, but the experienced and skilled practitioner does not usually use hypnotherapy in a direct attempt to treat the symptoms as such. Instead, we focus on treating the whole person and the *cause* of the symptoms. Once the underlying issue is addressed, the symptoms often spontaneously correct themselves. As Cervantes observed: 'Take away the cause, and the effect ceases.'

Unfortunately, there are many misinformed and poorly trained practitioners out there who seem completely unaware of the necessity to treat more than just the presenting symptoms. These days, schools and training seminars of all sorts are turning out alleged 'hypnotherapists' and 'NLP (Neuro-Linguistic Programming) practitioners' who are taught only how to use hypnosis in a superficial manner to dismiss symptoms of deeper problems. These people merely attempt to relieve clients of their symptoms with total disregard for their underlying origins and psychological function. From 'fast phobia cures', to scripted 'visualizations' and 'mind-management' cognitive strategies, trainees are taught how to offer the quick-fix, concentrating almost entirely on treating only the symptoms of the people who turn to them—often so desperately—for help. What these practitioners fail to recognize is that focusing only on symptom relief can be a considerable and often a grave error.

Louisa was a hard-working mother of three and a busy sales rep. Although she was friendly and sociable, her smiling countenance hid an undercurrent of anxiety and fear. For as long as she could remember, she had struggled with these uncomfortable feelings, doing her best to accept them as part of who and how she was, and she had somehow managed to soldier bravely on.

When she came to see me, it was because her job, and therefore her livelihood, was in jeopardy. Louisa was dependent on her car and on her ability to drive that car in order to carry out her work, yet she had developed a terrible, almost crippling fear of driving. She just could not bring herself to get behind the wheel of her car and drive. At first she had managed to maneuver around this by asking her daughter to drive her to her appointments, but her daughter had begun working and could no longer do this. So Louisa had signed off sick, while what she was really experiencing were anxiety and panic attacks connected with driving.

According to Louisa, the problem had started two years previously when she was passing through a particularly difficult time and was in the process of divorce. Following her husband's car down the slip road and onto the freeway, she had difficulty merging with the fast-moving flow of traffic and saw her husband's vehicle speeding away in front of her. Suddenly and without warning, Louisa had felt her legs involuntarily kick out and her muscles stiffen; they just seemed to lock and freeze. Her limbs felt like they were working independently of her, and Louisa felt completely powerless to do anything about it. She just wanted to get out, but she couldn't. Almost instantly she became terrified that she was no longer in control of her vehicle. Her breathing became shallow, her heart pounded, and dizziness clouded her mind. Panic swept through her, and Louisa barely managed to steer the car onto the hard shoulder where she scrambled out, gasping for breath. Sweating and scared, she knew she had only narrowly avoided a serious accident.

Eventually she managed to call a friend on her cell phone. About three-quarters of an hour later, the friend arrived with his wife, who drove a much-shaken and confused Louisa back home. After that experience, Louisa managed to drive only with great difficulty and only because her job depended on it, and she assiduously avoided driving on the freeway under any circumstances, often adding hours to her journey. Soon she found herself experiencing more acute anxiety and panic while behind the wheel, and then feelings of anxiety when merely thinking about driving. Those terrible, frightening feelings just seemed to spring out of nowhere, taking over to the point where, eventually, she was unable to drive at all.

Louisa's doctor had routinely prescribed the antidepressant medication Seroxat (paroxetine) in the hope that it might settle her nerves and allow her to drive in a calmer state. But this only seemed to worsen her driving anxiety, making her feel even shakier, so she discontinued its use. On reporting this to her physician, Louisa was switched to another medication in a further attempt to address her problem with chemicals, but this, too, proved ineffective. Her driving anxiety had now escalated to the point that she could no longer get behind the wheel of a car. Even the thought of driving filled her with fear.

When Louisa first came to me, we began by looking at the foods she had been eating, and I encouraged her to eat a more balanced diet consisting of whole foods, to reduce and finally eliminate coffee and caffeinated drinks, and to take a supplement of the amino acid taurine, which has been shown to be beneficial in reducing anxiety.

As she talked, Louisa disclosed that she had visited a hypnotherapist about two years previously for help dealing with claustrophobic feelings that had long bothered her. After a series of sessions with this practitioner, she seemed to have responded fairly well and had reduced, though not completely eliminated, her claustrophobic fear. The problem was that the hypnotherapist had focused merely on symptom removal, using well-known NLP techniques and positive suggestion in hypnosis. As is unfortunately so often the case, he had entirely neglected any investigation into the reason for her symptoms.

Understandably, Louisa had not made any connection at all between the claustrophobia for which she had been treated by the hypnotherapist and the anxiety and panic attacks triggered by driving. To her, the two seemed totally unrelated.

In our hypnotherapy sessions, Louisa was gently guided into the deep state of hypnosis known as somnambulism. This is similar to the sleep-walking state, but unlike the sleep form, the person in hypnosis remains fully aware, relaxed yet in control at all times. Now her fearful feelings took her back many years through the tunnel of time to the origin of her problem—so far back, in fact, that in this state of hypnosis her mind returned to her mother's womb. There her subconscious mind recounted how she heard angry shouting; how she felt agitated, unsafe, and in danger, and how she had automatically been flooded with powerful feelings of anxiety and fear. Instinctively she found herself kicking out, her little muscles stiffening as if they were locking and freezing.

The awful feelings of anxiety swept through Louisa as the unborn child struggled to free herself of her frightening feelings—she needed to get out, but there was no way out. These, of course, were exactly the same *feelings* that had swept through her when following her husband's car onto the freeway.

A little later, Louisa was taken back to an experience with her big sister where, as an infant of three years old, she was trapped in an ottoman, her sister sitting on top shouting, 'I hate you!' as Louisa kicked out, her muscles once more stiffening and locking as she again experienced that sense of danger and those terrible feelings of fear and anxiety. Her sister's shouts produced feelings of rejection that combined with the feelings of being trapped, of claustrophobia, and of powerlessness—reinforcing those feelings that had become embedded within her subconscious when she was in the womb. There just was no way out.

When Louisa's husband sped away from her, leaving her once again feeling rejected and trapped, surrounded by the danger of fast-moving vehicles pressing down on her, that event triggered the old subconscious program, so she was again flooded with similar feelings. The events experienced by her infant self had created the anxious, claustrophobic feelings and the need to kick out with her feet and legs as she had the first times those strong feelings arose.

But here is something that may not be obvious at first glance: In the beginning of her adult problems, Louisa's symptoms were feelings that presented as claustrophobia. These symptoms became stifled by misguided hypnosis that focused merely on removing the symptom but completely ignored the underlying cause. Stripped of its ability to send its message (via claustrophobia), Louisa's subconscious was forced to manufacture even more dire symptoms to get her attention: this time, crippling anxiety, panic attacks, and the leg-kicking that had almost cost her her life while driving.

Once the causal experiences from her past were uncovered, Louisa was gently guided into using her wiser adult mind to reach back in time, as it were, and reassure her younger self that she was in fact safe, that she could relax through the shouting and emerge safely from the womb, that she would be safely released from the ottoman, and that no harm would come to her. Her subconscious mind now knew the truth that her younger mind had not been able to process or understand as it passed through those traumatic events: She was safe and she would remain safe.

As soon as this understanding was established at the subconscious level that part of the inner mind that had become stuck relaxed its grip. Louisa was no longer compelled to slavishly follow the old, redundant programming. Her panic attacks and fear of driving simply fell away, and she became free to calmly drive anywhere she wanted—including on freeways—knowing that she was safe and in control and that she would remain so. Her life returned to normal.

What had happened to Louisa was that in visiting the previous hypnotherapist and focusing only on the symptom of claustrophobia, a process known as 'symptom displacement' had occurred. Because the subconscious mind had been denied the ability to express itself through the symptom of claustrophobia, it found another way to manifest its unresolved difficulties. By treating only the symptoms of her presenting issue, the hypnotherapist had done this woman a great disservice. While the claustrophobia became somewhat reduced, its *cause* remained unaddressed and intact. So the creative subconscious mind had found an even more powerful way to attract Louisa's attention—one that almost killed her.

Louisa's case also illustrates another interesting fact. Amazing though it may seem, in the extremely deep level of hypnosis called *somnambulism*, it is not at all uncommon for a person to regress back to a pre-birth experience. The mother undergoes some traumatic event—perhaps a violent argument, a fall, or some kind of shock—and her body is automatically flooded with powerful catecholamines—the 'fight-or-flight' hormones. These then pass through the placenta and into the fetus, causing the unborn child to feel those same fearful feelings but without the ability to understand why, to make any sense of them, or to do anything about them. In the womb, the baby can hear sound, attaching an emotion and a meaning to it. So even before birth, a person may have already experienced fear causing the feeling of being unsafe to become embedded prenatally.

Most often though, such sensitizing experiences happen sometime later, after birth, usually before the fifth or sixth year of life (although sometimes—as is common with phobias such as fear of flying, for example—they can take place much later than this). In these ways, the seed of fear is planted and the program installed. The program is easily reinforced by subsequent events that bear a similarity to the experience that created the fear program originally. Although lying dormant for some time, sooner or later these programs become activated, triggered by a later experience or symptom-producing event, making themselves known in the form of disruptive energies that confuse and confound: acute anxiety, panic attacks, depression, compulsions, phobias, or behaviors that are simply meant as coping mechanisms, intended to distract the person away from their uncomfortable inner feelings: overeating, alcohol, drugs, gambling, pornography, nail biting, skin picking, hair pulling, and so forth.

This is the process that can lead to years of debilitation and misery, affecting a person's self-esteem and robbing them of the simple joy of existence. But paradoxically, it is also the process that can propel the individual forward, drawing them into the freeing process, the chi of change, that brings with it growth and personal development.

In the deep trance state of hypnosis, we can rapidly trace back and return to the cause itself, uncovering the origin of the problem, and then help the subconscious reinterpret those experiences that have been so poorly processed. In so doing, we rewrite the faulty program, unblock the chi, and restore harmony. When this readjustment is combined with the proper nutritional support, the person is able to live as they were intended to: in a freer, more authentic, and more life-affirming manner.

Chapter Four

Anxiety and Panic Attacks

'Our Age of Anxiety is, in great part, the result of trying to do today's job with yesterday's tools and yesterday's concepts.'
~ Marshall McLuhan

Who among us has never felt anxious? Anxiety seems to be built right into the fabric of existence. Indeed, some degree of anxiety may even be helpful, keeping us on our toes and giving us the edge that can push us to function at our optimum level. A certain amount of anxiety is normal and healthy. To expect a life completely free of anxiety is to ask life to be something other than it is.

But sometimes anxiety can be just too forceful and last far too long. There are times when it springs out as if from nowhere, hitting us like a truck or yanking the rug from under us, shaking us up and filling us with fear. When this happens, we know it is not simply those natural, anxious feelings that we all must sometimes experience. This is Anxiety with a capital 'A'. It's the kind of anxiety we will be talking about in this chapter and the next.

If you have been experiencing lots of anxiety and can see no obvious reason for it, you're certainly not alone. In fact, you might be surprised to learn just how common anxiety actually is.

Today anxiety has become the most common type of mental distress disorder in the U.S. (Anxiety and Depression Society of America, 2012), as well as in the U.K, where I live (Office for National Statistics Psychiatric Morbidity Report, 2001). In America today, anxiety disorders are thought to affect 40 million adults or fully 18 percent of the population, and as many as one in eight children. According to the U.S. National Institute for

Mental Health, those with anxiety disorders are six times more likely to be hospitalized for psychiatric disorders. One of the most common forms anxiety takes—social anxiety disorder—is estimated to affect an enormous 12 per cent of the population, making it a risk factor in the development of a whole range of difficulties, including those involving alcohol, substance abuse, chronic overeating, and depression. It can even lead to an increased risk of suicide (Sareen et al. 2005).

Personally, I consider such figures to be much too low, and I am not alone in this. Other experts (such as Dr David Baldwin, professor of psychiatry and head of the Mental Health Group at the University of Southampton) believe as many as one in five people experience some form of anxiety disorder.

Perhaps the official figures are lower than the actual numbers because they fail to take into account the many people who suffer from anxiety but do not seek treatment. Some people do not see anxiety as something the doctor can help with, and many others are too shy, ashamed, or afraid to seek help, so they remain beyond the statistics. Recognizing this, the World Health Organization (2009) has estimated that as many as 57 per cent of people suffering from an anxiety disorder do not receive treatment.

But if you suffer from anxiety, there's a good chance you won't care too much about statistics. You care about the awful way it makes you feel—tense, irritable, and on edge; how it takes your breath away and makes your heart pound, drying out your mouth and sending you rushing to the bathroom; how it interferes with your sleep, giving you that constant worried and worn-out feeling; how it stops you from relaxing and fills you with dread.

Let me assure you that you were not put here to live your life in this anxious state—it is simply not your true nature. You are not losing your mind, you are not mentally ill, and as we have already seen, you are by no means alone. Millions upon millions of people worldwide suffer from some type of anxiety disorder, and the treatment of anxiety in its various manifestations forms a very large part of my work as a therapist.

There is another thing of which I am certain: You really can get better.

Anxiety and its treatment is such a broad topic that I have divided it into two chapters. In this chapter we will look at two of the main reasons why people consult the therapist—anxiety and panic attacks—and we will also take a look at social anxiety, something that affects so many people in today's fast-paced society. In the next chapter, we will discuss some of the other guises anxiety may assume; how a person's disturbed luan chi can manifest itself in different forms, from performance anxiety and common phobias to sexual dysfunction and post-traumatic stress disorder. And we will see that the one common denominator in every form of chronic anxiety is irrational fear.

In every single instance, anxiety exists because of a fear of the future that is based on information from the past. We are, to paraphrase Marshal McLuhan, 'trying to do today's job with yesterday's concepts'. The fact that something unsettling has happened to us in the past has conditioned us to believe that it will happen again in the future and that, just as in the past, we will find it difficult to cope with. This prevents us from doing 'today's job' properly—it prevents us from enjoying life in the now.

Because of this, every form of anxiety is predicated on two little words: what if. 'What if this happens?' 'What if that happens?' 'What if I lose control?' 'What if I panic?' 'What if I cannot sleep?' 'What if I make a fool of myself in front of other people?' 'What if I cannot perform well in bed?' In this way, fear flows through the luan chi, the energy suffused with information that screams out: 'You are not really safe! Something bad is probably going to happen! Be on guard!'

This should not come as too much of a surprise. As we saw in

Chapter 2, fear is usually present in almost every difficulty that brings a person to the hypnotherapist, and as we have also seen, anxiety is one of the main issues with which clients present. Indeed, so interconnected are these two emotions that anxiety and fear are often used as synonyms for each other. Yet there is a difference.

Fear is the short, sharp shock response to a legitimate stressor—such as the sight of a raging bull coming towards you. It's the feeling you would get if you found yourself in an earthquake. It's a natural survival mechanism, entirely useful and not designed to last for very long. In fact, it is meant to end just as soon as it has done its job and withdrawn us from the dangerous situation. It is essential chi, a feeling sent by the subconscious mind in order to protect and keep us safe.

Anxiety shares many similarities with fear, but it has one crucial difference: It persists after the threat or stressor is no longer there. As such, anxiety is irrational. According to one definition: 'Anxiety is a mental disorder when it is more intense than is justified by the actual threat.'(Lickey & Gordon, 1991)

While fear has a logical reason to exist, anxiety does not. It exists beyond logic, lingering on when there is no logically justifiable reason for its existence. Sometimes hyper-anxious feelings can last and last, becoming chronic and incapacitating, affecting a person's ability to work, socialize, and live a normal life, with much time spent in a worried and over-vigilant state where the worst is always lurking just around the corner.

When we experience these irrational feelings over a period of time and they show no sign of abating, we have what can be termed an 'anxiety disorder'. As our subconscious mind continues to transmit information that is faulty, energetically instructing us that we are in danger when we are not, we are forced into a position of uncertainty and tension. When we are in a stressful situation or are under the cumulative pressure of stress, the mind can easily turn anxiety into panic, bringing on a panic attack, or triggering other worrying physical and emotional responses.

Anxiety then is a form of distorted chi. Our subconscious is transmitting information that is faulty and producing a negative energy that is uncalled for and unneeded.

Those anxious, panicky feelings and sensations are the mind and body's way of preparing us for dangerous experiences by putting us on 'red alert'. The purpose is to ensure our safety by keeping us vigilant and prepared for trouble, priming us and holding us on edge so that we can flee from or ward off danger. But the mind has it wrong when it creates this alert and keeps it going in the absence of a genuine threat. When that happens, the false warning itself creates a disturbance and threatens our well-being. Once again it comes down to perception. It is the subconscious mind's perception that something bad is about to happen—not that something bad is actually happening—that fuels anxiety.

For some people, anxiety appears in a rush and when least expected. They are feeling carefree when anxiety suddenly knocks them off their feet, sending them into a tailspin. For many other people, it is as if they have spent their entire life in a worried, jittery state. They feel there never was a time when they did not feel on edge. Having lived this way for so long, it is not unusual for them and for those around them to believe this is just who they are, that it is part of their natural disposition.

For those who have never experienced chronic anxiety, it is difficult to imagine the extent of the misery and terror it can produce. Often people try to disguise it, condemning themselves to a life filled with unshared feelings of foreboding, dread, and fear.

Is anyone really born this way? Is anxiety something genetic? Although some evidence suggests that genetic factors may make a person more prone to anxiety (Tsuang & Stone, 2004), other evidence overwhelmingly suggests that stressful life events can cause alterations in brain functioning, predisposing a person to anxiety and depression (Cowely, 1991). My years of professional experience support this latter view, though I also know that anxiety can pass from mother to child in the womb.

But just as events of a stressful nature can produce negative alterations in brain activity, the reverse is also true. By realigning the mind at the subconscious level and altering its programs, we can create fresh neural pathways in the brain, transforming it in a positive manner. This ability of the brain to reorganize itself and to undergo change, both physical and functional, is known as neural plasticity, and it is nothing short of amazing.

But to understand the mind's role in creating (or removing) anxiety, we have to go beyond the workings of the brain itself. We need to go to the life experiences and environmental influences that impacted our development. We have to reach back in time to those events that helped shape our brain and our mind because these are the things that continue to influence how we interpret and react to what happens in the present.

Even if anxiety is so embedded that it seems to be part of our innate personality, this is never truly the case. I have found that even in instances where a client was born feeling anxious, by reaching far enough back, we can find a time when anxiety was not present and when feelings of safety and well-being were all that existed. Let me illustrate this with an example.

Roberto was a young man of dual heritage who came to see me because his life had been spiraling out of control due to chronic anxiety and panic attacks. For years he had been taking powerful anxiolytic and antidepressant drugs prescribed for him by different doctors. He had visited a psychiatrist, a clinical psychologist, and two alternative therapists and had tried cognitive therapy, counseling, NLP, acupuncture, and Reiki, but nothing had provided significant relief. By the time he arrived in my office, he was desperate. He still lived in an almost constant state of apprehension and anxiety, worrying when and where the next panic attack might strike.

So fearful was he that a panic attack might strike when he was away from home, leaving him vulnerable and defenseless, that he dreaded going out of his house. Roberto had developed a condition called agoraphobia. He was able to visit my office only with the greatest difficulty and had to be accompanied by both of his parents.

In the deep state of somnambulistic hypnosis, Roberto returned to the experience of his birth and to the feelings that accompanied it. All he felt was an unwelcome pressure and then harsh lights that pained his eyes and strange, unfriendly-looking figures wearing masks and green coats. He seemed to have been plucked screaming from the warm, comfortable darkness, and then he felt a sharp shock of pain, as if being attacked, which made him scream out even more. All he could see were colors, bright red and orangey-brown mingling in with the green, and he was filled with an awful fear that sent shock waves flooding through his little body, shaking him to the depths of his being.

What had happened? Roberto's mother had experienced difficulty in giving birth, so he had been delivered by caesarean section, cut from the safety of his mother's womb and abruptly transported into a strange new reality full of uncertainty and apparent danger. Orangey-brown was the color of the antiseptic iodine wash the doctor had used to swab his mother's belly, and red was the color of the blood that bathed him. No wonder he was afraid.

This was the origin of the program that would later translate into chronic anxiety; the initial sensitizing event that would eventually produce his awful panic attacks. Who could blame Roberto for believing he had been born with anxiety? In a very real sense, he had.

Yet anxiety had not existed prior to his birth. There was indeed a time in his mother's womb when he felt warm, safe and anxiety-free. In the deep trance state of hypnosis, he went back to that safe time when the life force of chi flowed freely. The program that produced Roberto's anxiety was embedded in his subconscious as a consequence of his traumatic birthing experience; it had nothing to do with genetics, nor was it native to him. This is a point worth reiterating: Chronic anxiety is not native to anyone. It has to be acquired through a process of sensitization; it is something learned on life's journey.

As he grew, Roberto would encounter other experiences—subsequent sensitizing events—that reinforced the anxiety, driving the program deeper until it felt like a part of him, the lens through which his life experience was filtered and perceived. Once we located the origin of the program, we were able to neutralize it and to work our way through the series of subsequent sensitizing events that had served to reinforce Roberto's anxiety. Today Roberto is free to enjoy his life much more fully. He rarely looks back on his previous, anxious existence.

Of course, not every person born through caesarean section will go on to experience chronic anxiety and panic attacks, just as not everyone scratched by a cat will go on to develop a cat phobia. It all depends on the way the individual interprets and responds to the experience.

Anxiety is not always the result of our own direct experience; it can also be absorbed vicariously, through observing others. Our brains are naturally programmed to instinctively recognize how other people feel. It's part of our inbuilt survival process. To be able to read the emotions of others through body language and facial expressions is important. It is an ability we share with other animals, such as apes and dogs (Nagasawa, 2011), and is something we have been aware of for quite some time. Writing in the 19th century, Charles Darwin devoted an entire book to the subject (1872). To know if people are happy or angry to see us, for example, allows us to modify our behavior and act appropriately. We begin this process as infants, intuitively honing our ability to interpret what others are feeling, subconsciously learning how to read even the subtlest of messages.

Through this process, anxiety may also be learned. Children in particular can subconsciously model their attitudes and responses on the behavior of another person, a relevant other. In psychology this is known as 'emotion contagion'. How we feel can be negatively influenced and learned from other people, especially at an early age.

Sometimes anxiety is learned through the process of association, in which an otherwise neutral stimulus—an object, setting, or normal bodily sensation, for example—may become associated with fearful feelings until the neutral stimulus itself can trigger the fear response at any time. (Association of a certain emotion or reaction with a neutral stimulus is known as a 'conditioned response'.)

Lance was a portly and distinguished-looking man in his mid-fifties with two grown-up children and a third in college. He came to see me because of the intense anxiety he had been experiencing. His panicky feelings seemed to spring from nowhere and were now seriously affecting his ability to socialize or even visit with his children and grandson. In the beginning, Lance had tried to shrug it off, telling himself it was just one of those things and would soon clear up, but his anxiety only worsened over time.

The clincher had come when he and his family were invited to the wedding of his close friend's daughter. Lance's anxiety had been so great that he had failed to attend, begging his wife to plead a bout of food poisoning as an excuse for not being there. The lie allowed him to avoid the wedding but left him filled with feelings of self-disappointment and shame. Anxiety was seriously affecting his life, so he finally was determined to do something about it.

With gentle probing, we discovered that while feelings of generalized anxiety had been lurking in the background for many years, they had remained more or less under control.

Lance recalled a time in his twenties when he experienced intense anxiety bordering on panic while returning home late at night from the office, but he had managed to dismiss this as a one-off and did not remember being bothered like that again. Interestingly, many of Lance's recent anxiety attacks had also happened at night, the first one taking place following a heated argument with his youngest son, a teen who had arrived home late reeking of alcohol.

As the hours had passed and his son still had not returned, Lance's worry had exacerbated. He sat in the living room, the lights off as though he had gone to bed. When the boy finally tiptoed in, shoes in hand, Lance sprang up and angrily confronted him, but as he did so, he found himself gasping for breath and clutching his heart as if about to die. Lance had been rushed to the hospital, where doctors found nothing physically wrong with him. They explained to Lance that what he had experienced appeared to be a panic attack.

The second attack happened some weeks later at the gym as Lance was furiously pedaling away on a stationary bicycle. Suddenly panic had gripped him, and he struggled to the corner of the gym where the stretching mats were. There he lay, gasping for breath on the floor, covered in sweat, his heart pounding in his ears.

After Lance related all this, he was guided into a state of somnambulistic hypnosis, where he quickly found himself back at the age of five, playing with his older brother in the bedroom they shared. Suddenly his breathing changed, becoming shallow and labored. He gasped for breath. His heart raced, and he was covered in sweat. In the memory Lance had revisited, his brother had him trapped under a thick duvet and was refusing to let him out.

It was supposed to be a game, of course, but for little Lance, it was not. This was a matter of life or death. Before long his brother opened up the duvet and released him, but not before the experience had embedded itself deeply in the little boy's mind.

The associations were now installed at the subconscious level. The darkness and the hot, sweaty feeling he had experienced under the duvet—of themselves quite neutral stimuli—when combined with a state of heightened emotion would become triggers waiting to go off at some future time, once more filling him with panic. In another individual, such an experience might have been the precursor of claustrophobia, but each person responds in their own unique way, and Lance had escaped that particular difficulty.

As he grew, Lance's associations were reinforced by various experiences, subsequent sensitizing events where he again felt great anxiety. Years later, he found himself in the 'darkness' of his living room involved in a 'heated' confrontation with his son. In his highly charged emotional state of anger, the ancient program of panic was fully activated, making his heart race and forcing him to hyperventilate as he gasped for breath, fearing he would die. Later, in the gym, as Lance pedaled on the stationary bike, the sweaty sensations and elevated heart rate alone set things off, triggering yet another anxiety attack, the previously latent subconscious program now completely active and functional.

Why had it taken so long for the program to fully manifest? That is anyone's guess. No two people are alike; no two people will react in an identical way to any of life's situations. An experience that one person might easily brush off as nothing at all might be the initial sensitizing event that eventually snowballs into panic attacks, depression, addiction, or a phobia for another person. Perception, meaning, and the importance we attach to it determine the effect any experience will have on an individual. Because of this, each person responds subjectively in their own unique way and in their own time.

As Lance's case demonstrates, the subconscious mind has little comprehension of time, and programs can remain inactive for years before being triggered. For Lance, the troublesome program became active later in life, although it had hovered in the background for years.

Anxiety and worry seem to go hand in hand, and for many people the two are synonymous. When we feel anxious, it is almost always because we are worrying that something bad will happen. Worrying, in fact, is a way of coping with anxiety. It is an attempt to prepare ourselves for difficult experiences we think await us in the future. As we saw with Lance, anxiety is most often triggered when we are in a situation bearing some resemblance to a previous unsettling experience, or when we connect with some element similar to one that had once disturbed us, though we may not be consciously aware of the trigger. The anxiety reaction can occur because of an event that happens in real time, or one that is simply imagined.

Let's take a look at how this happens. When we perceive any kind of threat, we do so through our senses. Something suddenly frightens us, and the information is sent careening along two different paths in the brain.

The first path is the shortest. It operates below conscious awareness, at the unconscious level. When we become startled, for example, our brain automatically sends a message to its fear center, located in the amygdala. The amygdala goes into red alert, rapidly informing other parts of the brain—and the body-mind complex—of potential danger. Adrenaline and other hormonal neurotransmitters are released, and everything is primed for action: We experience the overriding impulse to flee or to fight.

If we are in real and significant danger (when being attacked by a predator, for example), and if there is no option to flee or to successfully defend ourselves, we might automatically 'freeze' in an instinctive last-ditch effort to convince the predator we are dead, so that it might turn its focus elsewhere. This is the origin of the expression 'frozen with fear'. All this is part of our primitive alarm-and-defense system, intended by nature to ensure our survival. And all of this happens in a trice, often before the conscious mind is aware of having seen or heard anything. Before our conscious mind knows we are afraid, we already are.

The second path is activated only after the conscious mind has become aware of the threat. At this point, some of the information coming from the senses is sent to the brain's sensory-cue-processing center, the thalamus, and from there on to the cortex, which analyzes the sensory information. Now the mind is called upon to make a vital decision: Does the situation require an ongoing fear response? Do I need to remain on red alert, or can I just relax and move on?

As we saw in Chapter 2, the subconscious rapidly performs a search of our referential index—our filing cabinet of past experiences, perceptions, and learnings—to determine how to respond to what is happening. If it decides an ongoing fear response is justified, it quickly feeds this information back to the amygdala. Then the body-mind complex remains on red alert as the adrenaline, cortisol, and other hormones continue being pumped and anxiety continues being generated, ensuring we remain in a highly vigilant state, ready for action.

The physical sensations we experience from ongoing anxiety result from these powerful chemicals flooding through us. If you have ever experienced high anxiety or panic, you know these sensations only too well. They might include any of the following:

Rapid heartbeat and palpitations
Increased body temperature producing sweating and flushing
Respiratory changes—with shortness of breath or shallow breathing
Muscle tension

Nausea, sick feelings in the stomach and gut
Pain or discomfort in the chest and heart area
Dizziness
Tingling, pins-and-needles sensation
Paleness or pallor
Urgent need to run to the toilet
Dissociation, disconnection from the body
Eyes widening
Sense of being out of control

All these feelings have useful survival value and a good reason for existing. For example, the size of the pupils grows so that more information can be absorbed through the eyes, making us more aware and prepared to deal with the danger. The heart rate is elevated and the breathing changes so that oxygen-rich blood can be rapidly pumped around the body and into the muscles that need it to successfully fight or flee the threat and so on.

Where once the body operated almost without our notice, a person experiencing acute anxiety is hyper-aware of their body's functioning. The strong, almost overwhelming sensations can frighten anyone who does not understand what is happening. It's as though the body has taken over and the person is no longer in charge. This feeling of helplessness, of things spinning rapidly out of control, can fill even the bravest soul with feelings of terror.

In a way, the person in the throes of great anxiety or panic is absolutely right—the body has taken over. More precisely, the unconscious and subconscious parts of the mind have taken over, sending the sensations—or chi—through the body that they believe are needed for its safety. This can be upsetting to the logical, conscious mind, which likes to think it is in control and always running the show.

Our reflexes are innate and work hand-in-hand with our chi; they've been hard-wired into us as long as humans have been on

Earth. The purpose is our safety. The problem comes when this process loops back on itself—when the physical sensations and intense hormones continue and escalate, fuelling even more fear, to the point that panic happens. This can happen in the presence of an imagined danger, as well as a real one. The subconscious, remember, makes no real distinction between the real and the imaginary.

Fear, which lies at the root of anxiety, is designed to bypass the conscious, rational mind, which might otherwise slow us down with its methodical, logical processing and cerebral analysis. Nature, in her wisdom, knows that when it comes to immediate threats, we cannot rely on the conscious mind to make quick enough decisions. When we are in danger, the instinctual unconscious and feeling subconscious parts of the mind care only about protecting us, and the physical responses they generate are there to help get us rapidly out of the situation they perceive us to be in.

As human beings evolved in a world filled with physical dangers, we needed a survival mechanism that was enormously swift. Our unconscious mind had to do its work by speedily asking and answering those four basic questions: Do I quickly withdraw from it? Do I fight it? Do I eat it? Do I mate with it? The subconscious mind, in turn, had to be able to inform the unconscious mind quickly as to what was dangerous, fightable, edible, or mate-worthy.

The problem, as we've seen, is that in rapidly searching our experiential databank, our referential index, the subconscious is flipping through not what actually happened in the past, but its stored perception, its interpretation of what happened. What the subconscious is really doing is searching for *meaning*. In order to give an appropriate response, it needs to make sense of what the experience it is now being called upon to deal with actually means. (The need for meaning is fundamental to the human psyche and we will examine this more in the concluding chapter of *The Chi of Change*.)

When in the past we encountered an unexpected, uncomfortable, or frightening experience that upset, hurt, or embarrassed us, this memory and the meaning we attached to the experience are stored as information in our subconscious databank. This becomes a template, so to speak, against which the subconscious compares what it perceives to be similar experiences in the present moment.

If our referential index used an alphabetical system, negative experiences would be stored under 'D' for 'Danger!' and 'A' for 'Avoid!' The information runs like a piece of programming in the giant computer of the subconscious mind, ready to be activated at any time, as needed. It is primed to spring into action and fill us with feelings that propel us into whatever action the subconscious believes is needed to 'save us' in the current similar situation.

And this would be fine, were it not for the fact that the subconscious often attaches incorrect meanings to past experiences, which then generate incorrect assumptions about current situations. What is actually quite safe can be perceived as a threat, triggering the same sensations and hormonal reactions that an actual threat would bring about. As we saw in the case of Louisa, who almost had a car accident when this happened, an unmerited fear reaction at an inappropriate time can actually create danger where none existed previously.

While the experiences that influence our beliefs and form our subconscious programming often happen in childhood, they can also occur later, at any time in life. Always, the experiences that have the greatest impact, that create the programs most firmly embedded in our subconscious, are those that are connected with the greatest degree of emotion. Almost without exception, these sensitizing experiences take us by surprise, happening when our mind is in a state of altered focus, perhaps upset or even filled with joy, innocently daydreaming or in a situation where we feel more vulnerable than usual.

These experiences are not always negative. For instance, when we powerfully fall in love for the first time, it creates a subconscious program attaching us to that person. This is beneficial if the love is reciprocal and the relationship turns out to be a good one, because the programming bonds us deeply to the other individual. But the same programming will be problematic if the relationship doesn't work out and we have to let go and learn to love someone else.

A perceived danger does not necessarily need to be physical in nature. It can be the threat of love withheld or withdrawn, the fear of abandonment, the fear of humiliation and so forth. For example, if a child is forced to stand up in a classroom and respond to questions for which they have no answer, causing feelings of foolishness and humiliation, this could easily create an adult fear of standing up and talking in front of people. The very thought of public speaking might fill such a person with panic.

This is how the past can control us subconsciously and rob us of the present, subsequently hamstringing our future. Fortunately, there is a solution. Using advanced hypnotherapeutic techniques, we can work directly with the subconscious to rewrite the faulty program that serves us so poorly. It is not necessary to let a poorly informed subconscious mind control us. With our conscious mind, we can choose to correct the false impressions by feeding new information to the subconscious, breaking the hold of the programming based on mistaken beliefs, and this is most effectively done in hypnosis.

Sheila was a wiry-looking, red-haired lady in her early forties who came to me because of long-standing feelings of anxiety. She lost no time in describing herself as a 'born worrier'.

'All my life I've lived on my nerves,' she said, 'but these days it's getting even worse. I find myself getting panicky when there's nothing to be panicky about. I can't really remember a time when I felt relaxed. I always feel tensed up. I don't even know if I'll be able to relax enough to go into hypnosis,' she sighed. 'But I want so much to change.'

'It's good that you want to change,' I responded. 'If you really didn't want to, there would be very little I could do to help you, but sometimes we want something so much that we actually try too hard. You don't need to be relaxed to enter hypnosis; that's a bit of a myth. All you have to do is to want it and allow it. So what I want you to do is to stop trying, and simply follow my instructions. I'm sure you'll do just fine.'

Soon Sheila surprised herself. She easily drifted into deep hypnosis where she went back to her first day in preschool. She was just four years old. Her mother had told her they were going out and that she was going to have a lovely day and meet some new children who would become her friends, but she hadn't mentioned she would be leaving little Sheila for a few hours, something that had never happened before.

When her mother left the preschool, Sheila was filled with fear and anxiety. She was also angry, as if she had been betrayed. Why had Mommy abandoned her in the midst of all these strangers? Didn't she love her enough to stay? Would she ever really come back for her? What would happen if she didn't come back? All of these thoughts raced through the child's head, the luan chi flooding her body and brain.

That was all it took for Sheila to become sensitized. She had become heir to the experience that psychologists call separation anxiety. The anxiety program was installed in the computer of Sheila's subconscious mind. In itself, the experience might have produced no real difficulty, its effects perhaps fading away with time, but soon there were other experiences that reinforced the program, anchoring it even more securely. Subsequent sensitizing events included her parents' divorce when Sheila was six years old, her unhappy experiences in secondary school where she was bullied, and her grandmother's death. As the subconscious program became more empowered, Sheila began to feel unsafe and wary, her mind on constant alert. She was filled with a generalized anxiety and the feeling that it was just a matter of time before something bad would happen.

Again, it is important to remember that not everyone passing through similar experiences will be affected in the same way. An initial sensitizing event also needs other subsequent sensitizing events for it to be affirmed and empowered as a program. What for one person turns out to be an important, traumatizing event might be of no real consequence for another person, something that is forgotten about and dismissed almost as soon as it is over. The difference, remember, lies not simply in each person's innate disposition, but in their perception of the experience and the subjective meaning they assign to it.

Anxiety, then, is always connected with feelings of fear and foreboding. The greater our fear that we will be overwhelmed and unable to cope, the greater our anxiety becomes. In the disordered state of chronic anxiety, the luan chi carries distorted information in an all-too-powerful and energetic way throughout the mind-body complex, frequently with devastating consequences. At its extreme, anxiety can cause debilitation, forcing the person to withdraw into a life of virtual seclusion or to become physically sick.

But is anxiety itself a sickness? A mental illness? Surely anxiety is no more a sickness than losing one's balance is a sickness. After all, what is anxiety if it is not a loss of our emotional and mental balance? To deny chronic anxiety the term 'mental illness' in no way diminishes its impact on the sufferer. The pharmaceutical industry, of course, is only too keen to promote anxiety as an illness that can be treated with costly prescription drugs.

In our fast-paced modern world, people visiting the doctor and complaining of anxiety are routinely prescribed anxiolytic medication, antidepressants, and beta-blockers. The most widely prescribed anti-anxiety medication is diazepam, brand name Valium, a drug belonging to the group known as benzodiazepines. Benzodiazepine tranquilizers are powerful psychotropic drugs that, besides Valium, include Ativan (lorazapam) and Xanax (alprazolam). Such pharmaceuticals are meant to be taken for only a brief period of time—as an emergency plaster or Band-Aid, so to speak.

Yet doctors continue to prescribe, and a high number of people continue to take, these psychotropic drugs on a regular, long-term basis. Indeed, it is not at all uncommon for me to be consulted by people who have remained on such drugs for ten years or more. Put quite simply, they have become addicted.

Where once these tranquilizing benzodiazepines were considered to be relatively harmless and non-addictive, we now know the reverse is true. Long-term use exposes people to multiple risks besides addiction, including poor mental and physical health, impaired cognitive function, and depression. They are a factor in road traffic accidents and falls involving the elderly.

Still, many doctors continue to prescribe these pharmaceuticals because they do not really know what else to do. A minority might eventually refer patients on for counseling or for some form of cognitive behavioral therapy. This can help patients manage their symptoms, but the majority of people presenting with anxiety will not even be offered these things. They will instead be handed a repeat prescription for drugs.

Anxiety is simply not a medical matter, but as long as it is treated as such, people will be offered medical 'treatment'—and that usually means pharmaceuticals. This, in spite of the fact that randomized control trials clearly show that, in the long-term, therapy is more effective than drugs (Howard et al. 1986; Smith, 1977 & 1982).

Jacob was in his early thirties and the youngest partner in a law firm when he came to see me. He had been diagnosed by his doctor with generalized anxiety disorder (or GAD). Talking with him, I soon saw he also suffered from social anxiety—something we discuss later in this chapter. He just didn't feel comfortable mixing with other people. He had also experienced two panic attacks in the previous six months, and since then his anxiety had grown to such an extent that Jacob was reluctant to leave his home in case he might have an attack outside, where he would be vulnerable. His doctor had prescribed an antidepressant, which he had obediently taken, but which paradoxically seemed to have only increased his anxiety.

In his initial session with me, Jacob confided that his first panic attack had happened on a train station platform. He was late and rushing to catch his train when suddenly he felt like he could not breathe. Soon he became dizzy and covered with sweat. He feared he might pass out. For Jacob, it felt like he was dying there on the platform, amidst dozens of strangers. He was overwhelmed with panic.

This frightening experience had left him shaken to the core. If he had felt anxious before, he now felt decidedly unsafe and no longer in control. This had happened once, but what if it happened again? What if he again lost control while away from home and surrounded by strangers? What if he blacked out or fainted in the street or in a crowded place?

Such thoughts are characteristic of anyone who has experienced the terror of a panic attack. The fear of losing control and of what might happen because of this lies at the heart of most panic attacks and is at the core of acute anxiety.

Panic disorders often first manifest themselves between late adolescence and the mid-thirties, and this was the case with Jacob. Yet for a panic attack to be triggered, the ground has first to be prepared by an underlying anxiety. It may also be made fertile by stress.

In Jacob's case, a hectic and stressful life had left him little time to self-nurture, and so we began by discussing how he might eat in a healthier way and perhaps take some additional nutrients, at least in the beginning of his therapy. I also encouraged him to begin a program of exercise. Hypnosis revealed that the initial sensitizing event or seed of his panic had been planted years earlier through an experience he had while in college. Ill-at-ease socially, yet desperately eager to fit in and be accepted by the other students, he had taken the recreational drug ecstasy (MDMA) in a club, which induced an experience of intense paranoia. His hands tingled, his head swam, and he broke out in a cold sweat as his heart pounded and he gasped for breath. In spite of being shaken by the experience, he had soon recovered and was able to consciously dismiss the incident, although he made sure he never took ecstasy again.

Years later, on the train station platform, he had a flashback of the same panic and fearful sensations. In his conscious mind, he never linked the two completely separate experiences, because their context was so different, but his subconscious, feeling mind had found little difficulty in doing so. It had simply connected the hot, sweaty feeling, the pounding heart, and the breathlessness brought on by his rushing for the train with the similar sensations he had experienced in the club.

In therapy we were able to revisit Jacob's younger experience and rewrite the program, but we were able to do more: We traced those same feelings of needing to be accepted to an incident in Jacob's childhood. When this initial sensitizing event and subsequent reinforcing events had been properly reprocessed in hypnosis, Jacob experienced healing at a profound level. His panic attacks ceased and his general anxiety faded away to entirely reasonable and normal levels.

So-called 'recreational drugs' such as cocaine, ecstasy, LSD, crystal meth, psilocybin ('magic mushrooms'), marijuana, and mephedrone, always carry with them the danger of an adverse reaction and are responsible for a good deal of lasting anxiety and emotional difficulty. Sometimes, as with Jacob, the really adverse effects manifest themselves only years later.

Each of us needs to feel that we fit in, that we are accepted by those who matter to us without being judged and found wanting. This need is fundamental to the human condition. As Aristotle pointed out, we are social animals, and when we feel excluded from the group, as if we are outsiders, it's easy to believe there must be a good reason for this—that there is perhaps something wrong with us.

Believing that there is something wrong with us is one small step away from one day behaving as if there is. Once again, perception is all. If we buy into the belief that we just don't fit in, that we are not really up to par, then we can become very self-conscious and experience real difficulty when with other people.

This brings us to one of the most common forms of anxiety, known as social anxiety disorder or SAnD (also known as 'social phobia'). In fact, so common is this type of anxiety that it has been estimated to affect around 12 percent of the population (National Institute for Health & Excellence, 2011; Bruce & Sayeed, 1999). SAnD is a difficulty that is equally common among men and women, and it typically begins in adolescence, often around the age of thirteen. Undoubtedly, social anxiety disorder (SAnD) is one of the most under-recognized—and therefore undertreated—psychological difficulties in existence today (Stein & Gorman, 2001).

While all of us may experience occasional times of awkward hesitancy and moments of bashfulness in the presence of others, social anxiety disorder far exceeds mere shyness and can become so incapacitating that it prevents one's living a normal life. Research shows that people with Social Anxiety Disorder are two to three times more likely than others to develop alcohol or drug dependence (Brady, 2001; Kendler & Gallagher, 1996). The World Psychiatric Association estimates that people experiencing social anxiety disorder are more likely to be single, attain lower levels of education, and endure other difficulties, such as depression. They may contemplate suicide, have fewer friends and acquaintances, and have an erratic work history with higher rates of absenteeism.

Social anxiety can present in a range of intensity and in a variety of guises. At the lower end of the scale, SAnD can simply mean awkwardness or difficulty in mixing socially and feeling out of place in certain situations such as at clubs, parties, work-related or family gatherings. For many, having to stand up and talk in front of others, make a presentation, or propose a toast at a wedding so fills them with panic that they would rather see a chasm open up in the ground and swallow them.

Curiously, a person might be very self-confident in other areas of their life but completely lacking socially. Woody Allen, the award-winning American film director, writer, actor and jazz musician, is known to actually vomit before going onstage, so acute is his anxiety. (If you're reading, Woody, then get in touch!) Entertainers such as Barbra Streisand, Kim Basinger, and the late Sir Laurence Olivier have spoken to the media of their social anxiety. The singer and entertainer Donny Osmond has likened his social anxiety to the feeling of being tied to a railway track with the train fast approaching. Again, perception is paramount. It really can feel that awful.

Truly, SAnD is no respecter of person or profession, affecting anyone from housewife to household name. Over the years I have treated quite a few celebrities for this particular form of anxiety. Readers might be surprised to know how many famous people actually suffer from some degree of Social Anxiety Disorder.

Once again, the origin of this challenging disorder usually lies in the early years. At some time the child was made to feel embarrassed or humiliated in front of others, or too much importance was ascribed to a successful performance or speech, so a program was implanted within the subconscious mind that now attempts to prevent the person from putting themselves in such a situation again. Using the language of anxious and fearful feelings, the subconscious tries to protect the person by making them steer clear of 'threatening' social situations. But the information contained in the chi is faulty and distorted. It therefore produces a distorted response totally out of proportion to reality.

No one was born to live a life riddled with anxiety and panic. These feelings are acquired, not innate. Fortunately, they can be successfully treated and resolved, and the systematic approach used in the best hypnotherapy is designed to rapidly accomplish this.

People with extreme anxiety often worsen their predicament with relentless self-criticism, telling themselves they should be able to 'snap out of it' and get over their 'silliness'. Most are unaware that the professional help they need is available, so they continue to live lives of nervous avoidance, with anxiety and fear always waiting in the wings, ready to pounce at any moment.

Self-criticism and self-doubt affect a good proportion of the human race, undermining self-confidence and generating an enormous amount of unnecessary anxiety. Yet I have found that people who consult with me because of severe anxiety and panic attacks—and also for depression—seem often to be extraordinarily hard on themselves. They are their own worst critic, relentlessly seeking a perfection that neither they nor anyone else can ever really attain. Often they easily overlook the shortcomings of others while focusing disproportionately on their own imperfections. In so doing, they create a sort of hyper-self-consciousness—an excellent breeding ground for nervousness and anxiety. They are rarely satisfied with their own efforts or achievements, which tend to generate feelings of tension and personal insecurity, no matter how successful they actually are.

The problem is, of course, that none of us is, or can ever be, perfect. Not only are we human beings incapable of perfection, but we also live in a world that is less than perfect. So perfectionists can never really feel satisfied or safe because they can never measure up to the demands they place on themselves. Nor can they control every aspect of their life, which makes it very difficult for them to feel secure. Because of this, the perfectionist is often someone who also has control issues.

It is certainly commendable to give our very best to the things we do in life, and to always strive to improve. To produce our best we need to reach for excellence. But if we are to maintain our mental and emotional balance, we need to understand that none of us can ever be really perfect—and that this does not mean we are really inadequate, worthless, or in jeopardy. Only when we are at peace with our imperfection can we become the person we were born to be: our authentic self.

No matter what we have passed through, no matter what criticism or uncomfortable feelings we have experienced in the past or may be experiencing in the present, if we are to live in peace with ourselves and with our world, we need to be gentle and forgiving of our imperfections and of the imperfections of others. When we have truly learned to do this, our chi flows so much more freely and we, in turn, flow more freely with life.

Chapter Five

Anxiety's Other Faces

'The thing always happens that you believe in,
and the belief in a thing makes it happen.'
~ Frank Lloyd Wright

In the previous chapter, we looked at acute anxiety, panic attacks, and social anxiety. In this chapter we will focus on some of anxiety's other faces, including sleeping difficulties, generalized anxiety disorder, phobias, sexual dysfunction, and post-traumatic stress disorder.

One sure way to instill a sense of anxiety in a person is through constant negative criticism. When we are children especially, negative criticism can hurt a great deal, sometimes casting long shadows that remain with us well into our adult years. Still in the process of forming their personality and establishing their identity, children are not yet equipped to take a step back and examine the nature and value of such criticism.

Positive criticism can make us question our behavior, acting as a useful corrective mechanism, but too much negative criticism can make us seriously doubt ourselves, producing a state of inner uncertainty in which anxiety can easily flourish. Once a pattern of self-doubt and anxiety has been firmly established, it can be extremely difficult to break. As adults, we tend to react to criticism in the way we did as nervous children. But in doing this we fail to see criticism for what it really is.

Criticism is feedback—but it is subjective feedback. It is other people's *opinion* of us and of our behavior, yet it can so easily influence our opinion of ourselves. When we are systematically criticized, especially in our formative years, it can make us feel as if there is something wrong with us. It is easy to confuse the action with the person. We may have made a mistake, or even acted badly, but this does not mean that we are bad, just as it does not mean that we ourselves are a mistake.

If from an early age we confuse what we do with what we are, we have already begun to stray from our authentic self, and our chi automatically becomes distorted. This distorted chi powers our feelings of anxiety.

As children and as adults, we do need to receive feedback, to be corrected when we get things wrong, and to learn responsibility for our actions. But we also need to receive praise when we get things right. Approval and positive reinforcement are deeply important to every child and, indeed, to every person. Humans have an innate need to be affirmed and to be genuinely loved. Especially in our early years, we need to be told that we are okay, that we are worthwhile, and that we matter. We need to be accepted and loved for who we are, not simply for what we do or what we accomplish.

The influential psychologist Carl Rogers, proponent of person-centered psychology, popularized the term 'unconditional positive regard' to identify this essential component in a person's healthy emotional development. With non-judgmental, unconditional acceptance, an individual is nurtured—released from the fear of being hurt, humiliated, or judged; free from the fear of damage to their self-esteem. The child grows and adapts to life in a natural, spontaneous manner, able to function and respond in an authentic and intuitive way to the challenges life can be expected to present.

This unconditional acceptance is a key aspect of love, and it is extremely important to the growth of the individual. It is essential to one's sense of security and emotional and mental balance, and to the free flow of our chi. Excessive negative criticism and a lack of positive affirmation can cause a child to grow into an adult whose life is punctuated by self-doubt, a compulsive perfectionism, and anxiety.

Cicely was an intelligent, mature woman with short-cropped, salt-and-pepper hair and a solemn, fretful demeanor. She consulted me because of her generalized anxiety and lack of self-confidence. In talking with her, I soon discovered that she did not suffer fools gladly and that she looked upon life as a serious business indeed. In our first session together, she said that all her life she had been wracked with feelings of anxiety and of never quite fitting in. Rising to become deputy head teacher in an exclusive private school, she told me she felt very much like a failure, that she could have risen further and made so much more of herself had her anxiety not held her back.

Cicely was an avowed perfectionist. She had never felt relaxed or confident enough to enter into a relationship; work had always seemed to take precedence over her personal life. Often she labored well into the night and on weekends, but she never felt that her work was good enough. Feeling she could never produce the excellence she demanded of herself, she held back, passing up career opportunities, keeping her head low and trying her hardest to perfect the work at hand.

For more than ten years, Cicely had been working on a novel. For over a decade she had been writing and rewriting, polishing and re-polishing, yet she never thought her manuscript good enough to submit to a publisher. There was always something that could be improved upon, something that could make it the perfect book she felt compelled to create.

When I enquired about her childhood and how she had done at school, Cicely's eyes glazed over. 'I wasn't very happy,' she told me. 'My parents were staunch Roman Catholics and quite strict with me. I know they loved me. They gave me everything I could want, and there was never any real disharmony at home. I don't think I had a bad childhood. I studied hard and did my homework, but when I got 90 per cent in an exam, my father would always say, 'What went wrong? What about the other 10 per cent?' It was as if no matter what I did, if I did not bring back

100 per cent marks, then it just wasn't good enough. And if *it* wasn't good enough, that meant *I* wasn't good enough.'

In hypnosis therapy, we returned to those hurtful events that had sensitized Cicely, compelling her to endlessly demand perfection, and in doing this we also uncovered a mass of unexpressed rage that lay deep within. It was an anger Cicely harbored towards her father for having bullied and criticized her so much. But this anger was in conflict with how Cicely believed she *should* feel. After all, hadn't her father provided everything she needed, paying for her private school education, tennis and riding lessons, ensuring that she had the very best of everything? Cicely knew that he loved her. He had never once raised his hand to her, and yet she felt enormously angry. As an adult she could clearly see that his remarks, like his attitude, had been intended to help her, to egg her on to do her very best, so Cicely's anger was mingled with guilt for feeling as she did. She believed she had no right to feel this way when her father had done so much for her with the very best of loving intentions.

Such feelings are by no means rare. In fact, the great majority of people who consult me for issues such as anxiety and depression have a strong need to deal with internalized feelings of both anger and guilt, and it is essential that these powerful emotions be addressed during the therapeutic process.

By returning to the origin of Cicely's anxiety and to the subsequent sensitizing events that reinforced it, then systematically reprocessing the perceptions upon which her anxiety was based, Cicely was helped to rewrite the program and to realign it more properly with her current reality. As she processed her anger and guilt, she was able to release herself from her perfectionist demands and move forward with her life in a much more affirmative manner. Working with specific ego states, she reached a state of greater inner harmony, finding a balance that had previously almost completely evaded her. Gone was the anxiety-ridden perfectionist; it had been replaced by another altogether brighter, lighter personality.

When last I spoke with her, it was at an end-of-year party held at a radio station where we both had been interviewed. I was delighted to learn that Cicely's book had been published and was already receiving a good deal of critical acclaim.

As we know, anxiety can present itself in many different guises and affect people in a host of different ways, and one condition that often goes hand-in-hand with anxiety is insomnia. Indeed, insomnia is itself an acknowledged risk factor for anxiety.

When we are fatigued from lack of sufficient sleep, this easily translates into feelings of increased anxiety, which in turn can feed back into our disturbed chi, further interfering with our ability to drift off into a restful, restorative sleep or to remain asleep for as long as we need to.

All of us can have difficulty sleeping from time to time, especially when away from our own bed, or when we have a lot on our mind. But true insomnia transcends this kind of occasional sleeplessness.

In today's unsettled economic climate and social upheaval, sleeplessness appears to be increasing exponentially. In fact, research conducted by the US National Sleep Foundation in 2012 found that fully 30 to 50 percent of people report experiencing sleeplessness, while a good twenty percent report suffering from ongoing, chronic insomnia.

The knowledge that we have to arise and face a new day with all of its challenges, as the clock ticks away at our bedside and we are still awake, can fill us with feelings of dread. The inability to easily fall asleep or to remain asleep and get a good night's rest is almost guaranteed to create feelings of anxiety and tension.

Too little sleep also elevates stress hormones such as cortisol, affecting the mood center of the brain, the hippocampus. Getting enough sleep makes the difference between an anxious, tired, foggy mind and a calm, alert, attentive mind that is tuned in to the world and to the self.

What causes insomnia? There is a multiplicity of possible causes. Sometimes the inability to sleep is brought about by the mind's reluctance to 'shut down' or 'switch off' for the night. Perhaps the conscious mind is simply restless and overactive. It may be dwelling on financial, work, or relationship challenges, or pondering the events of the day; at other times it may be focusing on upcoming events, or perhaps running around in circles going over the past.

Some people can easily trace their sleeping difficulties back to their childhood. They have had sleeping problems off and on for as long as they can remember. Others are at a loss to explain their insomnia; it seems to appear from nowhere, sapping their energy and sending them into a tailspin of anxious listlessness and restless fatigue.

It is helpful when experiencing insomnia to remember that, no matter how uncomfortable and fatiguing it might be, it will not kill you. Though it may contribute to stress and negatively impact health, no one ever actually died from sleeplessness. What is certain is that not everyone needs the proverbial eight hours of sleep, and lying there worrying that we are not getting enough can only complicate matters, aggravating and further increasing our sleeplessness. Exactly how much sleep each person needs is subjective. Some of us need more and some less.

Like every other behavior, insomnia always exists for a reason. When a person has experienced difficulty in sleeping for any significant period of time, it means that the mind is attempting to accomplish something it believes cannot be done in sleep. Strange as it may seem, if we cannot sleep it is because something within our own mind is attempting to do something useful—to analyze and process, to problem-solve, or to protect, for example.

Which brings us again to an important understanding: *All human behavior has a positive intent.* Disruptive and annoying though it may be insomnia is no exception to this rule. Even bad habits begin for a reason. Once we are able to discover why the mind insists on remaining active and alert in the waking state, and what it is hoping to achieve in doing this, we are in a good position to help it accomplish its objective or alter its approach, without depriving us of sleep.

Let me give you an example of what I mean. One of the more even personalities I have had the pleasure of working with in recent times was Alwyn, a man who had spent more than seven years under the most barbaric conditions in an Asian prison for attempting to smuggle hashish, or cannabis, out of the country. For the first couple of years of his incarceration, his life had been hell on Earth, and he twice tried to escape his reality by attempting suicide. Those early years were spent in a state of abject despair and depression. But then, strangely, Alwyn awoke one day to a different world in which there was a beautiful inner peace, a sense of all-pervading calm and inner stillness he had never before experienced.

At first he imagined this strange feeling was a temporary state, perhaps induced by a medicine he had been given by the prison doctor, but as the days passed, he was surprised to find that the state did not wear off. The sense of peace remained despite the volatility of his prison surroundings, becoming an inexplicable part of who he was and how he related to existence. He knew only too well that he had not become 'enlightened', but he knew too that something within him had changed. He had arrived at a place of acceptance.

Two years after his release from prison, this man arrived at my practice, where he said, in a soft voice, 'I am at peace with myself now, and the only thing that is in any way disturbing that peace is the fact that I cannot sleep.'

In hypnosis, Alwyn returned once more to that fetid, dark prison, to the rats and cockroaches and the concrete floor on which he was forced to lie. Crammed into his dingy cell were a dozen other prisoners—murderers, rapists, thieves—all lying head to toe with not the least bit of space between them. Filled with feelings of fear, his subconscious mind had made its decision: 'I will not let you sleep because if you do, there is a good chance you will be murdered and never awaken.'

From that time on, Alwyn had never experienced a full night's sleep. Typically he lay awake for hour upon hour. Such was the 'initial sensitizing event' that embedded the protective program of insomnia within Alwyn's subconscious mind.

In hypnosis, his subconscious mind was helped to see that vigilance was no longer necessary, that it could release its protective grip and allow him to drift safely asleep at night, and that, moreover, the hours spent in sleep are not wasted but can be used creatively to dream and bring about the restoration of energies needed for Alwyn to function properly and enjoy each moment of life.

Such an extreme case is rare, but I believe it illustrates a truth common to so many cases of insomnia: that behind the sleeplessness, the subconscious is busy working, doing its best to bring about something it sees as helpful. At the bottom of its behavior, there is always positive intent.

With sleep, as with so many other aspects of life, our expectations play a crucial role. If we lie down with the expectation that we will have difficulty sleeping, this can quite easily become a self-fulfilling prophecy.

But it may be that sleeplessness isn't all bad, if it allows us to do some serious soul-searching. Walking those pre-dawn streets of the mind, we can learn a lot about ourselves, which is perhaps why insomnia has been called 'the great educator'.

When insomnia is not caused by deep, unresolved psychological issues that need to be addressed in therapy, often all that is necessary for many people to regain the ability to sleep is to gain greater control of their conscious mind, to switch it off when appropriate. This can be quite easily accomplished by learning self-hypnosis together with a simple technique. The technique involves the power of imagination, and if practiced on a regular basis, it will easily transport the person into the tranquil realm of natural slumber.

Whatever its origin, be it simple habit or underlying psychological difficulty, insomnia can usually be successfully treated without medication, and those restless, anxiety-provoking hours of wakefulness can be replaced with Mother Nature's natural healing balm—a calm and restorative sleep.

Now we come to one of the most common difficulties hypnotherapists are called upon to treat—phobias. Phobias are by far the most numerous of all anxiety disorders. On the 'Fears and Phobias' page of my website (peterfieldhypno therapy.co.uk), I list over five hundred different phobias, and this list is by no means exhaustive; in fact, I am constantly adding to it. A person can be phobic towards almost anything, from spiders to snakes, balloons to buttons, water to wind.

All phobias are, by definition, irrational in nature, a fact that usually does not escape the person experiencing the phobia. But consciously knowing a fear is irrational and unnecessary in no way reduces its power. Fear is a feeling and, as we have seen, feelings come from the powerful subconscious—not the conscious, rational mind. All it takes is for our luan chi to be triggered, and its faulty information will cut through logic, flooding us with sensations of fear and discomfort.

As with so many emotional issues, the origin of all phobias lies in a person's past. Phobias are a conditioned fear. There are probably only a couple of fears that a person is born with. The fear of falling, the *Moro reflex*, which also encompasses the *startle reflex*, the fear of loud noises, is certainly one of them. And, because each of us comes into the world in an essentially dependent state, we are probably also born with the fear of abandonment. Practically everything else is learned, acquired on life's journey.

Among the most common phobias are those termed *specific phobias*—irrational fears of particular objects or situations. Such phobias are most often a result of a single, conditioned response. The person has had an experience that has sensitized them to respond to a specific stimulus in a fearful way. Simple phobias include such things as fear of spiders (*arachnophobia*), fear of the dentist (*odontophobia*), fear of stickers (*pittakionophobia*) and so on. (*Pittakionophobia* is a neologism, or new name, that I coined in 2009 [there being no suitable name in existence] for the fear of stickers, something I have successfully treated many times. The first part of the word *pittakion* is taken from the Greek word meaning 'label', and the second part *phobia* from the Greek word for fear.) People who suffer from specific phobias seldom have underlying psychological difficulties.

But there is another classification known as *complex phobias*. A complex phobia includes several related anxieties rolled up into one and is most often the result of a series of psychologically sensitizing events. An example of this is *agoraphobia*—the fear of leaving home or a familiar 'safe' area. This phobia was once defined as the fear of open spaces, but now the definition has been rightly broadened to include *any situation in which the person feels unable to quickly and easily reach a safe place* (such as in shops or other public places, in crowds, when travelling alone or on public transport, and so on). What the agoraphobic person is really afraid of are the feelings of panic that might arise in such situations, feelings that would leave them out of control and vulnerable. Indeed, it is estimated that around 50 per cent of people experiencing agoraphobia will have experienced a panic attack at some time, so interlinked are panic and agoraphobia (Brit. Journ. Psychiatry, 2006).

At its extreme, agoraphobia can have devastating consequences, forcing the sufferer to lead a life completely governed by fear, unable to leave the house, go to work, or socialize. Phobias such as agoraphobia may also be associated with other psychological difficulties, particularly depression. Complex though this phobia may be, with the right kind of hypnotherapy it can be successfully treated.

A complex phobia that most people have heard about is *claustrophobia*—the fear of being trapped or confined with no clear exit. This, of course, can happen even in the safety of home, in a small room or in a locked bathroom, for example, or when night falls, drawing things in. (Something that plays a role in some people's fear of the dark.) A common misunderstanding is that claustrophobia is only the fear of small, enclosed spaces, and indeed, such places can trigger this phobia, but for many people suffering from this condition, it goes well beyond this. A person can feel claustrophobic in a large theatre or auditorium, for example. For the claustrophobe, it is more accurate to say that *claustrophobia is the fear of being confined or trapped with no clear exit.*

There are other fears, such as the fear of driving (*aviophobia*) and the fear of heights (*acrophobia*), which though quite specific in their focus, may also come under the heading of 'complex phobias' because they are the result of a series of initial sensitizing events and so involve a number of psychological difficulties.

At some time or other, most phobic people have tried to rid themselves of what they recognize as an irrational fear, but still the fear remains. Most will have adopted avoidance as a coping strategy, but this merely increases feelings of powerlessness over the phobia. Understandable though the desire to avoid a fear-provoking situation or object might be, in doing so the person is strengthening the hold the phobia has over them. Avoidance isn't always an option of course. While it may be easy for the urban city dweller with a snake phobia (*ophidiophobia*) to avoid snakes, it's not so easy for the arachnophobe to avoid spiders or the aquaphobe to avoid water.

What happens with phobias, of course, is that the powerful

subconscious mind is once again attempting to perform its protective function. It has linked the phobic object or situation with some sort of danger, so to keep the person safe, it uses the feeling of fear to steer them away from such exposure in the future. Interestingly, research has found that a person is three times more likely to experience a particular phobia if a close relative also has it—another example of the power of emotion contagion.

Phobias can affect absolutely anyone. They are totally unrelated to intelligence, character, class, or educational background, and they can crop up in the most unexpected places. In my career as a therapist, I have successfully treated hundreds of people with a whole range of different phobias, including a commercial airline pilot who suffered from fear of flying, a driving instructor with fear of driving, a policeman afraid of crowds, and a good number of medical students who were afraid of needles or blood. In a nice piece of irony, some years ago I even treated a celebrated circus performer, a man whose profession it was to defy danger virtually on a daily basis, who told me: 'I am absolutely fearless—but I am afraid of clowns!' (A phobia that goes by the name of *coulrophobia*.)

Joy was a new mother of two lovely girls, twins just a couple of months old. She told me she was terrified of vomiting and of being around sick people who might vomit. Joy suffered from something called *emetophobia*—a very common phobia that I am regularly called upon to treat. The fear of vomit or of vomiting can prevent a person from eating away from home, from visiting restaurants, from mixing socially, travelling, and from doing so many of the things that the rest of us take for granted. In Joy's case, it was preventing her from taking proper care of her newborn babies. Her mother had taken over feeding the twins and many of the other maternal responsibilities, and this was causing Joy real distress. Not only did she feel that she was failing as a mother, but she felt unable to bond with her own children because of her fear.

In hypnosis, Joy returned to a time when she was a very small child with her brother in the bed next to her, who was retching and vomiting. He had eaten something that disagreed with him and was sick because of it. To the young girl's mind, her brother's retching and groaning made it seem like he was dying. The experience had left an imprint on her subconscious, conditioning her so that the fear response would be triggered at the mere thought of throwing up or of being around anyone who might be sick. Again, the subconscious was simply doing its job of protecting her from *perceived* danger in the only way it knew how—through feelings of fear.

Once the cause and the subsequent sensitizing events that had reinforced her fear were uncovered, the program could be systematically altered, and Joy's subconscious could rapidly let go of its fear response. It was simply no longer needed. While the post-phobia Joy did not like vomit any more than the rest of us do, she was no longer afraid of it and could lead a normal life, feeding and caring for her little girls and being a nurturing mother.

One of the commonest phobias hypnotherapists are called on to treat is the fear of flying (*aerophobia*). Unfortunately, this is a fear that unnecessarily stops untold numbers of people from travelling, preventing them from taking holidays, visiting family and friends, and engaging in business activities.

Rationally, of course, the person locked into a fear of flying may know very well that commercial air travel is the safest means of public transport in existence. They may even be aware of the research conducted by the United States Federal Aviation Administration, based on the accident rate of recent years, which concludes that a person would have to fly every day for the next 22,000 years before they would likely become a fatality in a commercial airplane crash. But phobias are not rational, so the odds in favor of safety do not mitigate the suffering. As we have learned, fear emanates not from the rational conscious mind but from the subconscious feeling mind.

Distressing though it is, this specific phobia can usually be completely cleared in just a couple of sessions. Once the initial sensitizing event and the experiences that reinforced it are located and the sensitivity to them neutralized, the subconscious program can easily be rewritten. The person is then freed to enjoy travel and flying in a way that was not possible before therapy.

Of the countless phobias I have treated, one particularly sad case impressed itself on my mind. Joe was a man in his fifties who was in urgent need of major surgery for a life-threatening condition. The problem was that Joe had a terrible phobia of hospitals and simply could not bring himself to enter one. He had tried counseling and had been treated by a psychologist, but nothing had changed. It was as though his fear of hospitals was greater than his fear of death. In fact, so great was Joe's fear that he had been unable to be with his mother as she lay dying in a hospital bed some years earlier. His incapacitating fear had alienated him from his sister, who had never quite forgiven him for failing to be with their mother at the end of her life. For years he had been wracked by guilt and remorse for not having had the 'courage' to do what he knew he should have done and in fact dearly wanted to do. What made matters worse is that he was at a complete loss to explain it.

I guided Joe into that deep state of hypnosis known as somnambulism, where he was transported back to a time when he was a boy of six undergoing surgery for appendicitis. Drifting up from the foggy state of anesthetized oblivion, he suddenly felt a sharp, burning pain as if his stomach was being ripped open. The raw pain seemed to consume him as he instinctively tried to scream out, but his mouth would not move. Nothing was under his control, everything felt frozen and paralyzed, yet he was acutely aware of all that was happening. Little Joe could feel everything. Helpless, flushed with fear and agonizing pain, the boy was unable to communicate his predicament to anyone. He could not stop what was happening to him. All he could do was to lie there in terror, filled with the most horrible agony imaginable.

After a short while, whether through the extreme pain or the eventual working of the anesthesia, the boy mercifully lost consciousness, and with unconsciousness came amnesia. His conscious mind simply repressed the experience, making him forget he had ever awoken during the surgery.

When we undergo general anesthesia, the anesthetist may introduce a chemical agent that completely paralyses the person, together with an analgesic that controls pain. The anesthetic produces unconsciousness; the analgesic removes the perception of pain, while the paralytic agent prevents the person from moving around during the operation, as they would, for example, in the normal sleep state. What had happened with Joe was that the anesthetic had proven inadequate to maintain unconsciousness, and so he had woken up during the surgery, but he had been rendered completely immobile, unable to move because of the anesthetic's paralyzing agent. As if this were not enough, the analgesic administered appeared to be insufficient to do its job. Joe was burning, on fire with pain.

Little surprise then that such a horrible event had left such an indelible mark on the little boy's subconscious mind. Determined never to allow him to be put in such a helpless, painful condition again, his subconscious had used fear to ensure that he remained safe—and safety meant keeping Joe far, far away from hospitals.

In the trance state, we were able to uncover and revisit this experience, then reprocess it, breaking things down and explaining them to the subconscious mind. Yes, little Joe would awaken, and yes he would feel terrible pain, but it would be over very quickly and he would survive; he would not die of the pain; his wonderful mind would take back control and guide him into a beautiful, calm unconsciousness, and such an extremely rare experience would almost certainly never happen again.

Once his subconscious understood and accepted this, it no longer needed to run the fear program in order to protect him, so it was able to realign itself; the program was rewritten, and his fear of hospitals faded away. He no longer felt afraid. All that now remained was for us to process Joe's guilt for failing to be with his mother at the end. This we accomplished in a single session, as Joe forgave that aspect of his psyche, or ego state, that was only trying to do its job and protect him. Recognizing that his mother, who loved him dearly, would have understood how his fear could incapacitate him, Joe could finally be at peace with himself, freed of his burden of self-directed anger and guilt—a wiser man who could move on with his life.

Several months after our sessions, Joe contacted me expressing his thanks. His surgery had been completely successful, and he was well on his way to a full recovery. The one thing he regretted was that he had not come into therapy before his mother had passed. Had he done so, he would have been there with her. The only reason Joe had not sought my help earlier was because he did not know such help was available. No doctor, psychologist, or counselor had ever mentioned it, so he had suffered unnecessarily almost his entire life from this incapacitating phobia.

In life there is always an element of danger. Planes can crash, boats can sink, and people can experience difficulties in hospitals as they can in crossing the street. Yet the probability of these things happening to us is really quite small. In order to live in a healthy, balanced way we have to be able to factor this in and still function in the world. When excessive fear stops us from doing so then we need to address our fear—which is where good hypnotherapy can be so very useful.

Generally speaking, specific phobias can be cleared within a couple of sessions, while more complex phobias (such as agoraphobia) and phobias that involve anger or guilt typically take a little longer, with five to six sessions being the average.

Yet another anxiety disorder that often presents itself to the hypnotherapist is that of sexual dysfunction or SD, a difficulty that can affect both men and women. For women, sexual dysfunction can manifest itself as desire or arousal difficulties, as pain or discomfort during penetration (*vaginismus* or *dyspareunia*), or as difficulty in having an orgasm. It is extremely rare for women to consult me regarding sexual dysfunction difficulties, perhaps because they usually and understandably prefer to work with someone of the same sex in this intensely personal sphere, and there are experienced female therapists to whom they can turn. For this reason, here I will be writing about the area in which I do have a good deal of professional experience: male sexual dysfunction.

For men, SD usually means the inability to have or maintain an erection (erectile dysfunction, sometimes called *impotence—a term no longer employed because of its connotation of failure*), something we briefly discussed in an earlier chapter when talking of Andrew, the man who had become a burglar in order to deal with it.

In addition to erectile dysfunction, SD may also present as premature or delayed ejaculation, or loss of libido. Sexual dysfunction is an issue that is far more prevalent than is commonly recognized, perhaps because this is a topic that few men feel comfortable talking about with friends or family. So common is it, however, that it is estimated to affect at least one in every ten men in their thirties and forties, and more than half of all men between the ages of forty and seventy (Araujo et al. 1999). Fortunately, this is another area in which the right kind of hypnotherapy can produce truly impressive results.

A man seeking an appointment with a hypnotherapist for SD is always well advised to first visit his doctor. This makes sure there is no underlying physiological reason for the difficulty. Although there can be both physical and psychological reasons for the condition, only when a medical doctor has given the patient a clean bill of health is it really ethical to proceed with therapy of a psychological nature.

Contrary to popular belief, the leading cause of erectile dysfunction is physical, not psychological. Diabetes, high blood pressure, thyroid or kidney problems, blocked blood vessels and atherosclerosis, prescription medications, drug or alcohol use, and heavy smoking are just some of the things that can produce problems in this area. Age-related erectile dysfunction, which is not connected to any underlying psychological cause, may often be effectively treated with the use of drugs such as sildenafil citrate (Viagra), tadalafil (Cialis), or the prescription drug vardenafil (Levitra).

In some instances, sexual dysfunction may be part of a bigger picture. It may be a call to action, asking the person experiencing erectile difficulty to examine a relationship, or it could be an aspect of underlying depression, but in many more cases it may be a form of social anxiety; certainly social anxiety disorder can often contain distinct elements of performance anxiety. The anxiety-triggered inability to experience or maintain an erection, or the premature ejaculation so many nervous young men naturally encounter during their first sexual encounters, can, for some, set up a program of nervous anticipation and anxious expectation that becomes a self-fulfilling prophecy. With sexual dysfunction, as with so many other difficulties of a psychological nature, 'The thing always happens that you believe in, and the belief in a thing makes it happen.' Through this kind of experience, sex becomes something other than a beautiful, sharing, and loving intimacy and turns into an anxious performance in which the man believes he will somehow be judged and perhaps found wanting.

Other men may have difficulty because at some sensitive time in their psychosexual development they were discovered in a compromised position—when masturbating, for example—and felt embarrassed or humiliated by the experience. Still others are prevented from achieving or maintaining an erection because the man's subconscious mind clings to the belief that the sexual act is inherently sinful, or that it will lead to him contracting a disease or fathering an unwanted child.

Perhaps the most extreme case of sexual dysfunction amongst the many I have treated was that of Amadeo, a soft-spoken and unassuming man of Mediterranean origin in his late forties. Though living and working in the United Kingdom much of his adult life, he was born in a rural wine-producing area of southern Europe, where his parents had raised him as a strict Roman Catholic, making him attend Mass daily. He also attended the local church school, where nuns had taught him. While perfectly healthy physically, Amadeo had never been able to maintain an erection when with a woman, nor had he ever had an orgasm while in the waking, conscious state. The only time he ever reached a climax was when he slept, in nocturnal emissions, so-called 'wet dreams'. For years he had been married, and his wife was the only person with whom he had ever attempted to have sex, but the marriage had never been consummated. Much to the disappointment of the couple, Amadeo could simply not experience or maintain an erection when needed. He had come to me because his wife had stumbled upon an article I had written on sexual dysfunction and had shown it to him.

In hypnosis, Amadeo quickly returned to his childhood and to various experiences that had deeply left their mark on his subconscious mind. At home, sex had never been spoken of. It was a taboo subject assiduously avoided, except for once when Amadeo was about six or seven years old and his father sent the neighbor boy packing. The lad had been thrown out of his family home and disowned by his parents for having a girlfriend. He had come at night with tears in his eyes, appealing to Amadeo's father to take him in and to give him work and shelter, but the door had been closed in his face with a flurry of moral indignation. Amadeo had been left with no uncertainty as to the reason why the 'sinner' had been turned away into the night—it was because of 'sex'.

As he grew, the young Amadeo was surrounded by negative messages regarding the evils of sex. Even the priest had preached sermons from the pulpit, his spit flying in fine droplets into the shaft of light that shone like a searchlight from the church window as he spoke of fire and brimstone and the eternal hell awaiting anyone who dared have sex outside of marriage or who committed the mortal sin of 'self-abuse'. In Amadeo's subconscious mind, sex had become synonymous with sin and anxiety. So powerful had this conditioning been that the boy, and the man, had never been able to overcome it.

Such long-term conditioning runs deep and cannot be undone in just a couple of brief therapy sessions, but I am happy to report that with time and the correct re-processing of his subconscious mind, Amadeo was eventually able to rewrite the negative programming and experience both erection and orgasm, enabling him to finally enjoy sexual relations with his loyal and patient wife.

Rarely are the sensitizing events that produce SD as pernicious and all-pervasive as they were with Amadeo. Usually the cause of sexual dysfunction can be traced to simpler, more mundane occurrences than the extreme and systematically conditioned sort he had encountered. In some cases, sexual dysfunction can be traced to a habituation to masturbation. The sensations experienced when masturbating—the pressure, angle and grip applied to the penis, for example—may have sensitized the man to a particular feeling, or set of feelings, that is simply not available through intercourse, making sex with another person feel less stimulating and therefore less arousing. The subconscious has become programmed to a certain way of feeling, linking this with a particular way of behaving. This can quite easily be corrected through the use of hypnotherapeutic reconditioning and by practicing a systematic modification of behavior.

When it comes to sexual dysfunction, it is always wise to consider a man's true sexual orientation. If a man is in fact not really attracted to women, if he is gay, it is natural that he will be unable to experience or maintain an erection with them. Sometimes it transpires that the man experiencing SD is in fact in denial about his true feelings, and when this is the case, the only way to end the sexual dysfunction is to end the state of denial. No one really chooses their sexual orientation, be it heterosexual, homosexual, bisexual or transsexual, and to attempt to conform to some preconceived idea of how a person 'should' be, instead of finding the courage to be what one is, is a certain recipe for disaster—in and out of the bedroom.

Another area that can lead to erectile dysfunction in men is an overdependence on pornography. In viewing porn, people are forced to use their imagination, depending on it to connect vicariously to some form of sexual experience they are not actually involved in. Remembering that imagination is the instrument of the subconscious mind, and that the subconscious is extremely powerful, it is not difficult to see how 'the real thing' can seem boring compared with the wild scenarios that have habitually fed and stimulated the imaginative subconscious libido. The intensity of emotion generated when watching porn can all too easily produce a conditioned response that prevents the man from achieving the same degree of excitation and feeling when with a real-life partner, and this can easily interfere with the man's ability to maintain an erection. This is an issue that can be successfully treated through the right kind of hypnotherapy. (We will be discussing pornography addiction more fully in Chapter 8 when we come to sexual addiction.)

Premature ejaculation, or PE, is another difficulty often brought to the hypnotherapist. This is another problem far more common than is generally recognized. When considering PE, it should be borne in mind that what might be premature for one man may be average for another because men may differ considerably in the length of time they take before ejaculation. Also, there may be quite a bit of difference in the length of time sexual partners wish the sex to last. This makes the question of exactly what is premature something of a subjective matter.

Understandably, premature ejaculation is an area in which research is difficult to come by. A survey made by the famous sex researcher Alfred Kinsey found that fully 75 per cent of men ejaculate within two minutes in more than half of their sexual encounters (Kinsey, 1948). Currently, just six and a half minutes is thought to be the average time before ejaculation in men between the ages of eighteen to thirty (Waldinger et al. 2005). But such figures really do depend on which expert one listens to. Some research cites an average time of three to ten minutes before ejaculation, while still other sources state that it is anywhere from fifteen minutes to one hour.

The causes of PE can be multiple, and again can very often be traced back to the man's younger years. Perhaps the man suffering from PE was accustomed, as a youth, to masturbating in a hurry, rushing things for fear of being disturbed. This would habituate him to climaxing quickly. Or it could be that his early love-making was rushed because he was afraid of discovery. Of course, PE may simply be the result of a generalized nervousness or anxiety because when a person is nervous and anxious, there is the likelihood of reaching orgasm too quickly, or of being unable to maintain an erection. For other men, genetics may play a part. Some men are hypersensitive in the area of the penis, which causes them to climax with very little stimulation. Whatever the cause, hypnotherapy can usually help most men experiencing PE to prolong the time before ejaculation, which increases their enjoyment and that of their partner in this most intimate of experiences.

Perhaps the most important thing to remember when considering matters of a sexual nature is that an individual's sexual activity is only a part of the person. Despite what some glossy magazine covers and 'glamour' photos might suggest, a woman's value does not really depend on her ability to conform to anyone's preconceived fantasy or stereotype, and likewise for a man. Whatever a man may be, he is so much more than an extension of his sexual imagination. Anyone whose identity rests largely on sexual performance may well need to do some serious introspection and a re-assessment of their own self-image. The really good news is that with the right kind of approach, the anxiety that causes sexual dysfunction can usually be cleared within a few brief yet intense sessions of effective hypnotherapy.

Next we turn to the anxiety disorder known variously as shy or bashful bladder, pee shyness, shy kidney, or to give it its medical name, *avoidant paruresis* (pronounced 'par-you-ree-sis'). While it is not uncommon for most people to have brief, isolated episodes of urinary hesitation in situations where other people are in close proximity, shy bladder is a form of social anxiety that goes far beyond simple shyness and is much more severe and potentially handicapping. In many cases, the person experiencing bashful bladder is completely unable to physically empty their bladder when others are in the vicinity.

There is also a similar condition that prevents bowel movement, stopping a person from defecating, called *parcopresis*. Although I will be talking specifically about paruresis here, the following information applies equally to both conditions.

In severe cases, paruresis can have highly restricting effects on an individual's life, making the person unwilling to journey far from home. Some sufferers find they cannot urinate even at home if someone else is nearby. Affecting men and women, paruresis is far more common than might be supposed. Although more research needs to be conducted, it is thought that around 7 per cent of the population suffers from this restrictive condition (Kessler et al. 1998).

Anyone experiencing difficulty in urinating or defecating should contact a doctor to ensure that there are no underlying physical reasons or medical conditions such as bladder or bowel obstruction, prostate trouble, or kidney problems. Once such things have been ruled out, we can safely say that the problem is psychological in nature and something that should respond to hypnotherapy.

Almost always, paruresis has its origin in the formative years of childhood although it might not manifest as a condition until much later. Usually it is the result of an uncomfortable experience in which anxious feelings were present while the person used the lavatory with another person or people in the vicinity (such as at school or in public bathrooms). This created a program in the subconscious, linking urination with anxious feelings, that prevents the person from freely going to the bathroom when others may be around. The good news is that both paruresis and parcopresis usually respond very well to hypnotherapy treatment, and most often the prognosis is excellent.

One of the most disturbing anxiety disorders is the condition known as post-traumatic stress disorder, or PTSD. This potentially incapacitating condition can produce both psychological and physical symptoms, the luan chi created by past trauma playing havoc with the person's perception and emotions, and therefore with their ability to function normally.

Post-traumatic stress disorder is a psychological condition caused by the subconscious mind's response to a major traumatic event, such as war, rape, a terrorist attack, a catastrophic accident, a natural disaster, an abortion, or the death of a loved one or friend. It is marked by emotional dissociation, flashbacks, a heightened startle response, and sometimes severe personality changes. PTSD is thought to affect around 30 per cent of all people who have been involved in a traumatic event (NHS Choices, 2010) or in any situation that has produced feelings of extreme fear, helplessness, or horror.

PTSD might appear to be something of a modern phenomenon, but it has actually been around for centuries. The Greek historian, Herodotus, wrote about it as early as 490 BC; Samuel Pepys, the English diarist, recorded his response to the great fire of London in 1666, providing an excellent description of his own personal encounter with the disorder, which was at the time unnamed.

During the First World War, the condition became known as *shell shock* because its symptoms were commonly seen in soldiers at the front. The physical shock from artillery was thought to have caused some kind of concussion that resulted in a physical malfunction of the brain. Later the name would be changed to *combat neurosis* before being designated post-traumatic stress disorder in 1980 following the Vietnam War, when the American Psychiatric Association entered the new name into its *Diagnostic and Statistical Manual of Mental Disorders*.

Today we recognize that PTSD can affect not only soldiers and military personnel but anyone who has experienced or witnessed severe trauma. It may even be seen in the family or close friends of someone who underwent a major trauma, a sort of 'trauma by proxy' so to speak. PTSD—especially this type—often goes unrecognized and undiagnosed.

Individuals differ in the way they develop the symptoms of post-traumatic stress disorder. While many experience the effects in a matter of hours or days, for others it takes weeks or even years before the symptoms appear.

Those unfortunate people who do not receive proper treatment can spend long years in a sort of nether world, hovering between reliving the traumatic experience and trying their best to avoid it. Often the person has blanks in their memory, recalling parts of the experience only too vividly, while repressing other parts.

Most often, people with PTSD relive aspects of the trauma

over and over again, and they do this in numerous ways. They may suffer from insomnia, intensely disturbing nightmares or realistic dreams. Feelings of *déjà vu* may occur and flashbacks happen, appearing suddenly, forcing them to re-experience the feelings of panic or helplessness that the trauma initially produced. Such feelings can be triggered when anything remotely similar to an aspect of the initial sensitizing event occurs, such as a car backfiring or a light flashing. It might happen in response to a symbolic stimulus, such as the appearance of the color red or the falling of shadows that goes unnoticed by the conscious mind but initiates a response from the subconscious. Or it might happen when the person's thoughts simply drift back to the traumatizing event for no particular reason at all.

Understandably, PTSD is a condition that can seriously affect relationships. The traumatized person can find it extremely difficult to experience strong—particularly loving—feelings for another person. The disturbed luan chi, consistently transmitting feelings of fear and trepidation, seems to block the finer feelings so that the person becomes distanced from others. When someone has been emotionally shocked or wounded, the subconscious may automatically attempt to protect them by erecting a barrier to emotion so further hurt may be avoided. Increasingly, options appear to close down as belief in the future diminishes, leaving the person with a depressed, pessimistic life view and perhaps pressing thoughts regarding death.

My client Harry was a young Canadian father of two boys. In our initial session, he told me that a few short years previously, he had been a carefree person, driving fast cars and enjoying life to the full. But now everything had changed. He had, in his words, become a completely different man. Gone was the light-hearted demeanor. Now each day was a struggle, with anxiety a constant companion. His nights were no better, with terrible dreams regularly disturbing his sleep, leaving him exhausted and on edge.

Harry was in a mess. Unable to concentrate on his work, he had lost his job. Then his wife had left, taking their sons with her. She could no longer put up with her husband's irritability, his erratic and moody behavior, or with his coldness towards her and the boys.

Our first step was to get Harry's eating right. For so long he had ignored this important aspect. In addition to eating healthy, whole foods, I recommended certain supplements that he could take that might help him to correct any imbalances and also support his nervous system, particularly in the initial stages of recovery.

In a deep state of hypnotic trance, Harry was safely taken back to the event that had caused his problems. He had been in a bank in Ontario, withdrawing money, when suddenly he found himself in the middle of an armed robbery. Three men wearing motorcycle crash helmets with visors that hid their faces were brandishing guns and screaming at everyone. Twice guns were pointed directly at Harry, and he thought he was going to die. For one brief moment, he had been left alone and had pleaded with the girl behind the cashier's window to quickly open her door and let him in, but she had refused. One of the robbers had raised his visor to wipe his face, and Harry had seen it. He now felt certain he would be killed. After all, if he lived, he could identify the man. In that moment, Harry's mind locked into the fear, programmed with the terrible sense of helplessness and despair that would govern his life for years to come.

In hypnosis, Harry was guided again through the intense, traumatizing experience, but this time his older, wiser mind could inform his younger self that although the experience would be frightening, he would survive it, and he would be safe. Harry relived the experience almost as if he were a spectator in his own life—worried, yes, but now certain he would get through it; he would be safe. In the hypnotic state, he recalled many things that had been completely lost to his conscious recall, and once more his life began to make sense. The nightmare was over, and now the healing could come.

Later we worked on Harry's anger towards the robbers for creating the situation, as well as on the anger he harbored towards his wife for leaving him. While his rage was understandable, Harry knew if he wanted to free himself of the past and move on with his life, he needed to forgive. It was not that the bank robbers deserved his forgiveness—after all, they had put him through hell. But Harry understood if he failed to forgive, he would remain their victim, shot through with rage and resentment, in emotional bondage to them and to the traumatic experience, firmly trapped in the past.

The last piece of the puzzle was to deal with the internalized feelings of guilt that Harry had been carrying around. In therapy, he came to see that his reactions had been entirely sane and perfectly natural given the insane and abnormal circumstances in which he had found himself. They were not the result of some character weakness or cowardice on his part.

As we know, the way the subconscious mind processes and perceives time can vary greatly from chronological, clock time. The subconscious can easily confuse past and present. In hypnosis, Harry's subconscious could be realigned to the understanding that the nightmare experience was fully in the past and truly over now; he had survived, so it could let go of its fear. Finally we focused on Harry's life outlook, working with various ego states and teaching him self-hypnosis so that he could relax at will and let go of whatever stress he might encounter as he moved forward with his life.

Because hypnotherapy is a brief yet intensive therapy, the entire process took only half a dozen sessions. When last I heard from him, Harry had been reunited with his family and was working in a career he truly enjoyed. He had become interested in Buddhism, which he was now practicing. What once had been a living nightmare had turned into the doorway to a deeper existence. His chi was freely flowing, and life had regained its sparkle. Harry's case is typical of those who experience post-traumatic stress disorder, typical of my approach to treating PTSD, and typical, too, of the human ability to recover from even the most difficult experiences, given the right approach.

Whatever form it takes, anxiety can have an extremely draining and damaging effect on the person experiencing it. It is essential that we do all we can to help our body-mind complex counter anxiety's harmful effects. A diet rich in toxin-free plant food—fresh vegetables, fruit, whole grains, beans, legumes, and a few nuts—can go a long way in keeping both brain and body in a healthy biochemical balance under the most trying conditions. With its usual generosity, nature has provided us with natural substances in our food that protect and help calm the nervous system, working to counter the harmful effects of the powerful hormones produced by anxiety and stress.

Research has shown that certain isolated nutrients such as GABA (Lydiard, 2003; Abdou et al. 2006), taurine (Kong et al. 2006; Zhang & Kim, 2007), and theanine (Kimura et al. 2007; Mason, 2001) act in a medicinal, almost pharmaceutical manner that aids in the reduction and management of anxiety disorders. GABA is a neurotransmitter, and it is also chemically an amino acid. It can be taken as a supplement, but it is poorly absorbed because of its difficulty in crossing the blood-brain barrier. However, GABA combined with niacin is available as a commercial preparation called *Picamilon*. Research shows that this form does cross the blood-brain barrier. If you or someone you care about is experiencing acute or chronic anxiety it may be wise to work with an appropriately trained nutritionist or health practitioner who can advise on such supplements and their dosage. Also, anyone experiencing anxiety would be well advised to avoid coffee and other caffeine-laden drinks because these can greatly accentuate anxious feelings.

Exercise is also a powerful antidote to anxiety. A substantial body of research indicates this (Broman-Fulks et al. 2004; Smits & Otto, 2000). Not only does exercise increase the feel-good endorphins in the brain, but it also increases serotonin and dopamine levels, calming things down and elevating one's mood.

What's more, in studies, exercise has been shown to be more effective than Prozac (Harvard Health Pub. 2011). Just a few minutes of brisk walking every day has been shown to elevate mood. The problem is that many people with a history of anxiety avoid exercise. Sometimes this is because the anxiety has drained them of energy, leaving them exhausted and lethargic. Other times it is because on some level we believe the sensations exercise generates (sweating, elevated heart rate, faster breathing) are too similar to those experienced in acute anxiety. As we saw with both Lance and Jacob in the previous chapter, for the person sensitized to anxiety, such sensations can be misinterpreted by the mind, triggering feelings of upset and panic.

Exercise 'grounds' us. It is extremely helpful in breaking the cycle of misinterpretation of bodily sensations that can trigger anxiety and in recalibrating the fear-bearing luan chi. Through regular exercise, an anxious person can learn to amend their responses to such sensations, desensitizing and weakening the false connections that might otherwise trigger a panic attack. Exercise 'reconditions' us, encouraging the mind to see that the sensations—whether experienced in exercise or in an anxious situation—are simply the body's natural response to the chemicals flowing through it. They are completely natural and not to be feared.

It is our fear and the *belief* that these sensations will in some way seriously hurt us that is the root of the problem. But rest assured, if you have ever experienced acute anxiety or a panic attack, you have probably already gone through the very worst that can happen, though you may not realize this.

And this really is an important part of the secret to

overcoming those frightening experiences. Instead of constantly running away from unpleasant feelings, we need to recognize them for what they are: physical sensations caused, for whatever reason, by a rapid release of certain hormones. Once we understand this, our fear becomes much more manageable. We can even learn to almost relax into the experience—floating, as it were, beyond the sensations themselves, knowing that they will soon pass and that no real harm will come because of them. When we allow ourselves to do this, we can regain control. We are on the road to recovery.

For all of these reasons, I usually recommend a program of regular exercise to anyone who has been experiencing anxiety. Of course, it is always advisable to visit your doctor for a general check-up before beginning any new exercise program. If you are not already exercising on a regular basis, begin slowly, and gradually increase the length and intensity.

So what, finally, have we learned about anxiety? We know it can manifest itself in numerous myriad of forms, from simple phobias to crippling panic attacks, and we know that anxiety's power lies in its ability to frighten. As all the case histories have demonstrated, we also know that whatever form it takes, anxiety can—with the right hypnotherapeutic approach—be successfully treated and conquered.

Chapter Six

Depression—The Medical Approach

'Since I was sixteen, I've felt a black cloud hangs over me.
Since then, I have taken pills for depression.'
~ Amy Winehouse

Before we begin our discussion of depression, here is an extremely important note: No one should discontinue antidepressant treatment without medical advice. Stopping such medication suddenly, or even too quickly, can trigger severe, life-threatening reactions in the body, and severe, psychotic reactions in the mind. There is nothing wrong with wanting to get off medication and to find a more natural approach to handling depression. (We'll talk about such approaches in the next chapter.) But unless such change is embarked on slowly and methodically, dire consequences can result. It is extremely important that the reader understand this.

Perhaps no condition is more guaranteed to suck the light out of life, to plunge one's inner world into darkness, than the collection of feelings we label *depression*. Few things can leave us feeling more hopeless and stuck, locked helplessly in the belief that we are powerless to change how we feel.

While all of us experience life circumstances that sometimes make us feel down, chronic depression is in a league of its own because of its ability to rob us of the joy of being alive. Depression is not the same as 'the blues' or the natural yet temporary feelings of sadness or grief that we all experience from time to time that can be most often directly attributed to difficult life events.

No, this thing called depression lasts, and then it lasts some more. With all the wonders of modern medical science and the enormous breakthroughs in our understanding of how the mind and brain work, depression appears at the top of the list when it comes to difficulties and blocks to our mental and emotional well-being.

Indeed, if fear is the emotion underpinning almost every problem that the hypnotherapist sees, depression is by far the most common issue (together with anxiety) that clients bring to therapy. So prevalent is it, in fact, that it is estimated that every single one of us will be affected by depression—either our own or someone else's—at some time in our life (Singleton et al. 2000).

Yet, as with practically every diagnosis of a psychological or psychiatric disorder, depression has no biological markers. The term itself tells us nothing of its cause. It is merely a label assigned to a group of symptoms—a diagnosis determined by the way we *feel*.

So what are the symptoms? Well, according to the World Health Organization, these generally include such things as low mood or mood swings; losing interest in life; not coping with things that used to be manageable; feeling exhausted, tired, restless, and agitated; holding pessimistic views of the future; loss of appetite or weight loss; sleeping difficulties; reduced self-esteem and self-confidence.

When our chi is flowing freely and we feel good, we have none of these symptoms. We can all lose our balance from time to time, but this does not mean that we are mentally ill or sick. It is far more helpful to see these disruptive feelings as forms of blocked chi, patent manifestations of a disturbed energy that is playing havoc with a person's emotional and mental balance.

Unquestionably, depression and its treatment is a wide and complex subject. As with practically all the issues discussed in *The Chi of Change*, it is a topic that deserves a book in itself, but here we must restrict ourselves to two chapters. In this first one, we look at the way depression is currently regarded and treated by the medical profession. I think you may be surprised and perhaps even shocked at some of the things you will learn. In the next chapter, we will focus on an alternative and, I believe, far better way of approaching and treating this collection of symptoms that we have chosen to label 'depression'.

Let us begin by becoming acquainted with the different classifications of depression that doctors typically use to diagnose and treat. Keep in mind that any diagnosis is based purely on *arbitrarily defined symptoms*. There are no lab tests for depression, so its diagnosis hinges on the individual's own subjective, self-reported experience and on the *opinion* and mind-set of the person being reported to (the doctor). Also be aware that each classification is simply a descriptive label. It tells us nothing about the cause of the condition. Diagnosis (assignment of a label) is part of a naming game used to categorize certain kinds of human experience and states of unhappiness. Above all, remember that a person is not a diagnosis: People are so much more than the name assigned to a collection of symptoms.

These days it is customary to divide depression into three main categories: mild, moderate, and major, all defined by the severity of the symptoms. The feelings that fall under the heading of major (or clinical) depression are difficult to imagine if you yourself have not experienced them or seen someone you care about do so. Such feelings can be truly incapacitating, making life almost unbearable, turning day into night, disrupting natural sleep and eating patterns, and making routine activities such as getting out of bed, washing, working, or going to school painful and difficult.

In centuries past, this kind of depression was known as *chronic melancholia*, but today it has been relabeled. Because such depression can be so seriously debilitating, anyone experiencing a persistently depressed mood that seems to last beyond a couple of weeks would be well advised to seek help without delay. Although it may take some time, major depression, with proper treatment, can most certainly be successfully treated—and so can mild and moderate depression.

Another classification applied to depressed feelings is called *dysthymia*. This is described as a chronic condition characterized by depressive symptoms that last for most of the day, occurring more days than not, for at least two years—less time in children below the age of fifteen. This classification is a label applied to symptoms less severe than major depression. It is estimated that dysthymia is two to three times more likely to occur in women than in men.

According to those who classify these things, the essential difference between dysthymia and a diagnosis of major depression is the duration and intensity of symptoms. It is thought that dysthymia often goes untreated because its symptoms have existed for so long that the sufferer and their family come to believe it is just the person's natural personality.

The kind of depression most often seen by the hypnotherapist, however, is so-called *moderate depression*, a less acute but nonetheless troubling form that is also known as *subclinical depression*. Moderate depression usually responds quite rapidly to the proper treatment, but as we will discover in this chapter, the proper treatment is not often forthcoming.

Bipolar disorder (formerly called *manic depression* and today often referred to just as *bipolar*) is another label applied to a form of depression that can play havoc with a person's life. Bipolar is characterized by massive and largely unpredictable mood swings that can take the person from an absolutely euphoric or highly agitated state to the very depths of despair. All too often, the condition is accompanied by recurrent bouts of prolonged and severe depression that leave the person feeling completely exhausted. Bipolar is often relieved by alterations in diet and behavior. Exposure to sunlight, or use of a full-spectrum daylight bulb or light table (Reeves et al. 2012), and taking supplements including EPA, vitamin D3, and magnesium have proven useful in alleviating this condition, as has regular exercise.

Yet another classification of depression that many people will have heard about is *postpartum depression*. This is something that an estimated 10 to 20 per cent of women will experience after giving birth (O'Hara & Swain, 1996; Gutzler, 2006). Its onset can occur anywhere from a few days to a few months after the baby is born. Although the fact is largely unrecognized, postpartum depression can also occur in men (Paulson, 2010; Roberts, 2010).

SAD, or *seasonal affective disorder*, is a particular type of depression that appears to be affecting more and more people these days, bringing ever-increasing numbers to the doctor. Seasonal affective disorder is connected with a lack of sunlight or daylight and is particularly prevalent during the winter months. A diagnosis of SAD is made after three or more consecutive winters of depressive symptoms. SAD often responds well to the use of a light box or light table. (People with macular degeneration, eyes that are very sensitive to light and those with diabetes who also have eye problems should check with a doctor or ophthalmologist before using light therapy.) Something called a 'dawn simulator' is also available and may prove useful to those experiencing SAD. This is a device designed to gradually increase the light in your bedroom as you awaken. Vitamin D3 supplementation has also been helpful in this area.

Whatever kind of depressed feelings a person may be experiencing, if the symptoms last for more than a couple of weeks, the first port of call should always be the doctor in order to eliminate any underlying physical reasons before looking for psychological causes. If you suffer from the symptoms of depression, you will probably need to explain to your doctor that you are there to determine if there might be a physical cause for your symptoms. If you neglect to say this, you might simply end up with a prescription for an antidepressant.

Depression and anxiety are now considered to be the most common psychological difficulties in the United States (Devane et al. 2005), and in the United Kingdom (Singleton & Bumstead,

2001), with children as young as three exhibiting what are considered to be clear signs of depression (Luby, 2010). It is estimated that one in ten people will experience serious depression or bipolar disorder (National Institute of Mental Health), and every tenth American over the age of twelve now regularly takes prescription medication for depression (Pratt & Brody, 2011; Wood, 2011). Depression statistics in Australia are comparable to those of the United States (Australian Institute of Health & Welfare, 1998). But depression is not restricted to Anglophone countries. 1 in 10 people in Europe have now taken antidepressant medication. According to the World Health Organization (WHO, 2008), depression is now the leading cause of disability in the world, with more people suffering from it than from heart disease, cancer, and HIV combined!

Beyond any shadow of doubt, in the twenty-first century, this thing called depression has reached truly epic proportions. So serious is the epidemic that the WHO has forecast that by 2020 depression will be the second-largest killer, after heart disease.

Who then can blame our doctors for feeling overwhelmed by the problem? All too often physicians find themselves automatically reaching for their prescription pads and quickly prescribing antidepressant and anti-anxiety drugs, as if they had no alternative.

We expect our medical doctors to take action, to *do* something. So they compassionately try their best to oblige, handing out pills and capsules as though depression were a disease, like malaria or meningitis, something that can be defeated by swallowing the latest pill, bolting down a neatly colored capsule.

The belief that emotional difficulties stem exclusively from some kind of medical abnormality or faulty biology that can be corrected by drugs has gripped the mind of doctors and patients alike. It has turned us into passive consumers of potent chemicals that supposedly have the magical power to help us deal with what are, essentially, difficulties in living.

And all of this is taking place with an almost total disregard for the individual's unique life journey. It ignores the multiplicity of personal experience, an individual's cognitive processing and behavioral patterns, their lifestyle and dietary habits, as well as environmental and social influences—all of which are undoubtedly at play in the formation and maintenance of those heavy feelings termed 'depression'.

Questions need to be asked: Do the claims made for these drugs really justify such widespread use? How effective are they in actually treating depression? Does their value truly lie in the alleviation of suffering, or is there something else at stake?

Here is the clincher question: Is it possible these drugs are being so commonly prescribed not to actually cure depression but to manage troublesome people? In other words, is this massive prescribing of antidepressants nothing more than a well-intentioned attempt at social management? Let's look at some facts.

It is easy to imagine that depression has always been part of the human condition, but this is not entirely accurate. In the past, a condition called *melancholia* was indeed diagnosed by doctors, but depression as we know it today was not. Only in the mid-twentieth century did depression become a widely accepted clinical diagnosis. The process of labeling and dividing it into sub-classifications continues to this day, embroiled in controversy, as doctors and researchers still debate which feelings, emotions, and symptoms should fall under the label. But while lumping unwanted human feelings and experiences together under a medical label and indexing them in a manual of 'mental disorders' may satisfy many in the healthcare industry, it does little to ameliorate anyone's suffering.

Having established depression as a medical diagnosis, researchers began focusing on medical ways to treat it. While several different theories were proposed, the one that gained favor was the psychopharmacological theory that depression might be caused by a chemical imbalance, an insufficiency of neurotransmitters, especially the 'feel-good' one, serotonin, and so the condition should respond to drugs that make more of this hormone available to the brain. This theory—and it remains a theory—was based on observations made back in the 1950s, about the same time depression was becoming a diagnosis.

Powerful pharmaceutical companies became really excited: if depression was seen as a chemical imbalance, they ought to be able to synthesize and sell chemicals designed to correct it. Very quickly they began investing in the development of drugs intended to boost available serotonin levels—and elevate their already massive profit margins. Presto—the chemical 'antidepressant' was born.

Soon drugs known as tricyclic antidepressants were being mass-produced and marketed. One such drug, Amitriptyline (marketed under various brand names such as Elavil, Tryptizol, Lentizol), a medication originally produced in 1961, is still widely used today. But before long it was discovered there were serious drawbacks with this class of drug. It came with a long list of dire side effects and could be particularly dangerous in overdose. Because of this, doctors ceased recommending it as a first-line therapy for depression, and alternative drugs, called selective serotonin reuptake inhibitors (SSRIs) and then selective serotonin-norepinephrine reuptake inhibitors (SNRIs) took their place. With a massive publicity push, Prozac was created and launched. Prozac, by the way, was not the very first SSRI to be developed—that dubious distinction belongs to a Swedish drug called Zelmid (generic name zemelidine), which was swiftly withdrawn from the market when it was discovered that it could cause death by paralyzing the respiratory muscles.

If an antidepressant were to sell and make really big money, a really big market would be needed to sell it to. Prozac came at exactly the right time, hitting the market when doctors and the media were obsessing over ghastly stories about Valium and benzodiazepine tranquilizer addiction. This new wonder drug promised to deliver, to calm things down or buck things up—without becoming addictive. This was precisely the same thing the benzodiazepines had promised when they replaced barbiturates.

With its vast resources, the pharmaceutical industry quickly set about creating and growing this market, engaging in an advertising and marketing blitz never before seen with prescription medication. *Interbrand,* the same advertising agency that handled the accounts for brands such as *Sony, Microsoft,* and *Nintendo,* was hired to give fluoxetine, the drug's generic name, a slick and sexy identity. They came up with the name 'Prozac' because it sounded snappy, upbeat, and positive. It had a kind of clean, professional ring to it, too.

National campaigns, all paid for by the drug's manufacturer, Eli Lilly, informed doctors and the general public of the dangers of this thing called depression and what to look out for. By the time Prozac was actually launched, patients were already requesting it by name. Articles appeared in magazines from *Newsweek* to *New York* magazine, *Woman's Own* to *Men's Fitness.* Soap operas featured 'clinically depressed' characters. Talk shows and TV programs were devoted to the subject of depression. Celebrities, movie stars, politicians, sportsmen, royalty, and rock stars—everybody was talking about it. In the shortest possible time, depression and antidepressants had become part of our culture, with SSRIs like Prozac appearing almost as a trendy lifestyle option.

Prozac was now the hottest pin-up pill in town and depression a routine topic on people's minds and lips. The Canadian poet and singer Leonard Cohen felt compelled to remark: 'The term clinical depression finds itself in too many conversations these days. One has the impression that a catastrophe has occurred in the psychic landscape.' In a very real way, it had.

The pharmaceutical industry is the second most profitable business in the world, surpassed only by the international arms trade. With its massive advertising machine working at full throttle, Prozac and its SSRI spin-offs rapidly became the drugs of choice for doctors and patients alike. One would be hard-pressed to find a general practitioner or family doctor in the United States or the United Kingdom who does not write out prescriptions for these drugs on a daily basis.

There is absolutely no question that the development of this market and the enormous profits it generates for the multinational pharmaceutical companies has strongly influenced our view and our very definition of depression. It has shaped our concept of the way depression should be treated.

With the advent of the supposed chemical fix that antidepressants promised to deliver, doctors no longer needed to ponder or deal with the causes of their patients' troubles. They could simply prescribe a pill, and patients could go away believing it would help them cope with their difficult, negative feelings.

But exactly how are these drugs supposed to work? As mentioned, the most common type of antidepressants operate on the assumption that the depressed patient has insufficient levels of that key neurotransmitter serotonin (and perhaps also of the neurotransmitters norepinephrine and dopamine), and that these low levels affect mood, causing feelings of depression. The SSRI antidepressants (such as Prozac, Zoloft, Citalopram, and Seroxat) and SNRI antidepressants (such as Venlafaxine or Effexor) are supposed to increase the level of these neurotransmitters available in the gap between neurons, giving them a better chance of re-activating the receptors on the next neuron or nerve cell, and in so doing, change the way the person feels.

Not even the pharmaceutical companies claim these drugs actually *increase* the amount of serotonin or norepinephrine in the brain, merely that they may allow for more effective use of what may already be there. The actual reason why the person might be lacking sufficient serotonin or any neurotransmitter—if they even are—is completely ignored, as are the personal circumstances, the mind's role, and individual life-style choices in all of this.

But here is the startling fact about the link between serotonin and depression, and why this biological model remains only a theory: The most sensitive studies have shown no lowered serotonin in sufferers from depression, and no research has ever found their serotonin levels to be abnormal. Perhaps it isn't surprising then that even to this day there are no biological tests that can possibly predict the way in which any person will respond—or fail to respond—to antidepressants.

While Prozac was originally approved and used solely for depression, to the delight of its purveyors, it soon began to be prescribed for a whole host of other difficulties: anxiety and panic attacks, obsessive compulsive disorder, premature ejaculation, obesity, anorexia and bulimia, chronic fatigue syndrome, drug addiction and alcoholism, migraine, arthritis, fibromyalgia, and so-called 'behavioral problems' in children and adolescents.

Regardless of the lack of evidence, the medical model presses on with its concept of pill-shaped psychotherapy. If the SSRIs and SNRIs fail to do the trick, then some other pharmaceutical agent will probably be tried on the patient. An old tricyclic antidepressant may be prescribed, together perhaps with beta-blockers, tranquilizers, or sleeping medication.

This is how drugs are used to manipulate depressed people. They are modern medicine's attempt to muffle a person's luan chi, the unsettling messages coming from patients' subconscious. While symptoms are the focus, nothing is done about the *cause*. The mind-body connection—the role the mind may have played in producing the condition—is given no thought at all. Depression is seen strictly as a matter of biology without consideration of an individual's history, current circumstances, or unique life story. It is a reductionist approach that is as ineffective as it is simplistic.

Pharmaceutical 'solutions' also have the downside of side effects. Prozac (fluoxetine), for example, is listed as having over forty-five negative side effects. The range includes nausea, headaches, insomnia, dizziness, fatigue, increased anxiety, aggression, sexual dysfunction, and vastly decreased sex drive. It is as if something in the mind-body complex, some instinctive wisdom, is rejecting this crass approach to the problem, screaming out not to do this. Similar medications fare little better.

Not every single person taking these medications will experience negative consequences, of course. But many will. There is no way of determining who will and who will not.

Terrible though these side effects (and the eventual withdrawal difficulties) may be, some people are prepared to put up with them, believing anything is better than the overwhelming feelings of depression. But in doing this, I believe they are mistakenly turning their back on the truth because depression is something other than a Prozac or Seroxat deficiency.

Just how effective are these costly drugs, anyway? The answer: not very. There is an abundance of solid research that runs contrary to the hype and myths perpetrated by the mighty pharmaceutical companies. This research flies in the face of the beliefs held by so many—family doctors, psychiatrists, and psychologists included—about how well these medications work.

The hugely negative side effects of antidepressants have been documented—in *fully independent* testing, free of the bias and influence of the multi-billion-dollar pharmaceutical industry. This testing has been unable to validate the claim that these medications in any way help those with depression. The astounding truth is that *antidepressant drugs work little better than placebos* –dummy sugar pills (Kirsch, 2009; Moncrieff, 2008; Johnstone, 2000).

If you have not heard of research that demonstrates so clearly that these drugs are ineffective, you are not alone. Even the majority of doctors are unaware of these facts. Research costs money, and so, too, does its publication, and those who have the money—the pharmaceutical companies—will not publish negative information that does not serve them. After all, they have their shareholders to answer to, and they are in business primarily to make money—not to cure ailments.

Here are just a couple of examples of what I am talking about. In a scrupulously conducted analysis of five completely independent research studies conducted in the United States, the United Kingdom, Canada, and Australia, researchers found the following: 'Meta-analyses of antidepressant medications have reported only modest benefits over placebo treatment, and when unpublished trial data are included, *the benefit falls below accepted criteria* for clinical significance'(Kirsch & Moore, 2004). (Emphasis added.)

In other words, the much-touted ability of these drugs to reduce the symptoms of depression depends mainly on their placebo effect—on the *belief* that they will work—and the placebo effect, in general, works 35 to 75 per cent of the time (Harrington, 1999). (The word *placebo*, by the way, is Latin for 'I shall please.')

In another study (Turner et al. 2007) published in the prestigious *New England Journal of Medicine*, researchers found that pharmaceutical companies have been selective in choosing which antidepressant studies they have allowed to be seen and which they have buried. The article states that the drug companies have published almost all the studies that appeared to demonstrate a benefit, but practically none of the many studies that showed antidepressants to be ineffective.

This extensive and thorough study reported in the journal scrutinized research—published *and unpublished*—into twelve different antidepressant drugs in more than seventy-four different clinical trials, involving over twelve thousand people.

The published studies were, of course, easy enough to obtain, but the unpublished studies were often extremely hard to uncover. In fact, so deeply hidden were they that the researchers only succeeded in locating and gaining access to their findings by using the US Freedom of Information Act and carefully combing through the U.S. Food and Drug Administration files.

Why were these studies buried? Because more than half of all studies into the efficacy of antidepressants conclude that they work not much better than placebos. To add to this grand deception, some of the studies that show negative results have been selectively published, but the negative results, according to the investigating researchers, were 'published in such a way that conveyed a positive outcome'. The studies were twisted to say what the drug companies wanted them to say—that the antidepressant drugs worked when they actually did not.

With the skewing of research data and aggressive marketing, combined with the myth that has been built around these drugs' efficacy, antidepressants are now a leading class of drugs sold in the United States and the United Kingdom, second only to cholesterol-lowering drugs—and this despite the wealth of independent research demonstrating that people who benefit from antidepressants do so largely because they *think* that the drugs are helping them.

While it is easy for doctors to dish out antidepressants, what they and their unsuspecting patients regularly fail to recognize is that withdrawing from these drugs can be far from easy. In fact, coming off these powerful psychotropic chemicals can be something of a nightmare, often producing symptoms that make the anxious and confused patient rush right back to the drug in an attempt to regain some semblance of stability. Reported withdrawal symptoms include increased anxiety, low mood, tingling sensations, pins-and-needles sensations, electric 'zap' sensations, general flu-like feelings, and pain.

But that's not all. SNRIs (such as Venlafaxine or Effexor) have the potential to produce terrible side effects and prove even more difficult to withdraw from than the SSRIs when 'treatment' is over. Suicidal thoughts and suicide attempts, auditory and visual hallucinations, electric shock-like sensations in the brain, acute anxiety, and aggression are just a few of the known withdrawal symptoms that may be experienced by people attempting to discontinue their use. A frightening state of affairs, I think you'll agree.

Many people who try to come off these medications will experience awful withdrawal symptoms that send them rushing back onto the antidepressant, just as any addict experiencing withdrawal might rush back onto their drugs.

Public relations departments in the pharmaceutical industry do not like the word 'withdrawal' because of its connotations of addiction. During a medical symposium convened to discuss the problem of withdrawal, they came up with a neat euphemism. 'Withdrawal' was softened and replaced with the term *'discontinuation syndrome'*—a clever linguistic deceit designed to obscure the potential severity of withdrawal symptoms and of antidepressants' tendency to impel patients to continue taking them. Eli Lilly, the manufacturer of Prozac, funded the symposium.

'Discontinuation syndrome', of course, is something the manufacturers of SSRIs are eager to have us believe happens only with abrupt cessation of their medication. Yet there are many who strongly disagree with this supposition. Countless people have found it very difficult to withdraw from these drugs, even when gradually reducing the dosage. Some of these patients are attempting lawsuits, alleging that they were not warned about the danger of addiction. I regularly meet people who, having been put on these drugs by kind and well-meaning doctors, have tried to withdraw, only to experience acute anxiety and feelings of depression that sent them scurrying right back to the doctor, who readily put them right back on the drug, sometimes at an increased dosage.

According to Dr Michael Banov, medical director of Northwest Behavioral Medicine and Research Center in Atlanta, about 20 per cent of people who take SSRIs experience 'discontinuation symptoms'. Many believe this estimate is far too conservative. In one impeccably conducted study of volunteers who had never experienced clinical depression but were placed on an antidepressant, it was found that over 85% suffered from a variety of withdrawal symptoms, ranging from increased depression and anxiety to agitation and insomnia (Moncrieff, 2009).

Another expert in the field, leading US psychiatrist and author Dr Peter Breggin, states categorically that difficult withdrawal from antidepressants is a common occurrence, with some patients experiencing withdrawal periods lasting several months or longer. Dr Breggin notes that when the person's condition grows worse, as withdrawal symptoms manifest themselves, both doctors and patients believe this to be evidence that the person 'needs' the drug even more, while in reality what is needed is simply time to recover from the withdrawal effects (Breggin, 2008).

An additional problem these so-called antidepressant drugs create is that they block the uptake of serotonin by other parts of the body that need it. The 'second brain'—the enteric nervous system, or gut—suffers especially because of this. We cannot block uptake in one area of the body and not in another.

In attempting to keep serotonin circulating at the synaptic level of the 'head brain', the antidepressant medication also blocks its absorption where it is needed in the gut, making less available for use there.

There is a reason why fully 95 per cent of all the body's serotonin is diverted to and found in the bowel (Doe-Young & Camilleri, 2000). Serotonin is essential to the gut, and a lack of it there soon causes problems both mentally and physically. Serotonin calms the digestive tract. An imbalance can easily cause physical symptoms such as constipation, diarrhea, and nausea—symptoms all associated with irritable bowel syndrome or IBS. Unsurprisingly, fully one-quarter of all people taking Prozac and other SSRIs experience such digestive tract problems.

Insufficient serotonin in the enteric nervous system also causes psychological problems such as anxiety, poor appetite, and sleep irregularities—all symptoms associated with depression. Deprive the gut, the second brain, of sufficient serotonin, and it really doesn't matter how much you make available to the head brain. Both body and mind will suffer.

But what might the medical response be if the chemical approach fails to work and the feelings of depression worsen? Well, there's always electric shock therapy. If the drugs don't do it, maybe the doctors can electrocute those feelings into submission—simply zap the luan chi into oblivion.

There is no doubt that the administration of electro convulsive therapy (shock treatment) is among the most controversial aspects of current psychiatric procedure still in use today. So dubious is electroshock therapy that a former president of Britain's prestigious Royal College of Physicians has warned doctors that it is a potential scandal waiting to erupt (Kendell, 1998).

Although it has been largely discarded as an ineffective modality of treatment in Italy (the country where it was first introduced in 1938) and is rarely used in Germany, Holland, and Austria, it remains very much in use in the Anglophone countries—the United States, the United Kingdom, Canada and Australia.

In my opinion, shock treatment is a dangerous and damaging procedure. With this treatment, the patient is first anesthetized and given a muscle relaxant. Electrodes are then positioned on the temple or temples, and an electrical current is passed through the brain, inducing an epileptic seizure lasting up to one and a half minutes.

The official line of the powerful ECT lobby is that it carries no harmful side effects and is a practically benign procedure with little or no long-term memory loss and absolutely no possibility of brain damage. But there is a whole body of convincing evidence to the contrary, causing one leading expert (Breggins, 2008) in the field to categorically state: 'There can be no real disagreement about its damaging effects.'

Scientific study after scientific study has demonstrated the harmful effects of electroshock to the brain, routinely causing brain dysfunction, cognitive (thinking) difficulties, permanent amnesia and both short and long-term memory loss (Scott, 2005; Rose et al. 2003; Service User Research Institute, 2002). This is the case even with so-called modified ECT and the supposedly newer and ostensibly more 'benign' forms of electroshock treatment (UK ECT Review Group, 2003). In fact, to call these treatments 'modern' is a misnomer, since they have, in fact, been around for a long time.

In one follow-up study of 347 patients given shock therapy (Sackeim & Prudic, 2007), it was found that electroshock had caused irreversible brain damage and permanent dysfunction. Memory loss, for example, was reported in fully 74 per cent of those having undergone this 'treatment'. The electroshock had not simply affected the short-term memory; it had damaged long-term memory, too. The research showed that many people were never able to recover normal memory function.

As if this kind of thing were not enough to put an end to this primitive form of treatment, there is also evidence demonstrating that ECT (shock therapy), besides being ineffective, can also cause or increase the risk of suicide, especially in the first week following treatment (Breggins, 2008; Teicher et al. 1990). Ironically, the proponents of ECT often justify its use by claiming it to be an effective treatment for patients who are a high suicide risk. In doing this, they are completely ignoring research evidence to the contrary.

The most thorough study available on ECT-induced suicide found an actual *increase* in suicide for patients who had been treated with ECT (Munk-Olsen et al. 2007). This extensive study, published in the *British Journal of Psychiatry,* covered five years of ECT administration to patients admitted to a Danish hospital. Although the authors were decidedly pro-ECT, even they could not disguise the tragic figures of those who had taken their own lives after having been subjected to electroshock.

The despair created by his memory loss and subsequent inability to write following ECT treatment is thought to have seriously contributed to the suicide of literary legend Ernest Hemmingway, who reportedly told his biographer A.E. Hotchner: 'What is the sense of ruining my head and erasing my memory, which is my capital, and putting me out of business? It was a brilliant cure, but we lost the patient...' Fighting for recovery, it is not at all unusual for patients subjected to shock treatment to find their emotional difficulties exacerbated by brain damage that cannot be rectified.

All too often, the bludgeoning of the human psyche with electric current creates a confused mental state that may temporarily pass for release from depression. But soon the depression re-emerges from the fog, leaving an even more damaged and bewildered mind in its wake.

As with the antidepressants, those who have vested interests in the continuation of shock therapy as a treatment for depression—it is a very lucrative business—are not exactly opposed to skewing the evidence and re-interpreting research in a way that is favorable to their financial profit. Expert psychiatrist Dr Peter Breggin said, 'I have rarely seen so much fabrication in the psychiatric literature as I have seen with ECT.'

How is ECT supposed to work? No one quite knows, but one theory is that—as is claimed with antidepressants—it elevates available serotonin levels. Just how it is supposed to accomplish this remains unexplained. Curiously, a clue as to how ECT might sometimes seem to work, at least in the short-term, is found in the case of a hospital where, unknown to staff, an ECT machine had been broken and did not work for a period of two years (Jones, 1974). Patients were routinely anesthetized, the electrodes attached, and the switch thrown. While the ECT machine appeared to be fully functional, it actually no longer delivered an electrical current.

Despite this rather important anomaly—an electric shock machine incapable of delivering any shock—absolutely no one, not psychiatrists, doctors, mental health nurses, or patients, noticed any difference in results. One thing they might have noticed, though, if they had been truly observant, would have been that no brain damage resulted from the anesthetized non-treatment.

There is a body of other evidence demonstrating that sham ECT procedures (where the patient has electrodes placed and is anesthetized, but receives no electric shock) are more effective than receiving no ECT procedure at all (UK ECT Review Group, 2003). Once again, the wonderful power of belief—the placebo effect—appears to be the explanation for why some people claim to have benefited from ECT. People believe that this draconian treatment works, so for some of them, it does. But the times it doesn't work, and the times it causes actual harm, far outstrip the value of any possible positive placebo effect. Moreover, the awful psychological blunting caused by ECT administration and the creation of a mental state too bewildered to register any nuanced emotion is much too high a price to pay for any temporary relief that electroshock might possibly afford.

We as a society, and the medical profession in particular, are sleepwalking our way through this crisis. We have bought into the belief that troublesome feelings and emotional difficulties are manifestations of a disease and that a chemical substance or an electric shock—a medical silver bullet—can cure us of feelings of unhappiness and despair.

Yet, as we have seen, the link between depression and a lack of serotonin or norepinephrine is extremely tenuous, and a deficiency may very well not be the actual cause of those troublesome feelings. Remember that no test has ever shown that depressed people have a lack of these neurotransmitters. At best, the serotonin-norepinephrine-depression link is but part of the story, and at worst, it is a red herring, delaying or precluding access to more effective treatment. If we are to focus on biological factors, then cortisol (the hormone produced in response to stress) is almost certain to be involved, and research needs to be done in this area.

Whatever temporary masking effects chemical preparations and electroshock strategies might promise, they can never take away the *cause* of a person's depressed feelings. But remember this important fact: If you or someone you care about is already taking antidepressants or other psychoactive drugs, abruptly stopping this treatment or stopping it too quickly is a very bad idea.

Understand that antidepressants, like all psychotropic drugs, bring about semi-permanent changes in the brain. It is imperative that withdrawal is done incrementally in order to allow the brain chemistry sufficient leeway to again become normal. Finding and working with a doctor who understands the problems that may be associated with withdrawal is the wisest thing to do, and I strongly urge you to do this if you are considering stopping the medication. This might require 'shopping around' a bit until you find the right practitioner.

A book that provides some really useful information that you might like to read and share with your doctor is Joseph Glenmullen's *The Antidepressant Solution.* It lays out the best ways to end dependence with a minimum of side effects.

In the next chapter, we will look at an alternative approach to depression and its treatment. It is an approach that sees depression not through a psychopathological lens, as a mental illness requiring medication or brutal electric shock, but as a form of psychological and behavioral shutdown that results largely from the way in which past experience has been perceived and processed. Depression is often further compounded by faulty cognitive habits and poor lifestyle choices that are being made in the present.

When we recognize the feelings generated by luan chi for what they are—important messages energetically sent from the deeper, inner self—then we can begin to use these feelings not to conform to some medical diagnosis or arbitrarily assigned label, but in order to get better. When we listen to what even our most difficult feelings are telling us, then we flow with the chi of change.

Chapter Seven

Depression—A Better Approach

'You largely constructed your depression. It wasn't given to you.
Therefore, you can deconstruct it.'
~ Albert Ellis

In the previous chapter, we saw how the medical model of depression appears in so many ways to be inadequate, falling far short of any real solution to the problem. My hope is that if you or someone you care about is considering taking antidepressant medication or undergoing medical treatment for depression, you or they will first read that chapter in the interest of making an informed choice.

In this chapter we will focus on a different, non-medicalized approach to depression, one I believe to be more humane as well as more effective. It is an approach that views depression not as an illness, but largely as an inability to see our choices and to come to terms with them.

What precisely does the word *depression* mean? It comes from the Latin *deprimere*, meaning 'to press down'. Pressed down is a good description of the feeling we have when we say we are depressed. It can feel as if we are carrying the heaviest of loads. If this were all the word *depression* meant, then the term would be reasonably accurate, but it has come to mean so much more. Depression is now viewed as a pernicious disease, one that is in the process of 'going viral'.

Without a doubt, the feelings generated by this thing we call depression can indeed be terrible. I am not for one moment attempting to minimize such feelings or the devastating effect they can have on a person's life. For the depressed person, these feelings are as real as real can be. I know this very well because I was once diagnosed with 'clinical depression' myself and hospitalized for it. What I am suggesting is that these feelings, pressing and difficult as they are, are not a disease and that there is no reason for us to treat them as such. A better way to view these feelings is as a form of distorted energy, based on faulty information. In other words, depressed feelings are serious disturbances in the person's chi.

As we saw in the previous chapter, depression is a relatively recent medical diagnosis. It is one that is being applied to ever-increasing numbers of people, and a whole mystique has been built up around it. To begin, let's extract depression from the disease model and free it of medical terminology by removing that little word *clinical* (as in *clinical depression*, meaning *major depression*). *Clinical*, after all, turns us into patients, and patients are by definition in some way ill. *Clinical* also has an austere, antiseptic connotation, distancing the condition from human emotion. Emotion is what sets us apart from machines and from cold-blooded states of being. It is an essential aspect of our chi, an important part of what makes us human. And, of course, emotions have everything to do with depression and with therapy.

This is the reason why I dislike the terms *clinical hypnotherapy* and *clinical hypnosis*, terms now much in vogue and promoted by so many hypnotherapy training schools. One cannot help but wonder what exactly 'clinical hypnotherapy' is and how it differs from 'hypnotherapy' itself. Perhaps it is an attempt to distance itself from stage hypnosis, hypnosis used solely for entertainment, and from the more esoteric practices to which hypnosis is sometimes applied, such as past-life regression. But I believe the term is confusing and does a disservice to those who turn to hypnotherapy for a solution to their emotional problems.

Hypnotherapists are *not* clinicians; they are people who possesses certain skills and understandings which, when wisely used, help another person better deal with aspects of life that trouble them. Here the emphasis is on one person helping another person. It is not at all one person as patient and the other as clinical authority.

When we use the term *depression,* rather than *clinical depression,* we have already taken a step in the right direction and are in a better position to see the condition for what it is: *Depression is our modern word for feelings of intense and profound unhappiness.* These powerful feelings can overwhelm the body-mind system, seriously affecting our ability to function in a normal manner.

Many who have accepted the depression label believe that practically everyone else is quite happy but they are not, so there must be something horribly wrong with them. They have given a *meaning* to their feelings that is not inherent within them but which turns feelings into symptoms of illness. Yet unhappiness—even at its most profound level—is not a medical condition; it is not a disease. Unhappiness is a psychological state, based on our old friend *perception.*

Once we see depression in this light, we are in a much better position to deal with it. If depression is a disease, then it needs a medical treatment, and such treatment is something external to ourselves—essentially beyond our own grasp. But if we see depression as a state of profound unhappiness, doesn't this mean we ourselves are in some sort of position to influence it?

We are not to blame for this thing we label depression—though as the psychologist Albert Ellis pointed out, we may have played our part in 'constructing' it—and it certainly does not mean we are weak or inadequate, but if these feelings are ours, then we *are* responsible for managing them. We may well benefit from professional help in tackling them, but it is we ourselves who need to act and actually *do* something about them.

If I am unhappy in my job, then I can look for another means of making a living. If I am unhappy with my living arrangements, I can look for different accommodation. If I am unhappy in a relationship, I can seek to alter or end it.

Such changes will come at a cost. It may well mean giving up something we would rather keep—a sense of the familiar, for example, or the way that family, friends, and others see us. It may mean an adjustment in the way I see myself, and it will mean finding the energy to initiate change, but it is within my power to do so. A medicine does none of these things. But I can.

What if we have absolutely no control over the cause of our unhappiness? What if it's because of a difficult family member or the death of a loved one? How can we change these things and turn from a state of intense unhappiness into a state of intense happiness?

The short answer is that maybe we cannot. Maybe there are some things in life that we have to learn to cope with, and maybe that means we will have to learn to deal with feelings of real unhappiness from time to time—and those times might last far too long for our liking. But this isn't the same as saying we are powerless or ill. Just because we cannot change certain facts does not mean we are powerless to change the *effect* that those facts have on us. This concept is at the heart of the best hypnotherapy.

Neither you nor I were put on Earth to play the role of victim any more than we were born to play the role of a label, regardless of whether that label has been popularized by the media or sanctioned by the medical profession and given the name 'diagnosis' or 'depression'. When we allow ourselves to become a victim or a label, we cease to be our authentic self. We then enter into a mind-set in which unhappiness becomes a pathological condition.

Perhaps we can begin to see now how this labeling compounds the profound unhappiness we have learned to call *depression*. When we turn 'severe unhappiness' into 'depression', we produce an alchemy that greatly reduces our ability to deal with it.

Thinking of ourselves as depressed, off we trudge to the doctor, head bowed and shoulders hunched under the weight of our own misery. We explain the way we have been feeling and how difficult it is for us to go on feeling this way. Within minutes, our compassionate doctor confirms our own diagnosis: We are suffering from 'depression'—basically because we tell him or her that we are. With the label sanctioned, out comes the prescription pad, and everyone feels a little better, even if no one really is. All the time the actual *cause* of the terrible unhappiness remains untouched and essentially unquestioned, as if it simply does not matter.

But the cause does indeed matter because the cause of our unhappiness determines the way it needs to be addressed. If we know the origin of our discomfort and distress, then perhaps we can do something about it.

But what is the cause of depression? Depression is undoubtedly heterogeneous in origin, which is to say that there are multiple factors and influences involved in its cause, just as there are multiple factors responsible for its continuation. And these differ with different people.

For some, the problem is physical. Adrenal insufficiency, thyroid malfunction, and diabetes, for example, can all produce feelings of depression. So can the weather—as is the case with people who get depressed during the winter season because of a lack of sufficient daylight or insufficient vitamin D in their bodies due to decreased sunlight. (If you suspect this problem, take a Vitamin D3 oil-based supplement, use a full-spectrum light bulb or light table, and see if your condition improves.) Sometimes other nutritional elements are lacking from our diet because we have been eating in a way that fails to provide what we need for physical and mental health, or are unable to properly assimilate the required nutrients. Or the foods we have been eating may be fogging up the brain, causing mood swings and affecting the way we feel.

Environmental toxins, too, can play a role. Mold, pollution, and food sensitivities may all be negatively affecting the way we feel. Cleaning mold from windows etc with a solution of soap, water and vinegar, using an air purifier—especially in the bedroom—and checking for food sensitivities (by systematically eliminating and then reintroducing items such as wheat, dairy, etc. and observing any changes in mood), are all wise steps well worth investigating.

Depression can be caused or influenced by early life events that have programmed us to respond to particular stimuli and to view life in a certain way. Depression can be caused or influenced by our present circumstances and by the people who play a pivotal role in our life. It can be caused or influenced by our lifestyle—the way we treat ourselves and allow ourselves to be treated. It can be caused or influenced by how we use our mind to process and think. And, above all, it can be caused or influenced by the way we cope with the feelings generated by all these things.

Because of this, a one-size-fits-all approach is not the best way to address depression. Neither is it wise to simply focus on our symptoms. As with so many other difficult feelings, we do well to heed the wisdom of that great Spanish writer Cervantes: 'Take away the cause, and the effect ceases.'

If something or someone in our current situation is causing our unhappiness, for example, it is up to us to change the circumstances. Difficult though it may be, there is always an alternative way, but this cannot be found until we face up to the problem and commit to taking concrete steps to deal with it. This might well cause some additional suffering in the short-term, but if a choice must be made between remaining stuck in a state of profound unhappiness or removing the cause, we must make the courageous choice and take action, or the unhappiness will only continue. In attempting to avoid dealing with what needs to be dealt with, we open ourselves up to greater misery. Remember

Carl Jung's words: 'Neurosis is an attempt to avoid legitimate suffering.'

If we are in an unhappy situation but can *genuinely* do nothing about it, then we are challenged with the responsibility of coping with it until time brings about change. We may have to wait a long time for this, so we'll need all the courage and stoicism we can muster. We'll need to nurture ourselves and take care of our own emotional needs. Here a close friend or understanding relative can be invaluable, helping us to bear the load and providing the emotional support we badly need. If no such person is available, then a counselor, perhaps accessed through our family doctor, can be of enormous help.

But often, search as we may, the reason for feelings of profound unhappiness cannot be found in either nutritional deficiencies or in what is happening around us. Everything in our life may be going fine, and we might have no apparent reason to complain, yet still we feel an overriding sense of melancholy and confusion. Our lack of ability to pinpoint the cause can intensify the feelings of despondency, adding a sense of guilt to the burden of difficult emotions with which we are already struggling. 'What reason do I have to complain?' we might think. 'I am much better off than so many other people.'

When our awful feelings of dejection have no obvious cause, it is to the subconscious, feeling mind that we need to turn. We need to determine why it is disturbing our chi and sending us such disruptive messages, these dark and draining feelings. Once again, hypnosis, with its ability to connect directly with the subconscious, allows us to do this.

Deep unhappiness and the despair it so often accompanies may have multiple causes, but one thing is certain: if the despondency is not being generated by present conditions and circumstances, then it is being generated by the past. In all probability, both are generating it.

Kolya was a successful visual artist whose work had already

been exhibited internationally when he came to see me. In his late thirties, but with a furrowed brow and receding hairline that made him look much older, his darting eyes gave him a fugitive look, as if he expected an unwelcome knock at the door that might arrive at any moment. Balanced on the edge of his chair, he quickly explained that he had been suffering from feelings of depression and low self-worth for most of his life and that recently they had become much worse.

'I know the cause of my depression,' he told me. 'It's my awful childhood, but I just can't shift it. It doesn't make sense. I should be happy now. Everything is going well, but inside I'm completely desolate. It feels like I'm falling apart and won't be able to hold it together for much longer.'

Kolya was in no way unique in this. Many people who visit the hypnotherapist already think they know why they feel so badly, but they just cannot seem to do anything about it. They feel helpless. 'I know I shouldn't feel this way, that there's no need,' they sometimes say. 'I have everything, but I just can't help it—I'm so depressed.' What they are forgetting is that words like 'should' and 'shouldn't' are quite meaningless in a world composed of what 'is'.

While people sometimes do have an idea of the kind of experience that may have started their troubles, remembering many of the difficulties through which they have passed—an unhappy childhood, a failed relationship, a traumatic experience, and so forth—is challenging. Few people know the *specific* incident that is at the origin of their troubles. People often tell me they know the origin, but in hypnosis a different causal event is often revealed.

Kolya was just such a case. He was the son of eastern European immigrants. His father, though hardworking, regularly came home drunk, and many times Kolya was forced to jump in when the man lashed out in anger at his mother. Sometimes his father failed to return home for days, spending night after night with one woman or another. Often the child was sent to the pub to beg his father for money to buy food for the family, and gradually the boy grew to hate his father. All of this Kolya was consciously able to remember, and these were the things he believed were at the root of his depression.

In the deep trance state of hypnosis, however, Kolya went back to an experience not with his father, but with his mother. As a child of four he was again sitting on his mother's lap, listening as she complained of her life, of how worried she was about their future, but that no matter what happened, she would never leave little Kolya. No matter how bad it got she would never allow anyone to take him away—she would die before she would be separated from her son.

The words 'take you away' and 'die' had had a horribly frightening effect on the small child, and powerful anxious feelings embedded themselves indelibly in his subconscious mind. While his father's behavior was indeed part of the story of his depression, the event with his mother was the initial sensitizing experience—lost to conscious recall—that had begun the program that would later manifest itself as feelings of overwhelming despair.

Then came those many experiences in which his drunken father was abusing his mother, the frightening subsequent sensitizing events that served to reinforce the program already embedded in the boy's subconscious mind. These confirmed his belief that life was indeed an unsettling affair, with plenty of reason to feel worried, anxious, and unsafe. Filled with rage at his father and with an unexpressed, subconscious anger towards his mother for frightening him and allowing it all to happen, Kolya the man felt torn apart.

He could not allow himself to consciously recognize his anger towards his mother, let alone blame her, because he well knew how difficult her life had been. He knew that she loved him and that he loved her. To criticize his mother or allow himself to feel anger towards her would mean, he felt, that he had betrayed her and all she had done for him.

For years Kolya had lived his life suspended in this state of inner conflict until, luckily, he discovered his talent for art. This gave him a glimpse of meaning, and with this glimpse came some degree of release. In art he found a way not only to express his feelings, but also to matter. But even his art had not saved him from the awful despondency and growing despair that seemed to follow him like dark clouds wherever he went.

Kolya's unhappy past had left him with deep-seated, unexpressed feelings of rage that continued to feed his inner turmoil. Such anger is not at all unusual in people who come to me with depression. In fact, it is quite rare to meet a profoundly unhappy person who is not holding onto some form of anger, whether or not they are able to identify it or admit this to themselves. 'Depression is rage spread thin,' said the Spanish-American philosopher George Santayana. My own experience in working with this condition suggests that this is at least part of the story. In all the many cases of profound unhappiness I have seen, I do not think there has been a single one that was not connected with the perception of unfairness or unkindness.

Consequently, anger—and its twin, guilt—usually play an important role in keeping the person stuck in depression, so both of these emotions need to be worked through in therapy.

Sometimes, though, the anger has become so conflicted, as it had with Kolya, that the person is in almost complete denial regarding its presence. When anger becomes mingled with guilt, the two emotions become almost inseparable, like colors that have bled into each other. The denial of anger simply accentuates the feelings of guilt, deepening the inner confusion. Only when denial is ended and the anger and guilt faced and released, can the confusion and despair really be lifted.

Such was the case with Kolya, and because of this it was not enough to go back to those difficult, historic, sensitizing events, neutralize their effect, and rewrite the subconscious programming. We also had to work through the accumulated anger and guilt that were contributing so much to his unhappiness. This phase of the treatment employs Ego State Therapy, which we talked about in Chapter 1, and involves talking with various parts of the personality or psyche in order to restore inner balance and end internal conflict.

In addition to the hypnotherapy sessions, Kolya also began a program of regular exercise and temporary nutritional supplementation, including additional EPA (the fatty acid shown to be beneficial for people with depression) in his diet. He understood and accepted the fact that a body-mind constantly fed the wrong things can be neither balanced nor happy. He soon became more aware of the foods he was eating and adjusted his diet to a more wholesome one that provided all of the nutrients necessary for his inner stability. I also encouraged him to spend as much time as possible outdoors.

As he moved through the process, Kolya's feelings of deep, prolonged unhappiness lifted. As part of his therapy, he learned cognitive skills that would help him to continue moving forward with his life: how to recognize old negative thought patterns, to challenge unhelpful thinking, and to separate thoughts and presuppositions from facts. In our final session, he learned how to hypnotize himself and how to use self-hypnosis to relax, manage stress, and even to access aspects of his creative subconscious mind that he could draw upon in his work and in his life.

Would you be surprised to learn that this entire process took only six sessions, from start to finish? It did. In fact, it is quite unusual for any series of hypnotherapy treatments to take longer than six or seven sessions. We really do not need endless sessions of talk and exploration in order to bring about real change. In Kolya's case, the six sessions were spread out over a period of eight weeks. People vary, of course, yet this is about the average length of time it takes to move through therapy for complex issues such as depression.

Today Kolya approaches life with a much more stable and positive attitude, and I am pleased to report that he continues to produce the wonderful art that is so much a part of his life—dispelling the myth that, in order to create, an artist needs to be tormented.

As we have seen, the way we attempt to deal with life's difficulties (and the uncomfortable feelings they can produce) is directly related to how we learned to deal with experiences and feelings in the past, especially in childhood. Unquestionably, early life adversity—or more correctly, our *perception* of this adversity—creates a response pattern that can easily predispose a person to feelings of depression.

Suzanne was a demure and reserved woman in her early thirties who consulted me because of the chronic depression that had affected her for as long as she could recall. She was dressed in the drabbest of browns, her wispy and prematurely grey hair hiding half her face, her whole countenance bespeaking dejection and despair. I had been recommended by a member of her family whom I had previously treated, and she quickly admitted she had come to see me as a last resort, everything else having failed—something, by the way, that I hear on a quite regular basis from people who consult with me. My therapy room is often the station at the very end of the line.

For years Suzanne had been in psychiatric treatment for depression. Twice she had been 'sectioned'—forcibly placed in a mental hospital against her will—before she had reached the age of twenty-one. The doctors had tried just about everything short of a lobotomy in order to 'cure' her depression. She had run the gamut of antidepressant medication, anxiolytics, neuroleptics, and mood stabilizers—the list went on and on. She had undergone countless sessions with psychologists, psychiatrists, and counselors. She had even been subjected to two separate series of electro-convulsive therapy (ECT) sessions. The shock treatment had destroyed parts of her memory—she could no longer recall attending her mother's funeral, for example—but it had not alleviated her awful depression. Nothing seemed to work.

At our first meeting I explained to Suzanne that I was never going to ask her to go into a hospital because I did not believe her to be sick, nor would I ask her to take drugs or to undergo any form of electric shock therapy; I was not, after all, a doctor, and even if I were, I would still not ask this of her. I also explained, as I do with every new client I meet, that although I specialize in helping people to change, I could not change *for* her. It was she who needed to take responsibility for her own change. I would help and guide her and be there for her as she went through this process, but she needed to play her part and do whatever was necessary in order to bring positive change into her life. What I was really doing, of course, was asking Suzanne to stop viewing herself as a helpless victim of an illness and to begin to accept responsibility for turning her life around.

As I talked with Suzanne, it soon became apparent that she had not been eating well. She regularly skipped meals and rarely ate breakfast, often grabbing whatever snack was readily available during the daytime, and generally eating micro waved processed meals or take-out food for dinner. This is by no means unusual. Often people who are depressed have little appetite and little inclination to cook, so they all too easily skip meals. Feelings of profound unhappiness can either deplete a person's appetite or increase it to such an extent that the person binge-eats in an attempt to distract themselves from the pain.

Our first task was to draw up a guideline for better eating. Like Kolya, Suzanne had no difficulty in understanding that what she put into her mouth she also put into her mind. I asked her to do her very best to eat according to the clock so that even if she wasn't feeling hungry she would eat something at specific times during the day. It did not need to be a full meal—the quantity of food could be small—but it did need to be something nutritious, and she did need to eat at regular intervals.

I also recommended that in the beginning of her treatment she add some nutritional supplements known to improve the mood of people experiencing depression. This would give her a boost and ensure she had all the nutrition needed in order for her mind to function effectively. For most people, eating a balanced array of different foods delivers everything needed for a healthy body and mind, but for people experiencing difficulties such as depression, it can be helpful to add particular supplements, especially in the early stages of recovery. Additionally, I encouraged her to use a full-spectrum daylight bulb at home in the room she generally spent most time in.

In hypnosis, the ground was prepared for our hypnotherapy sessions, and Suzanne was rapidly able to reach the deeper levels of hypnotic trance, easily entering the somnambulistic state necessary for uncovering the causes of her difficulties. In this state, Suzanne went back to an incident that had happened when she was just a baby. As she was left sleeping in her crib, something had touched her cheek and suddenly awakened her. Her little eyes opened to the sight of a crane fly, or as we call it in England, a 'flying daddy-long-legs'. In this half-awake/half-dreaming state of consciousness, and with nothing to tell her otherwise, this new creature had appeared as menacing as a monster. It filled her with terror, and there was no one there to protect her.

So the little girl cried and cried, as babies often do. But for Suzanne, she was not simply crying because her nappy needed changing or because she wanted food—she was crying out in sheer panic. She was screaming out in order to save her life, but there was nobody to help her. It seemed, for all the world, as if she had been abandoned.

Later our therapeutic sessions would uncover the fact that Suzanne's mother was a rather remote figure who did not believe in 'pampering' children and would not allow her husband to do so either. If babies cried, they could be left to get on with it; they would soon tire themselves and fall asleep. For her it was all part of the process of growing up. Her mother failed to grasp that when a child cries it is always for a reason: The child is in some way distressed. It is critical that the distress and the child be treated with respect and kindness and not be ignored. Yet no one entered Suzanne's room, and the frightened baby was left alone with the monstrous insect until it finally went away. Eventually, the exhausted infant did fall asleep, forgetting all about the experience—at least at the conscious level.

Small and insignificant though this initial sensitizing experience may appear to the mature, adult mind, it was extremely powerful and important for the mind of this infant new to the world. Neurologically, the frontal cortex is almost totally lacking in the infant—as we discussed, it does not become fully developed until a person reaches their early twenties—and because of this, a baby is unable to properly interpret external stimuli. The infant depends on the mother or some other person to do that. In our earliest years, the adult in charge of us acts as our frontal cortex, assuming the executive function on our behalf. It is the adults who help us to interpret and form our sense of reality.

Of course, flying insects have been around since babies have been around. Suzanne could not have been the first child to be awoken by one. Why, then, did this experience traumatize and sensitize her, yet not affect every other little baby who has had a similar encounter?

We could hypothesize endlessly: The child might have been dreaming of something scary, and this might have set the stage for the entrance of a frightening monster, her sleepy eyes feeding back half-processed information that her sleepy mind incorporated into whatever insecure feeling had already been generated in dream. But this is guesswork. The actual reason why little

Suzanne reacted in such a way is not very significant. What is relevant is her *perception* of the incident. Her cries and her distress were unanswered; she was alone and without protection.

As we have seen, it is our perception of events and the meaning we assign to them that matters. As Epictetus pointed out almost two thousand years ago: 'People are disturbed not by the things that happen, but by their *opinion* of the things that happen.' Little Suzanne's perception was that she had been abandoned. (The fear of abandonment, remember, is one of the very few primary fears that a child is born with.) Abandonment means loss and the perception of loss is so often at the root of the feeling we know as sadness. The sadness seed had been planted, and it was this seed that would later grow into Suzanne's depression. The neural pathway that led to sadness and insecurity had been established, and soon that pathway would be even more powerfully established by repetition.

Still in the trance state, Suzanne's subconscious mind then took us back to another disturbing event. At the age of three, she was playing alone in an upstairs room while her mother prepared food in the downstairs kitchen. A gust of wind slammed the door shut on her finger, and the little girl screamed and screamed. The time it took for her mother to arrive seemed to Suzanne to be an eternity. She was helpless and alone and again she felt abandoned. The shock and pain of this experience served to reinforce the program already embedded in her subconscious mind by the incident with the insect. As far as Suzanne's subconscious was concerned, she was abandoned and alone in a scary, uncaring world in which even familiar, inanimate objects could cause her pain and represented danger.

Such 'small' and unrelated experiences are sometimes all that is necessary to install and energize subconscious programs. When reinforced by subsequent experiences, they can later produce many difficulties of a psychological nature, including depression.

It is unlikely that these experiences alone would have been sufficient to sensitize Suzanne's mind to the extent that her unhappiness would force her into a mental hospital. The human mind is wonderfully resilient. It has a marvelous elasticity and is capable of handling all manner of traumatic events and regaining its balance. Had no other difficult experiences happened to Suzanne in her formative years, perhaps she would have managed to shrug things off as she grew, and perhaps nothing would have come of it. She might well have led an entirely normal life, free for the most part of insecurity, fear, or extreme unhappiness.

Unfortunately for Suzanne, this was not to be the case. As she continued her journey into adulthood, a series of subsequent sensitizing events magnified her depressed feelings. In hypnosis she returned to other experiences, to feelings of rejection and failure. Her parents divorced, and she was used as a pawn in the break-up. She then moved to a new home and went to a new school where she had few friends and was bullied. All this compounded her difficulties, turning her further in upon herself, reinforcing the negative programming until everything seemed to implode. She could no longer cope with life and was admitted to the mental hospital and to treatment by well-meaning doctors who used powerful psychoactive chemicals and massive jolts of electricity to try to shock her out of those despairing feelings, the symptoms that had qualified her for an official diagnosis of 'major depression'.

Once we had uncovered these critical sensitizing events, Suzanne was helped to re-interpret and reprocess them on the level of her subconscious mind—in so doing, altering their meaning and effect. After clearing the negative programming, we continued the hypnotherapy process, systematically working through Suzanne's fear, anger, and guilt. She learned how to use her mind to better manage her thoughts and feelings and to systematically challenge her old thinking habits and negative thought patterns so that she could respond to life in a more joyous, affirmative manner. This empowered Suzanne even more, ensuring she would remain on an even keel as she moved forward with her life. Her cognitive skills improved, and she used the self-hypnosis I taught her to relax and deal with stress. Eating well and exercising regularly, she needed no medication and no more barbaric jolts of electricity. The darkness had lifted.

Today Suzanne is free of the depression with which she was diagnosed and is leading an active and rewarding life working with children with learning difficulties in one of Britain's largest cities. It is a job she loves. In spite of, or perhaps because of her past, she now has a depth of understanding and empathy that she brings to her work and that radiates into all aspects of her life—a life that has new meaning.

Suzanne's story again illustrates how early life adversity—be it actual or imaginary—can seriously affect our psychological state as we grow and become adults. Above all, it illustrates the importance and power of human kindness, and how this quality, more powerful than the strongest of drugs, can prevent so much unnecessary suffering.

As an interesting (and I think telling) side note, I once recounted Suzanne's story to a psychiatrist whom I was treating. His response was, 'Goodness! I hope I wasn't the one who sectioned her.' Although the psychiatrist had personally experienced the positive benefits of my hypnotherapy sessions, he expressed no desire to learn hypnosis for his patients, preferring to continue treating people in the way he had been trained. I sometimes hear his voice when I meet someone who has spent time in a mental institution: 'Goodness! I hope I wasn't the one who sectioned her.'

As we have seen, both Suzanne and Kolya found meaning in their lives, and with this came greater balance. When life has lost its meaning, a deep and abiding unhappiness seems to automatically seep in, as if to fill the vacuum. To find meaning, we have to find a way to matter, or to put that more accurately: We have to reach the point where at last we see that we *do* matter.

The meaning that Suzanne found, like the meaning Kolya found, cannot be *your* meaning, just as it cannot be *my* meaning, because meaning cannot be transferred from one person to another. Each of us has to find our own sense of meaning in life, and that meaning may change, just as *we* change as we move through the years that are invisibly laid out before us. We will be talking more about the importance of meaning and how we may find it in the final chapter of *The Chi of Change*.

For a long time now, science has been attempting to locate a specific gene, some chromosomal linkage that might be responsible for depression. None has been conclusively shown to exist. While some preliminary studies suggest that a chromosome may perhaps be implicated in severe recurrent depression in people of European ancestry (Breen & Todd, 2011), this line of research has still produced very little in the way of evidence.

Even if a genetic link is finally shown to exist, this does not mean every person born with a genetic predisposition will inevitably go on to experience intense and profound unhappiness. Genes need to be triggered in order to find expression. Nature may play its part, but it is nurture that really packs the punch.

Researchers in the field believe depression depends upon both genetic and environmental factors. Although genes carry information and instructions, they need to be activated or 'switched on' for their DNA blueprint to produce an effect. Such activation is dependent upon interaction with the environment, especially on conditions we are exposed to from conception to adulthood.

Likewise, our neural pathways are developed by the experiences we pass through and by our response to those experiences. Environmental stimuli and our reaction to them can actually affect our genes—and every other part of our body-mind complex—influencing the production and release of the neurotransmitters essential for our balanced emotional and mental functioning. Too much stress, for example, can interfere with our inner ecology, producing excessive amounts of cortisol, overwhelming the body-mind and disturbing our chi. When stress accumulates over a long enough period of time, we become overloaded. This can lead to a 'systems shutdown', a breakdown of our health at all levels: physical, mental, and emotional.

If we were raised in a caring and supportive environment where we felt safe and valued, where we could process our experiences in an affirmative manner, we created positive neural pathways we can freely and frequently access. Such an environment is far less likely to activate any genetic predisposition to depression that a person may have been born with.

If, however, we were raised in an abusive or non-supportive environment, if during our formative years our perception was that we were not nurtured, that we were unsafe or were treated badly or unfairly, or if we were traumatized by events, then this will have its effect on our body-mind in a detrimental manner. The negative experiences (or stresses) coming from our environment may very well switch on any negative genetic tendencies and establish unhelpful neural pathways, while subsequent experiences further entrench and enhance our difficulties. In this way, stress—childhood stress in particular—can easily increase the likelihood of our experiencing depression.

But here is a very important point: It is not necessarily stress that is the critical factor so much as it is our *response* to that stress. If we believe we can do something about it, then stress is far less likely to trigger or lead to despair than if we feel we are helpless over it. It is when the cause of our stress lies constantly beyond our ability to influence that we become overwhelmed. We feel powerless. When this happens, we just give up, and emotional or physical shutdown is the result. I believe this understanding is key to recovery from the profound state of unhappiness we call 'depression'. In accepting its catch-all label, we become its victim. We are blinded to the fact that we *can* influence our own feelings and life circumstances and that *we can learn to do this*. We are not powerless.

From my own personal experience I know that the only thing a depressed person really wants is for the darkness to be lifted, the ordeal to end. The overriding need is to get through this day, which feels like interminable night. The future, if ever it comes, will just have to take care of itself. In fact, the profoundly unhappy and despairing person often finds it difficult to think about or even to imagine a future. Our options seem either to have all closed down, or to be so numerous and confusing that the fear of choosing the wrong one can overwhelm and bring us to a grinding halt.

It is the demands that the present seems to make, the confusion it produces and the risks it seems to entail that keep the person locked in the darkness of depression. It is as though all of life's possibilities have been exhausted; the positive things and good times, such as they were, are all left behind. And this overpowering sense of loss brings with it deep melancholy and fatigue. In this state the person feels abandoned to the vagueness of it all, stuck in the loop of a past that is poorly processed and only partially understood, which continues to obscure whatever light and hope the future might once have promised.

In my early twenties, I myself experienced a prolonged period of what my doctors and I took to be clinical depression. Desperately unhappy with my life, I found myself adrift in a world that seemed both meaningless and unfair. I entered the depths of despair, the darkest of abysses. For me, it was as if time had stopped. Day had become night, night had become day, and both were an endless drudge. It felt as if the light and the color had been drained from my life. I was adrift at sea without rudder or compass. With a future so obscured that it seemed to oscillate between the unthinkable and the impossible, and a past that was permeated with both unexpressed rage and guilt, I found myself sinking into a terrible grayness, a foggy existence that appeared to be both empty and pointless.

Everything was filtered through this unhappy, grey lens. I believed that because I was depressed, I must be mentally ill. After all, wasn't depression a form of mental illness or disease? I believed that it was. I had been taught that it was. I gave myself that label and made no distinction between it and the person I was.

In this state of profound unhappiness and confusion, I had absolutely no difficulty convincing my doctor that I should be hospitalized. We were, after all, products of the same belief system, so all I had to do was tell him how desperately unhappy I was feeling in order for the diagnosis of 'major clinical depression' to be made and a bed arranged in the nearest mental hospital. Again, such is the power of belief—it can even get you a bed in a hospital and three meals a day, all paid.

Being hospitalized for depression was, for me, one of the great turning points in my life—but not because of any treatment I received. In fact, other than a few obligatory pills that I soon found myself covertly disposing of (yes, it was possible) and a couple of group sessions with an 'art therapist', there was no treatment. There was merely confinement within a mental hospital, some psychological testing, and chats with a couple of psychiatrists, one of whom I considered to be remarkably limited and narrow in his thinking and who easily became outraged whenever I challenged him. 'You are the patient and I am the doctor!' I recall him telling me once, the veins on his neck bulging as if they were about to explode. It has been said that there are two kinds of teachers. From one kind we learn what to do, and from the other we learn what not to do. From that psychiatrist I learned what *not* to do—and perhaps more importantly, I learned what not to *be*. It is a lesson that has served me well, both in my role as psychotherapist as well as in life.

Although I saw other patients drugged to the hilt and still others attempting to recover from the terrible effects of electroshock treatment, I myself was fortunate enough to narrowly escape such assault. Yet through this experience, something in me awoke to the reality of it all. Before any treatment could begin—and very much against the wishes and tactics of my psychiatrist—with the help of a friend I managed to get myself discharged.

It was a turning point because that experience awakened me. It allowed my eyes to open. In that hospital I saw more clearly than ever that I was no more mentally ill than those doctors who were attempting to manage people like me—and the same appeared to be true for most of the other patients on my ward. As far as I could see, none of us were really mentally ill but all of us *believed* that in some way we were.

Conquering depression was not simply a question of changing my thinking—it was a question of changing my *believing*. When I understood this, I began to get better.

I had awakened from the illusion and understood first-hand how these things we label 'depression' and 'mental illness' could come to define a person, seriously affecting their ability to function authentically. I had understood how these labels confine and proscribe and act as a block, a door slammed closed in the endless process of becoming. Moreover, I had understood how this door was jammed shut and sealed by *belief* itself, and with this understanding, the darkness at last began to lift. I could finally begin to accept responsibility for my own unhappiness and for my role in it.

As that wonderful American mythologist Joseph Campbell observed: 'It is by going down into the abyss that we recover the treasures of life. Where you stumble, there lies your treasure.' The paradox is that sometimes we need to wander in darkness so that the light might at last startle and awaken us from our sleep-walking.

I now see depression from an entirely different perspective: Sadness is not sickness, no matter how profound or incapacitating it may be. Difficult and painful though it is, the experience of those unhappy, despairing feelings can be a springboard to a fuller, more meaningfully lived life. Our darkest and most painful moments can clarify and light our way forward if we have the courage to face and learn from them.

The insight that my experiences brought left me with the conviction that no experience is ever really wasted, that each is an opportunity for learning and greater growth. This conviction remains with me today.

Recently, I met with Jonathan, a young man of twenty-seven who has been diagnosed with 'clinical depression'. He has also been experiencing panic attacks and wrestling with an awful fear of death. (Fear of death is something called *thanatophobia,* not to be confused with the fear of dead things, *necrophobia.*) At our first meeting, he told me that the following day he had an appointment with a psychiatrist, arranged for him by his family doctor, which of course I encouraged him to keep. (That his GP had arranged such an appointment is by no means the norm. In fact, only a fraction of patients judged by their doctor to need psychiatric help are ever referred to psychiatrists.) Jonathan's family doctor had prescribed the usual chemical antidepressants, but Jonathan was sagely waiting before starting to take them until talking with the psychiatrist.

On our second meeting, I enquired how the session with the psychiatrist had gone. With a long sigh, Jonathan said, 'I was really disappointed. The psychiatrist just sat there hardly speaking, and at the end he just gave me a prescription for some pills.' No other treatment was suggested, no further referral made, merely a prescription for antidepressants scribbled out and handed over by this mental health professional. It is a story I have heard countless times before. 'Here, kid, take this, it'll make you feel better...'

Again, is this really the best we can offer? I know we can do so much more for Jonathan and for all those others who are experiencing these very real emotional and mental difficulties. We *can* do something about depression by doing something about the *cause* of it— uncovering the origins; correcting sensitivities and nutritional imbalance; reprogramming and realigning mind and brain, and then establishing fresh, new skills that enable the person to take back control and assume responsibility for their life.

Through this healing process, which does not need to take years but usually only weeks, we can bring about a lasting state of inner balance and health, provided the person is willing to fully cooperate and take responsibility for their own life and its meaning.

I have briefly mentioned that I do advise supplemental nutrients for many of the people who visit me carrying the label of depression—these include EPA (Bourre, 2005; Martins, 2009; Parker et al. 2006), vitamin D3 (Hogberg et al. 2012; Hoag et al. 2011), vitamin B12 (Teimer et al. 2002; Lindenbaum et al. 1998), folic acid (Zhao et al. 2011; Teimer et al. 2002), magnesium (Chouinard, 1990; Giannini, 2002), and SAMe (Mischoulon, 2002). I must emphasize, however, that no amount of supplementation can ever compensate for an inadequate, unbalanced diet, nor can supplements ever take the place of good, healthy fresh food. Nutritional supplements are best used only in the preliminary stages of recovery, to give a boost where needed, or when it has been shown that the body is incapable of absorbing sufficient amounts of a certain nutrient through food. (The most accurate way to determine this is through blood analysis.)

When we are experiencing periods of profound unhappiness, it is easy to neglect our eating and to ignore the important role it plays in the way we feel. We might not feel like eating, but it is critical that we do eat on a regular basis—if necessary, eating even a small amount simply because the clock tells us to. We cannot forget that food and the air we breathe are essential for life; they are how we bring chi into our body.

Of course, persistent unhappiness can also tempt a person into habitually using food as an escape, as an attempted distraction from their feelings. But this only makes the situation worse. We will talk about using food as a way of dealing with difficult emotions when we look at overeating and weight management in Chapter 10.

The most sensible thing is to steer clear of processed foods and eat from a whole-food, largely plant-based menu, thereby ensuring that we eat in a manner harmonious with chi, taking in all the nutrients needed for excellent psychological and physical health.

Finally, we must not overlook the value of exercise in the treatment of depression. When we experience prolonged states of deep unhappiness, we can understandably become lethargic. Just about everything takes too much energy and feels like too much trouble. But taking to bed and pulling the blanket over our head won't work for very long. It will not lighten our mood or lift our despair. What is needed is movement, and exercise provides just the right kind of movement.

The positive effect of exercise on depression and on mental well-being in general is very well-documented (Blumenthal, 2007; Craft, 2004; Jasper, 2009; Salmon, 2001). Exercise increases levels of brain-derived neurotrophic factor (BDNF). A decrease in BDNF has been implicated in depression (Sinha et al. 2011). Exercise also releases an abundance of endorphins that function as neurotransmitters, eliciting those wonderful 'feel good' factors, sending them coursing through the entire nervous system. They free the chi and lighten the mood as they sweep through the mind and body. Exercise triggers important biological functions that go far beyond the physical realm, priming the entire body-mind complex in a positive manner, influencing how we feel and how we respond to life and its stresses.

In fact, exercise may be thought of as a non-pharmacological antidepressant—and an excellent, effective one at that! If you were to exercise for just thirty minutes a day, at least four times a week, you would be creating more of a positive effect on your mood than all the pharmaceuticals and SSRIs put together—and with no negative side effects.

If you have been experiencing a depressed mood and are not already exercising, simply begin with small steps, perhaps a five or ten-minute walk outside each day—fresh air is a wonderful, natural restorative—and then gradually build up from there. (If you have been doing little or no physical activity for some time, it's always wise to check with your doctor before starting an exercise regimen.) No matter the weather, no matter how little you slept, and no matter how you are feeling, *do it anyway*.

When all is said and done, perhaps living was not meant to be easy, but neither was it meant to be more difficult than it is. If you have been experiencing profound unhappiness that has lasted for far too long, then you really can get through it and even learn from it, emerging as a healthier, more rounded, and better balanced person. The darkness *can* lift and the color *can* return to your life, but this will only happen if you allow yourself to accept that you are so very much more than a label, a diagnosis, or a condition. No matter how overwhelmed you may feel, do not lose hope. With the right approach your depression can lift, your mood can lighten and your healthy chi can once more flow.

Chapter Eight

Habits—The Shackles of the Free

'Habit is stronger than reason.'
~George Santayana

We human beings certainly are creatures of habit. Each of us has habits of one kind or another, and not all of them are negative, of course. The habits of brushing our teeth, eating regularly, or even singing in the shower (which seems to lift the spirits) are all examples of good habits that serve a useful purpose.

In fact, if we look at the lives of successful people—successful in the sense that they reach their goals and lead balanced, productive, creative lives—we invariably find they have developed useful habits that play an important role in their success. It is next to impossible to live affirmatively without having a set of good, positive habits. As Aristotle pointed out, 'We are what we repeatedly do. Excellence is not an act, but a habit.'

Good habits strengthen the structure of our lives, supporting the chi, helping ensure its smooth running, and freeing us to direct our energies where they are most needed. With good habits working automatically in the background, we are free to choose where to focus our attention, and when we do this wisely, we can accomplish our goals.

There are also bad habits, of course, and it's this kind that has been called 'the shackles of the free' and that often bring a person to the hypnotherapist. Nail biting, procrastination, chronic cluttering, and overspending are all examples of habits that don't help us—they keep us stuck in the groove of mindless repetition, acting out behaviors we are better off without. Fortunately, this kind of habit usually responds very well to brief therapy and can usually be treated with a minimum number of hypnotherapy sessions.

But what *are* habits? Essentially, they are psychological processes that make us repeat certain behaviors in an automatic way, without much conscious thought. Our bad habits may be inconvenient and annoying, but, unlike addiction, they are rarely fatal. Habits are, in fact, a simple form of learning, where repetition has established neural pathways that mostly function below the level of conscious awareness and that get triggered by cues from the external or internal environment.

Though a habit may have started at the conscious level, habituation of the response occurs at the subconscious level. Because habits are driven mainly by the subconscious, feeling mind, they are notoriously difficult to break using willpower alone. Willpower, you will recall, is a function of the conscious, thinking mind, but as we have seen, this part of our mind can really struggle when attempting to exert its influence over the subconscious.

Whatever habit we might engage in, it is usually triggered not because we think, but because we *feel* like doing it. That's the thing with habits—they don't require thought; they are a conditioned response that bypasses the logical part of the mind.

If we were to use all the resources of our conscious mind to summon all of our willpower and use it to actually stop engaging in our bad habits, the worst that might happen is that we would feel uncomfortable, as if something were awkward or out of place. If we persisted and tenaciously worked our way through this feeling, the habit would eventually become extinct, and we would be free of it. It would simply fade away as a function of time and a simple lack of repetition.

All too often, though, in order to get rid of that awkward feeling and ease our sense of discomfort, we find ourselves subconsciously falling back into the old behavioral pattern. Our mind daydreaming or focused on something else, we can all too easily return to our old ways. When we try to explain this to ourselves, we might call this 'force of habit', and we would be quite right: Habit does indeed have a force; it really can throw its weight around.

Of course, this is not to say that willpower alone cannot put an end to a bad habit. Many people have indeed used willpower in order to do so, and they have been successful in their efforts. But for many others, breaking a habit can be very difficult indeed, and if we have repeatedly tried but failed, our self-esteem can take quite a bashing. It is important to remember that even if we have not succeeded in ending a habit yet, this does not mean we ourselves are a failure. A behavior, after all, is simply a behavior; it is not who or what we are.

When our habits are helpful, nothing needs to be done and we rarely think about them. We take them for granted. But when a habit begins to interrupt the smooth flow of our life, it can grow into a real problem, making us socially inhibited, affecting our sense of well-being, and wreaking havoc with our self-image. A bad habit can even affect our health. When this happens, we need to realize that something has to be done about it—and quickly.

But we really do not need to wait until our health or self-esteem is seriously affected. If we cannot seem to end an unwanted habit, hypnotherapy may be just what we need to turn things around and set ourselves free.

One of the most common habits that people bring to the therapist is that of biting their nails, a practice that goes by the rather convoluted medical name of *onychophagia*. Some people also have the habit of chewing the cuticle or skin around the nails, a behavior known as *dermatophagia*. With both these behaviors, people can so disfigure their fingers that they bleed. If not properly cleaned and allowed to heal, they can even become infected.

Nail biting belongs to a category of habits called *body-focused repetitive behaviors*, or BFRBs. There are two other habits that also come under this heading: compulsive hair pulling or *trichotillomania*, and compulsive skin picking or *dermotillomania*. These are all habits an experienced therapist sees on quite a regular basis.

With nail biting, people may have tried everything possible in order to end the habit—using willpower, painting their fingers with bitter-tasting concoctions, and wearing gloves or brightly colored rubber bands on the wrist to draw the subconscious behavior to the attention of the conscious mind—yet they continue biting. Often they resort to hiding their hands and fingers from view, keeping them tucked away in pockets or under their arms, or, in the case of women, sometimes concealing them beneath false acrylic nails.

Misha is a young fashion model who came to see me because she had been biting her nails since childhood, and it was really getting her down. She needed to end her habit because it was affecting her work, but she just couldn't seem to do so, no matter how hard she tried. Misha couldn't really remember when her habit had begun, but now it had become so entrenched that she found herself biting practically every day, especially when her mind was elsewhere, when reading a magazine or watching television, for example.

In hypnosis we first determined that her behavior was a simple habit and not a cover for a more serious psychological issue, and then we used a simple program of positive suggestion in order to alter the behavior.

Deep in trance, Misha was taken back to the first time she bit her nails. She was a teenager, a part of her nail had broken and she used her teeth to even it out. The feeling of biting down and the texture of the nail, all felt quite satisfying—a welcome distraction from the boredom she had been feeling—and she found herself engaging in this nail biting behavior more and more regularly as time went on, particularly when she was feeling bored or stressed. With repetition, the behavior seemed to become automatic, and she found herself biting her nails when she wasn't even aware of it.

What was needed now was simple behavior modification. As we have seen, in the trance state of hypnosis, the subconscious becomes open to positive suggestion, making it much easier for it to acquire new learnings, develop new ways of responding, and alter ways of behaving.

In the trance state, Misha's subconscious mind was given the suggestion that from now on, as soon as her hands moved towards her mouth to nail-bite, her arms would feel very heavy, like she was trying to lift a ten-pound weight. Before her fingers reached her mouth she would feel a little jolt that would immediately bring the behavior to the attention of her conscious mind before any biting or disfiguration occurred. She would then lose all inclination to bite, automatically lower her hands, and continue with whatever she had been doing. This was to be an automatic response: as soon as her hands approached her mouth to bite, the suggestion would be activated. (Implanting a suggestion in the subconscious in this way, designed to influence future behavior, is called *post-hypnotic suggestion*.) Misha left with a copy of my *End Nail-Biting Now!* CD which would reenforce suggestions given during our session, and I asked her to listen to this recording on a regular basis until we met again.

Our second and final session was one month later, and I was pleased, though not at all surprised, to learn that the nail gnawing had stopped completely. Already Misha's nails were growing out to a healthy length. The nail-biting behavior had become extinct. In this final session, Misha was taught my system of self-hypnosis, which enabled her to enter the trance state in a matter of seconds whenever it was safe to do so, and she learned how to use her self-hypnosis in order to let go of stress and relax whenever she needed to.

Misha's treatment is typical of the hypnotherapy approach that may be used with habits that do not have any profound psychological cause, behaviors that are not symptoms of any deeper issue, but that have simply developed from a process of repetition. (At the very beginning of treatment, the therapist determines if this is the case.) Often compulsive nail biting, like thumb-sucking, is among the easiest of habits to deal with. When the subconscious is addressed in the state of hypnosis, the automatic behavior can usually be easily eradicated primarily by the use of suggestion therapy. If the nail biting or thumb-sucking is not a manifestation of disturbed luan chi or a cover for some deeper, psychological or emotional disturbance, but simply a habit, then it can usually be successfully taken care of in just one or two sessions of brief hypnotherapy, as was the case with Misha.

The well-trained and experienced therapist will, of course, always check to determine which category the habit falls into so that the possibility of *symptom displacement* is avoided. Symptom displacement is when one symptom takes the place of another. As we saw in an earlier chapter with the woman who developed panic attacks while driving, it is not wise to remove a habit that is serving some useful psychological function only to have it replaced with something that might be a good deal worse.

Habits such as compulsive hair pulling and habitual skin picking, both body-focused repetitive behaviors that experienced therapists commonly see, *can* be deeper-seated and therefore more challenging. In these cases, their treatment is also more complex, often requiring a more extensive therapeutic approach. Whereas nail biting and thumb-sucking may be the result of simple habit, these and other BFRBs are sometimes driven by deeper emotional difficulties that remain unresolved at the subconscious level unless addressed directly through hypnotherapy.

In these cases, the habit is usually caused by an underlying anxiety, often accompanied by an elemental sense of anger, an inner tension that seeks release in what is essentially a self-harming behavior, and so something more than simple suggestion therapy is called for. Advanced hypnotherapeutic strategies are usually able to bring this release at a more profound level, freeing the chi and helping the person to move on with their life, freed of the compulsion.

Another habit that the therapist is often called upon to treat and that usually responds well to hypnotherapy is the habit of teeth grinding or *bruxism*.

It is rare for me to see a person with teeth grinding, compulsive hair pulling, or skin picking who is not also carrying some degree of internalized anger towards themselves. The experiences through which the person has passed, commencing often at a much earlier age, have somehow blocked the chi, creating a program of anxiety that can only seem to find release in these behaviors. These habits are usually made worse during times of stress, when pressure is added to the anxiety and anger, and the need for release is magnified.

Sometimes the behavior is carried out at the conscious-awareness level. The person is aware of their behavior but cannot resist the impulse or urge—much in the way that a compulsive overeater cannot seem to resist that cake or biscuit—but more often the behavior happens when the person is focused on something else, where the conscious mind is distracted and the subconscious more or less takes over.

Teeth grinding, especially in the early stages, usually occurs while the person is asleep and therefore consciously unaware of the behavior. Some people may awaken with an aching jaw yet only later realize what is happening; perhaps they are informed by a partner who has heard or seen them grinding, or by a dentist. In severe cases, if the condition is left untreated, the teeth can become cracked or so worn down by the grinding that root canal treatment or even extraction is required.

The medical response to teeth grinding is usually to advise some kind of mouth guard to cushion the grinding, but many people find these things uncomfortable and difficult to sleep with, and, of course, they function purely at the symptom level while doing nothing to address the underlying drivers, the reason for the grinding. Alternatively, some form of psychotropic medication may be prescribed—again attempting to silence the person's disruptive chi.

With hypnotherapy, we can work not only on modifying the behavior itself, in the beginning perhaps teaching the mind to redirect its energy so that it is the hand that automatically clenches and not the jaw, but we can also uncover the *cause* of the grinding and do something about the mechanism that continues to drive the potentially damaging activity. With this treatment, many people find that in just a few sessions the habit simply fades and they are permanently freed from this unwanted and potentially damaging behavior.

When most people think of habits and hypnotherapy, they automatically think about hypnosis being used to stop smoking. Indeed, hypnosis can be extremely effective with regard to this habit.

In the United States, as in the United Kingdom, one person in five is a cigarette smoker, and smoking is responsible for about one in five deaths annually (Centers for Disease Control and Prevention, 2004—2005). Unquestionably, it is the leading preventable cause of death, with smokers dying an average of thirteen to fourteen years younger than non-smokers. For every single person who dies from a smoking-related disease, twenty more suffer at least one serious illness from smoking (CDC 2000). Yet two-thirds of all smokers report that they want to give up smoking (Substance Abuse and Mental Health Administration, 2010).

There is absolutely no question that smoking is bad for us, so why do we persist with this self-harming behavior? Why do we insist on attempting suicide in this slow and hesitant way? It seems to be one of those special behaviors that straddle the line between habit and addiction, but which one is it?

The answer is both. When we light a cigarette, an astonishing number of chemicals are released. In fact, cigarette smoke contains in excess of four thousand different chemicals, from arsenic to cyanide, and at least sixty-nine of these are known to cause cancer. (These harmful chemicals are listed on my website: peterfieldhypnotherapy.co.uk.) The best way to view smoking then is to see it for exactly what it is: *a delivery system for toxic, cancer-causing chemicals.*

Though cigarettes contain all of these damaging chemicals, only one of them appears to be physically addictive, and we all know which one this is—that old devil, nicotine. The rest of the addiction is psychological, which is why good hypnotherapy is so very effective in helping people to deal with it. What few smokers realize is that nicotine remains in the system for only a short period of time. In fact, it takes only about forty-eight hours for nicotine to exit the body almost completely, and when it leaves, with it goes the physical addiction.

Nicotine replacement therapy—be it with gum, patches, inhalators, or sublingual lozenges—simply keeps nicotine circulating in the body with the hope that by gradually reducing the dosage and altering the means of nicotine delivery, the habit can be broken. And indeed, there is no denying that this approach has helped many people to withdraw from the physical addiction and to quit smoking. But what if you've tried these things and you still continue to smoke?

The better and more effective way to stop smoking is through hypnosis. Speaking as an ex-smoker myself—in the past I smoked as many as seventy cigarettes a day—I know that the only way a person can remain a smoker and continue to ignore the damage smoking is doing is to live in a state of denial.

The smoker is someone whose subconscious mind has been conditioned into accepting the belief that they *are* a smoker. Nature certainly didn't intend that any one of us should be a smoker; no one was born to live that label. But through repetition, it has become part of the person's identity, accepted as such by the subconscious, and because of this, the subconscious will do everything necessary to support and manifest this identity—and that means making sure that the person continues to smoke. Being a very astute part of our mind, the subconscious cleverly leaves it to the conscious mind to justify and rationalize this essentially irrational behavior and to come up with logical-sounding excuses for it to continue in its ways.

For a person to become a non-smoker and remain a non-smoker, the subconscious has to accept and *believe* that he or she is a non-smoker, and with hypnotherapy we can help the mind accomplish this.

How effective is hypnosis in helping someone to stop smoking? I find that everyone who has truly decided to stop can stop with hypnotherapy, and hypnotherapy can certainly make the process of stopping a great deal easier. *New Scientist* magazine reported the largest-ever comparison study of ways to stop smoking (Mathews, 1992). This comprehensive meta-analysis statistically combined the results from more than 600 different studies and covered 72,000 people from the United States, Scandinavia, and other countries. It found hypnotherapy to be the most effective way of stopping to smoke—at least five times more effective than willpower alone. According to the authors of the report, 'Most techniques turned out to be hopeless. Hypnosis, however, came out as the most effective anti-smoking technique.'

Perhaps the single-most important element in successfully stopping to smoke is the genuine desire to do so. This, of course, is something no therapist can provide. I ask smokers who come to me, 'Have you *decided* to stop smoking?' I also say, 'If you have, I can help you make it a reality. But if you haven't, there's not much I can do.'

We therapists do not practice mind control. The decision to

stop smoking and to stay stopped resides with the smoker. A degree of willpower is necessary to become a non-smoker. Once the decision is made, however, hypnosis can make it remarkably easy to end the smoking habit, assisting the ex-smoker to remain free for the rest of their life, and this can be accomplished with the absolute minimum of withdrawal symptoms and in a manner that feels almost amazingly easy and surprisingly effortless.

A habit that a good number of people experience but rarely discuss is the embarrassing habit of wetting the bed while sleeping, or *nocturnal enuresis.* Bed-wetting is the most common urological complaint in early childhood, with 95 per cent of bed-wetting children remaining dry by the time they reach the age of ten (Bennet, 2005). This condition is something that can cause real distress and great feelings of embarrassment when it occurs later in life.

The first thing to do, of course, when faced with bed-wetting, is to visit a doctor to make sure it is not caused by any underlying physical problem. There is absolutely no need to be shy about doing this. Doctors are as accustomed to dealing with such matters as gardeners are to tending plants. Once medical reasons for the behavior have been ruled out, we are faced with a condition that clearly is psychological in nature, and one that usually responds well to hypnotherapy.

In therapy it is essential that any anxiety, distress, or underlying insecurity that might be triggering the behavior is properly investigated and processed. It is also essential that any subconscious 'secondary benefit' of the behavior is uncovered and addressed. If the bed-wetting serves some useful psychological or practical purpose—such as excluding an unwanted partner from the bed, for example—its positive intent will ensure its continuation, and the behavior will end only when the subconscious believes the person is completely safe from threat. Successful treatment of bed-wetting also involves creating a greater degree of control over the behavior by calling it to conscious awareness before urination takes place. Unsurprisingly, given its capacity to reach the subconscious mind, hypnosis can prove a valuable asset in the treatment of adult enuresis.

Procrastination, or the tendency to postpone doing what really needs to be done, is yet another habit that brings people to the therapist, and this is an area where hypnotherapy can also be of great benefit. While some forms of procrastination can be ascribed to simple laziness—we can all put off doing the dishes until the morning because we feel too lazy to do it now, for example—for many people, chronic procrastination is a habit that can easily become a major problem, seriously affecting work and relationships. Some people put things off so indefinitely that promises are broken, important deadlines missed, and golden opportunities lost. When the habit of procrastination becomes chronic, causing regular disruption to the smooth flow of things, something clearly needs to be done about it.

To effectively treat the habit of chronic procrastination, we need first to understand why a person procrastinates. There are, in fact, several reasons for this, but the one element underlying many of them is our old friend, *fear*. It is often the fear that we are not quite good enough—the fear we call self-doubt. Fear is the sly inner saboteur that comes in various guises, all of which persuade the chronic procrastinator to postpone and delay. Examples include: fear of failure, fear of success, fear of disappointment, fear of being controlled, fear of relationships, fear of change, and fear of poking one's head above the parapet.

Harry was a successful man who worked in a large executive recruitment agency. It was a position he had stumbled into almost by accident. Having taken a temporary administration job when still in his twenties, Harry had quickly proven a valuable asset to the firm, and he rapidly found himself assuming a larger role with more and more responsibility. His new duties included connecting with clients, negotiating contracts, and handling bigger accounts.

For some time, all went well. Harry worked the phones, sought out qualified personnel, met and dined with prospective clients, arranged placements, and signed lucrative contracts. But gradually the smoothness started to give way to something more laborious; routine activities began to feel like chores, phone calls were left unmade, emails were delayed or unsent, and the desk became cluttered with unanswered mail and Post-it notes.

'I don't know what's happening,' he told me. 'I'm quite the perfectionist. I like to dot my *i's* and cross my *t's*, but these days I can't even put pen to paper. I just seem to find reasons to delay, and then I put things off so much that it's too late to do anything about them. I should be making phone call after phone call, arranging meeting after meeting, but I'm doing almost everything other than what I really should be doing. I don't think I'm lazy by nature. I really don't understand it.'

'The kind of procrastination you describe has little to do with laziness,' I assured him. 'It usually has to do with fear. There's something holding you back, stopping you from doing what needs to be done in a timely fashion.'

In hypnosis, Harry travelled back to a younger time and to an event that had imprinted itself on his subconscious mind. He was in primary school, and the teacher had asked the class what they wanted to be when they grew up. Little Harry had cheerfully piped up, 'I want to be an airplane pilot!'

'Ha!' sneered the teacher. 'They don't let people like you wash planes, let alone pilot them.' At that moment, something in the boy became stuck. This was the initial sensitizing event that planted the restrictive seed of self-doubt deep within his subconscious mind, the origin of the limiting belief that would repeatedly surface. Later this programming would be reinforced by numerous subsequent sensitizing experiences, working silently and invisibly below the conscious level, telling Harry that he could go so far, but no further.

And this was the basis of his procrastination. It was this limiting belief that had been causing Harry to continually put things off. By allowing things to remain undone, inevitable disappointment could perhaps be delayed or even avoided. If he didn't begin, he couldn't fail. Here were self-doubt and fear, masquerading as habit—and it all remained at the subconscious level, tucked far away from the conscious mind's awareness.

In hypnosis we were able to rewrite this limiting script, helping Harry's subconscious mind see that he *could* succeed, that he was allowed to be whatever he wished to be, do whatever he wished to do, as long as it was in line with his own conscience and inner wisdom.

In no time at all, Harry was back up to speed, making the contacts, cultivating relationships with clients, and bringing in so much fresh work that, even in the midst of a recession, business kept increasing. When last I heard from him, he told me he was leaving the organization to start an agency of his own. With his fearful limiting beliefs removed, there seems to be no holding him back now.

As we saw with Harry, the seeds of chronic procrastination are usually planted at an early age, often long before the postponing behavior becomes troublesome.

There may be several reasons driving serious procrastination. Let's look at some of them now:

Perfectionism—When we equate performance with self-worth, then procrastination seems to offer protection from failure. This can produce an 'if I don't start, then I can't fail' attitude.

Anticipating the Worst—When we focus only on disaster as an outcome of our activity, procrastination seems to protect us from anxiety: 'If I delay, then maybe I'll avoid catastrophe.'

Insecurity in Relationships—When we feel others will only

accept us if we perform well, procrastination appears to protect us from rejection: 'If I don't begin, then I can't be rejected.'

Self-Judgement—When we judge ourselves too harshly, procrastination seems to offer protection from feelings of self-loathing and shame: 'If I don't begin, then I can't beat myself up.'

Inflexibility—When our self-image is rigid, procrastination seems to protect us from having to change: 'If I don't begin, then I can remain as I am.'

Powerlessness—When we feel overwhelmed, procrastination appears to protect us from feelings of helplessness: 'If I don't start, then I won't sink.'

Loss of Control—When we feel that we are being dominated—incessantly nagged at by a partner, family member, employer, colleague, for example—procrastination can act as a form of resistance, giving us a sense of greater freedom: 'If I don't start I can't be controlled.'

Notice how so many of these reasons for procrastinating have to do with self-doubt and fear. The paradox is that although intended to spare us from discomfort, procrastinating actually adds to our discomfort. The subconscious mind has a positive intent—to protect and keep us safe—but when it makes us procrastinate, it is going the wrong way about it.

People bring many other habits to the therapist. Such things as the habit of becoming glued mindlessly to the television, drinking endless cups of tea or coffee, cracking knuckles, or becoming impatient, for example—but no matter the habit, with the proper application of hypnotherapy, it can usually be successfully and quite rapidly treated. (Impatience, by the way, may also be more than a simple habit and can be connected to unprocessed anger and other unresolved issues that need to be addressed in therapy.)

In letting go of a bad habit, it is always best to put some other, more positive activity in place, something that can fill whatever space has been created by the loss of the behavior. Giving up watching hour after hour of mindless television might mean we need to find a new way of being informed, relaxing, or socializing, for example.

With hypnotherapy from a properly trained hypnotherapist, almost anyone can end an unhelpful habit, install more positive patterns of being, and move forward with life in a much freer and more active way.

Chapter Nine

Addictions—An End to Shame

'It's all right losing yourself, as long as you can get yourself back.'
~ Mick Jagger

In the previous chapter we looked at habits and their nature and what we can do about them. Now we come to a far more powerful and potentially devastating adversary: addiction. As you read, keep in mind that in talking about addiction, I am focusing on the psychological aspects, not on the medical. I am not a medical doctor, and anyone engaged in a substance addiction should certainly consult with a medical doctor for help and advice in addition to considering hypnotherapy.

There really is no getting away from it: We are living in an addicted world. Addiction is all around us, an inescapable part of our modern society. It comes in many forms, from addiction to substances like alcohol or drugs to addictive behaviors such as gambling or compulsively viewing pornography. For ease of reading, in this chapter I will refer to both substance addiction and behavioral addiction as 'addictive behavior.'

If you have not been addicted, chances are you know someone who is or has been (though they may not have disclosed this fact to you). From popular celebrities who grab the headlines to family and friends, no one seems immune.

And all the evidence points to the fact that addiction is beginning at a younger and younger age, with preteens and adolescents becoming the fastest-growing sector of society to fall prey. Far from being a harmless phase, we now know addictive behaviors that start in the early years usually have long-term effects well into adulthood. From glue sniffing to marijuana smoking, the consequences can be far-reaching.

What do we know about the state of addiction today?

Well, the bad news is that one in three of us are estimated to suffer from an addiction. The good news is that addiction *is* treatable. If you are addicted, it will take courage and determination, but *you can recover*. You can leave the shame behind and move forward into a much better life.

But what, essentially, is addiction, and what is the difference between a habit and an addiction? Although there are similarities, habit and addiction are very different in the degree and manner in which they affect a person's life. Disconcerting and uncomfortable though bad habits may be, unlike addictions, they are rarely life threatening. Whereas a habit is a behavior that may be quite hard to give up, there is almost always an element of conscious choice about it. When it comes to addictions, the story is different.

With addiction, conscious choice has given way to physical and/or mental dependence. One can become addicted to (dependent upon) a substance or a behavior. No matter how the person tries, they feel driven to engage—and more so over time. It's as if their conscious mind has no control over the process. Good intentions, promises and oaths seem to fall by the wayside, as they find themselves doing things they have firmly made up their conscious mind not to do.

Once dependence has been established, with it come multiple changes, biological and psychological. These do not occur in someone who is not addicted, even though the non-addicted person may use or abuse the same substance or engage in the same behavior. Moreover, in order for people to end an addiction, they must go through a process that can be a lot more uncomfortable than the one involved in simply ending a habit. They must almost always pass through a process known as *withdrawal*.

Withdrawal can be physical or psychological or both, but one thing is certain: It can feel very unpleasant and even painful. So our natural tendency is to avoid it. The fear of the unpleasant, painful feelings that occur when withdrawal is attempted is an important factor in causing a person to continue with or rush back into an addictive behavior. Once more, the feeling of fear is at work. This feeling is carried in the luan chi, the energy and information that the addicted person would rather not have to deal with, and so the person remains addicted.

In fact, feelings are at the very core of all addictive behavior, just as they are at the heart of all that makes us human. When addicts begin their journey into addiction, the substance or activity brings wonderful feelings that contrast sharply with the feelings they experienced before. These new and intensely pleasurable feelings were the result of changes that occurred in the pleasure circuitry of the brain and body.

Traditionally, addiction has been viewed as a weakness, a simple lack of willpower and self-control, and many people continue to hold this view. Yet neurobiologists are beginning to understand that addiction has almost nothing to do with a shortage of willpower. To understand why, it's necessary to take another brief look at biology.

In addition to the amygdala (the area of the brain involved in processing emotion), there are other parts also involved in addiction. These areas are the same parts that process subconscious thought, known variously as the medial forebrain bundle (MFB) and the mesolimbic dopamine system (MDS). Repetitive use of psychoactive substances or repeatedly engaging in behaviors that stimulate and excite this area creates problems with the frontal cortex portion of the MDS, the part responsible for making decisions.

As we have seen, the frontal cortex, responsible for decision making, is not fully developed until we reach our twenties, which explains why we are more easily influenced—positively or negatively—when we are young, and why teenagers are especially prone to respond to media messages and peer pressure or to engage in drug use and other risky behaviors.

If we used these brain regions effectively as we grew up, receiving good guidance from parents and teachers, we will have established strong neural pathways and will be more likely to make wise choices. But if our upbringing was authoritarian (teaching us to just follow orders), or if it was too liberal and lacking in structure, or if it was chaotic and unpredictable, we will not have established positive neural pathways. This makes it more difficult—though certainly not impossible—for us as adults to make wise choices. For this trend to be reversed, new neural pathways that support positive behaviors must be created.

When we are addicted, we no longer choose: We simply feel compelled. The pleasure circuit begins in the amygdala and travels on to the temporal lobes of the brain—the median forebrain bundle or 'pleasure pathway'. But this pathway is not restricted to the head-brain; it also involves the whole of the nervous system because, as we have seen, there are neurological receptors in the stomach-brain and throughout the entire body-mind complex. This same pleasure circuit is at work with drugs, alcohol, sugar, chocolate, caffeine, and all other pleasing things. It is involved in any behavior that provokes feelings of intense pleasure—sex, a win on the horses, or a manic shopping spree, for instance.

When first we engage in an addictive behavior, it stimulates and excites us. It causes the release of feel-good beta-endorphins in the frontal cortex. It also instantly triggers the release of the powerful neurotransmitter *dopamine,* which has a euphoric stimulant effect that is highly addictive, and it is this potent neurochemical surge that gives us those euphoric sensations and ecstatic feelings of well-being that we call 'a high'. Given a big enough cocktail of dopamine and endorphins, stirred perhaps with a dash of serotonin, most of us would quite happily dance on the deck of the Titanic, listening to the band play *Nearer My God to Thee* as the ship sinks beneath the waves.

Such a dopamine-rich cocktail produces a powerful force, a combination of feelings that corrupt and distort the chi, turning it into a kind of high-octane fuel that courses through the body-mind complex, delivering those euphoric sensations. But such feelings are all too short lived. Soon they are replaced by other feelings, ones that contrast sharply with the ecstatic sensations now lost. It is this lost sense of euphoria that, in the beginning at least, the addict attempts to recapture.

The difficulty arises with too much repetition. It is too much repetition that makes habit a cousin to addiction—the great difference being that while one is simply a pest, the other is a tyrant. Habits can bother us, but addiction lords over us, abolishing choice and making us its subject.

When we feel happy and balanced within ourselves; when our body chemistry is normal; when we are living in a healthy fashion with good nutrition, plenty of sleep, and other good habits in place; we are less likely to crave this kind of euphoric escape. We enjoy the moments of natural euphoria that occasionally arise—the glass of wine with a meal, the massage after a long week, the high from a program of exercise, the bliss of sexual intimacy. But because we are stable within ourselves, having these experiences does not drive us to repeat them *excessively* in order to get that rush of endorphins that comes in their wake because we are already feeling good and happy to begin with, our chi flowing freely.

For people unaccustomed to feeling happy, healthy, or balanced, the situation is different. The neurochemical rush and the sensations created by the surge of dopamine, especially, produce a euphoria that powerfully contrasts with and transports them from their otherwise uncomfortable state. This euphoric state is one that the person who is suffering may easily be driven to crave, to want to experience again and again, compelling them to drink, or drug, or gamble, or shop, or exercise, or have sex constantly. This overindulgence—this excessive repetition—creates an overload on the body's pleasure circuitry, making it require a bigger jolt of the substance or behavior for the euphoria to be felt.

This process is called *habituation*: a person needing increasingly more of a substance or behavior just to get 'that feeling' again. The excessive repetition results in habituation, which then results in *dependence*: the feeling of profound *need* for the behavior or the substance. This is the mechanics of how people become addicted, and why people who are troubled or unhealthy are more vulnerable.

The euphoric sensations produced by the addictive behavior come as a welcome relief, an antidote to emotional discomfort and a way of feeling very differently within. But those ecstatic feelings are all too brief. Just as soon as the effect of the drug has worn off or the shopping spree comes to an end, that great feeling is lost. Since the sense of loss is so often at the root of sadness, the person feels worse than they did to start with, before they took the substance or participated in the activity. Soon they are driven to engage in it again, attempting to push back the feeling of sadness and loss they experience when the euphoria isn't present. All too quickly, the substance or behavior that once brought euphoria is now needed simply in order to function: The person is addicted.

Let's review the mechanics of addiction, using a little more scientific language, for the sake of accuracy: In the beginning, the budding addict just experiences pleasure in the substance or the behavior. But with excessive repetition, something more sinister occurs. Constant use of the pleasure neural pathways—the 'hedonic highway' (Austin, 2006)—causes the dopamine receptors to close down because they cannot cope with the constant deluge of dopamine. Now, what used to cause the 'high' doesn't seem to work anymore. The person has to increase the addictive behavior—thereby shocking the dopamine receptors into responding—in order to again feel the pleasurable sensations. Tolerance begins to develop. This is called *habituation,* and it is how dependency begins and grows, as more and more of the substance or behavior is required to produce the same effect. And each time the person engages in the addictive behavior, they further damage their dopamine delivery system, that part of the pleasure circuit that was simply not designed to undergo such massive over-usage.

If the addict persists, they eventually arrive at a state where it is impossible to experience pleasure like before, no matter the amount of the substance used or behavior engaged in. This is a state known as *anhedonia.* And once severely damaged, the dopamine delivery system almost never returns to normal. (Though a severely damaged dopamine delivery system may never become completely normal in its functioning, given enough respite and time, it can regain a good deal of its capacity.) With this dysfunction comes all manner of awful consequences.

But it is not only dopamine and endorphins that are involved in addiction. Our old friends serotonin and norepinephrine, together with a variety of other neurotransmitters (such as GABA and adrenaline) are also part of the picture. The biochemistry of addiction is a complex business. The simple part is seeing what addiction does in a person's life.

Addiction gnaws away at the self-esteem, eroding one's foundations—if we can't feel good about ourselves, it is difficult to feel good about anything. The quality of life declines as the addiction consumes more and more of the addict's attention. Responsibilities become difficult to handle, commitments difficult to keep. Sooner or later, the addict loses the respect of family, friends, and co-workers. Relationships, home, job, and even one's life eventually becoming sacrificed on the altar of the addiction.

Personal history, environment, family, health, and the individual's cognitive processing patterns (habits of thinking) all play their part in addiction. All these factors need to be addressed as part of the recovery process.

Researchers are now postulating that perhaps addiction has a genetic component. This may cause certain people to metabolize substances differently than other people do, making some of us more susceptible to becoming addicted. Geneticists have identified regions on chromosomes that may be involved in the addiction process, but much remains to be learned in this area (Li et al. 2008). It is difficult to identify any single gene connected with addiction. Any connection is likely to involve not one but a host of different genes (Nestler, 2000).

But even if there is a genetic connection, this does not mean that every person who has such genes will inevitably succumb to an addiction. The cocaine addict did not become a cocaine addict without repeatedly snorting or smoking cocaine, just as the porn addict did not become addicted without repeatedly viewing pornography. Genes need to be activated in order for their information to find expression, and this is where, in the beginning of the process at least, an element of choice exists.

As we have seen, then, through the process of repetition, the addict builds up a tolerance to the feel-good response produced by the behavior or substance. Where once only a little was needed to produce that euphoric feeling, now the person needs much more, and they have a burning compulsion to satisfy that need. Sooner or later, no matter how much they indulge, they just cannot recapture that great feeling. Yet now they are hooked on the behavior and no longer know how to function without it.

Addiction means we are no longer responding in a normal manner, and we have, in fact, lost control. It is relatively easy for an addict to be in denial where this is concerned, ever dependent on the next fix, ever just trying to keep their head above the water.

We know we are addicted when a certain behavior becomes central to our life, when it's something we feel driven to repeat. The conscious mind attempts to regain control, trying, with logic and reason, to run the show. Summoning all one's willpower, a really determined person may go for days, weeks, or even months without engaging in the addictive behavior, but sooner or later the compulsion becomes too much, often returning with a vengeance, or as if the person had never stopped. As we have seen in the cases of other emotional disturbances discussed in this book, the conscious mind seems to have little defense against the powerful feelings carried in the chi, generated by the subconscious. For healing to occur, the subconscious must be addressed and nutritional deficits corrected, as imbalances in the body can generate or exacerbate the craving for a substance or behavior.

Even though the negative and often calamitous consequences of addiction are plain to see, when we are addicted, we may feel powerless to stop. It's as if we are riding on a runaway train that has lost the use of its brakes. What began as a minor excursion, a little adventure, or a mere distraction has taken us over, becoming our way of life.

Sooner or later, the express train of addiction transports the addict to a place where they can no longer deny the problem. It interferes too much with the smooth running of life. The need for the substance or behavior is too great—and with this realization comes a feeling that serves only to worsen the situation and add to the already heavy load: the feeling called *shame*.

It is shame that makes a person hide their addiction, bringing with it manipulation and deceit; shame that further erodes an already shaky self-esteem and damaged self-image, tearing at the very fabric of the personality. And in the early stages at least, it is shame that prevents the addict from seeking treatment—or from sticking with the treatment—they need to recover.

This sense of shame increases the burden, the feelings of powerlessness, of anyone hapless enough to stumble into the snare of addiction. Shame is different from guilt. Guilt is an appropriate feeling when we have done something that hurts someone else or ourselves. Guilt can be good in these situations:

It can motivate us to make corrections to our negative behavior. Guilt is the feeling we get when we believe we have been unfair, our response to things we have done but wish we hadn't. Shame differs from this. With shame, we do not feel remorse for what we have done; we feel remorse for who we are.

Julian was a stout rugby enthusiast who came to me because he had trouble sleeping. In taking his case history, I realized he also had an alcohol problem. Julian was regularly polishing off at least six cans of beer a night in addition to drinking half a bottle of wine with his dinner. On weekends he drank even more, admitting he sometimes drank to the point where he couldn't remember how he got home. I asked if he had ever taken a drink in the morning, a so-called 'hair of the dog that bit you'. 'Never!' he shot back. 'I'm not an alcoholic!' When I pointed out that the amount he was drinking could be considered excessive, he automatically rejected this. 'Oh, everyone I know drinks like me,' he said. 'Where I come from, it's normal.'

This is typical of addictive thinking. The person normalizes their addiction, rationalizing it as reasonable when it is anything but. It was obvious Julian was not ready to confront his drinking and, because he insisted he had come to me only for insomnia, I taught him self-hypnosis and a technique for moving from hypnosis into sleep that I believed would help him.

Two months later, Julian again visited my office, visibly shaken. 'You were right,' he said. 'My wife has left me, and I just came off a four-day drinking binge. I think I'm an alcoholic.' He looked like a broken man. Julian had hit bottom.

The idea that people must 'hit bottom' before they can begin to recover from addiction is an old yet valid one. This does not mean the addict must lose everything, ending up on the streets, in prison, or in a mental hospital, though for some this will sadly be the case. What 'hitting bottom' means is that the person has experienced something shocking and now sees the absolute necessity of changing the way they have been living.

Julian was ripe for change. He could no longer continue in the state of denial and was ready to do whatever it took to get better. In this preliminary session, I explained that when a person becomes addicted, a biological change takes place. It is possible to recover and go on to live a healthy and balanced life, but that way involves abstinence.

Though there are other models of recovery, such as controlled but continued usage, I am firmly convinced that the only way for an addicted person to recover is through total abstinence. In my experience we can search in vain for easier, softer ways but all to no avail. Those ways just do not last. With addiction there can be no half measures.

For the person still actively addicted though, the idea of never again accessing *that* substance or engaging in *that* behavior can produce feelings of anxiety. They feel it impinges on their freedom. But in fact, it does not: The recovering addict is *choosing* not to drink today, not to indulge in the behavior today. The recovering addict knows what a nightmare it creates each time they fall off the wagon. It plunges their body and brain chemistry back into chaos, revoking their freedom, and once again they are in the grip of the addiction. How much wiser it is not to even go there, to stay in the zone of balance and health. This sensible understanding is often expressed as, 'Just for today, I choose not to… (*fill in the addiction*).' It's sometimes called 'taking one day at a time.' We don't tell ourselves we can 'never' do something. We *choose,* for today, not to do it. This goes down much better with the subconscious mind, which naturally desires wholeness and freedom. It can accept a choice—it has much more difficulty accepting mandates and 'nevers'.

When people who are addicted realize the enormity of their situation, they are left with only two choices. They can either continue in their usage, each day digging their grave and hastening their inevitable demise, or they can choose to do whatever is needed, take whatever steps are necessary in order to end their addiction and take back control of their life.

Julian had finally understood this. He wanted to stop drinking alcohol; he just didn't know how. 'It's not important that you know how right now,' I reassured him. 'Think of the satellite navigation system in your car: The map comes with the journey. What's important is that you take the first few steps—and keep on taking them.'

I asked him if he would be prepared to go to a Twelve Step support group on a regular basis in between our therapy sessions. Attendance at such a support group is a condition I place on anyone coming to me for help with addiction, and I will explain more about them later in this chapter. Julian replied that he was prepared to do whatever it took to end his addiction, and he meant it. He would go to Alcoholics Anonymous, and I asked my practice manager to print out a list of AA groups and meetings in his locality.

In hypnosis we returned to Julian's younger years and to the acute shyness he had experienced growing up. Shyness is a form of fear, and fear is the emotion we feel when we sense we are unsafe. The child had felt unsafe and unsure around others, and this feeling was carried in his subconscious. As a child, he had felt he didn't belong, like he was on the outside looking in. This had made it difficult for him to mix with others or to form friendships.

Still in the deep trance state, Julian went back to the experience of his first drink and the feeling of elation it had produced. No longer the shy and introverted boy, he had been filled with a warm, confident feeling. His inhibitions melted away, and he felt like no matter what happened, he had no reason to care. He felt he could like himself and relax around others.

In his teens, alcohol was always there in one form or another, the social lubricant that took the edge off things and made life flow so much more easily. It was there when he socialized, pubbing and clubbing; there after rugby games, increasing the feelings of acceptance and camaraderie with his teammates; there at parties and weddings. As he entered adulthood, alcohol became almost omnipresent: there when he had company and when he was alone, there with food, and there when he felt bored or frustrated; there when he returned from work, needing to relax.

As we worked our way through therapy, Julian came to understand the choices he had made and why he had made them. Working with his subconscious mind, we re-wrote the scripts that had kept him running to the bottle as if it were a normal part of existence. Gradually we confronted the feelings of anger, guilt, and shame he had felt for so long but had tried so hard to hide. And we worked, too, on his self-esteem, so that he could come at last to the place where he could like and value himself.

Addiction, as we have seen with so much of our life and the way we live it, has a lot to do with perception. In today's world, alcohol consumption is not viewed as being anti-social in the way that drugs largely are. There is also a gender component involved in our perception. A man who drinks heavily may be seen simply as a 'bad boy' or a 'man's man' in the cavalier sense, whereas a woman doing the same is rarely viewed in this light. Likewise, the heavy drug user is often seen as fundamentally anti-social, while in certain milieu—the entertainment industry, for example—the perception may be that it is something 'cool' or 'hip'. One thing I have observed is that people who are especially concerned about their behavior being socially acceptable, about being 'good', seem to be more attracted to addictions like food or shopping, or to prescription rather than illegal drugs.

Julian's particular drug of choice was the socially acceptable and readily available one of alcohol, but it could as easily have been another substance or behavior. In this respect, addictions are like phobias: The name of the addiction isn't very important, just as the name of a phobia isn't important. Whether a person is afraid of spiders or of snakes, the underlying mechanism is the same. The same is true with addictions. It's as if addiction is the hook on which the name of the addiction—just like the addicted person—hangs. It is the similarities, not the differences, that bring these apparently disparate addictions together. They are all cut from the same fabric. For this reason, people in Twelve Step programs often visit one another's meetings: Overeaters visit the alcoholics' meetings, for example. These people understand that while their difficulty may seem to be with food and the meeting seems to be about alcohol, beneath the surface, there is no such distinction.

From my own personal experience with addiction, as well as from my professional work as a therapist, I know addicts often wrestle with feelings of inadequacy, self-loathing, and shame. Even the most rebellious and confident-looking addict harbors a nagging self-doubt that either prevents them from achieving or somehow undermines whatever accomplishments they might have achieved.

For many, there is also the feeling of somehow not belonging, of not fitting in, which creates a backdrop of anxiety, as if the person can never really relax or feel completely safe. Indeed, the feeling that one is an outsider, someone who just doesn't belong (and so is vulnerable), is extremely common among those who are addicted. Look deep enough into any addiction and you will always find some form of fear. Look deep and you will find anger, the product of a burning sense of unfairness or injustice, also.

These are feelings, carried in the distorted luan chi that existed long before addiction became a reality. In the beginning, the addictive behavior will have gone some way towards assuaging and temporarily anesthetizing these feelings, but then it will turn around and magnify them, often bringing feelings of paranoia and of greater alienation in its wake. But these feelings were there in one form or another, permeating the luan chi, before the addict ever became hooked on a substance or behavior.

As we saw in the chapter on anxiety, research has shown that people who experience on-going social anxiety are more likely to develop problems with alcohol dependence and abuse than others, and in my experience this holds true for any behavioral addiction. People who wrestle with feelings of real discomfort or anxiety when with others are at much greater risk of addiction.

Because of this, the addicted person has often become distanced and detached from other people. This is one of the reasons why I ask people coming to me for addiction treatment to also attend a support group of some kind: for the social value, the connection with other people that the addict can make there (Boisvert et al. 2008). Yes, there are times to be alone, to reflect and simply to be, but there are also times when we need to be in this world of people and to find our own place within it.

When we are detached from others, we become detached from ourselves. In saying that people are social animals, Socrates was pointing to a great truth: We were born to interact with our kind and to form groups—not in a sham or exclusively self-serving way, but in an honest and trusting way, sharing strengths and weaknesses, giving and receiving. This can only happen when we feel secure and safe with others. With their guaranteed anonymity, ethos of mutual support, and natural fellowship that fosters person-to-person trust, support groups provide just such safety.

In many communities, there are a variety of support groups—not just Twelve Step programs—that a person can choose from. Such groups are helpful because they provide an emotional support network, often in the absence of family and friends. There are also Twelve Step support groups for practically every addiction that there is. There are no dues or fees attached to most support groups, and none at all to Twelve Step groups, be it Alcoholics Anonymous, Narcotics Anonymous, Gamblers

Anonymous, Overeaters Anonymous, Sex Addicts Anonymous, Debtors Anonymous, Workaholics Anonymous, or any other offshoot of the original A.A. These groups are self-supporting through their own contributions. What this means in practice is that the hat is passed around at the end of meetings, and those who can afford it and wish to contribute drop a coin or two in. The only requirement for attendance or membership is the desire to stop the addiction. Volunteer group members, not professionals, run the meetings.

Though aligned with no religion, at first glance the Twelve Step program appears to have religious undertones, but this is not necessarily the case. It is an intensely practical program, and all that is required for participation is an earnest desire to end the addiction. Atheists and agnostics can be as equally at home in these groups as the most devout. An excellent book that many may find helpful in this area is *Waiting, A Nonbeliever's Higher Power,* by Marya Hornbacher.

I should mention that for those who have considerable difficulty with the Twelve Step approach to recovery, there are many support groups—particularly online—that take a more secular approach to addiction healing.

Should you find yourself balking at the concept of Twelve Step meetings, the important thing is to honestly figure out why: Do you sincerely disagree, at a soul level, with some of the principles you're being asked to accept, or are you in truth resisting because you don't want to give up your addictive substance or behavior? Or are you simply not prepared to do everything necessary in order to end your addiction?

If you really do fall into the first category, I advise you to seek out another support group that is not based on the Twelve Steps. Doing a Google search for 'non-twelve-step support group', for instance, yields many search engine results—and sources of support—the addict may find useful. The important thing is to find on-going support as you launch into the life-changing process of freeing yourself from addiction.

Equally as important as forming a sense of belonging is the addicted person's need to have *meaning* in their life, because without this the addict's life is empty and chaotic. In the past the addict has looked to addiction to provide not only distraction or numbing anesthetic, but also to provide some kind of meaning. The rituals associated with the addiction form an important part of this; indeed, such rituals are very often an attempt to invest structure and meaning where none really exists. Which brings us to a great truth underlying all addiction: Regardless of whether the addicted person is consciously aware of it they have been living a life that lacks a sense of *meaning*.

In recovering from addiction, a person must take a long and serious look at what they truly want out of life—what they need to be whole—and at the life they are, in fact, living. And then they must decide that they *need* to change.

Good therapy can help an addicted person to change. It can greatly assist in returning the individual to an authentic, more natural state. It can, in the common parlance of addiction, help 'get the monkey off your back'. But as the American comedian George Carlin astutely pointed out: 'Just 'cos you got the monkey off your back don't mean the circus has left town.' If each one of us is a work in progress, the circus is something that can never really leave town. In one way or another, its tent is always pitched somewhere within the boundaries of the self. In that circus are fearful tigers of the mind, scary balancing acts, and clowns with the most bizarre sense of humor imaginable. Meaning acts as the powerful ringmaster of this circus, keeping the acts in check and ensuring that our feet are firmly planted on the sane side of the tent.

This is the time to get honest about what we want out of our time on Earth. No other person can answer this question for us. We each must independently determine what will give our lives purpose and joy. Then we need to forgive and learn to again love ourselves enough to take steps towards living a fulfilled, meaningful life.

In therapy we systematically work our way through past sensitizing experiences and neutralize faulty programming; we talk with those parts of the person that are at war within and help negotiate a peace. The addicted person learns how to monitor unhelpful thought patterns, challenge faulty thinking, and develop coping skills; they learn how to manage and let go of stress, but there is one thing therapy cannot give a person. It cannot give a sense of meaning to their life. This is something that each individual must discover or create for themselves. (We will look more closely at meaning and at how this might be accomplished when we come to the final chapter in this book.)

A good support group offers on-going companionship for the journey of recovery and, for many, it can serve as a portal that leads on to the discovery of a greater sense of meaning in life. A support group can be a good place to meet new friends, at various stages on their own journey of recovery, who are not dependent on any addictive substance or behavior and who can help the recovering addict reinforce the positive habits that abstinence requires.

Is it possible to recover from an addiction without therapy and without attending Twelve Step meetings or other support groups? Yes, of course it is. Think of the many smokers who stopped smoking without nicotine replacement or therapy of any kind. Likewise, there are drinkers who have stopped drinking, drug addicts who have stopped using, and gamblers who have successfully stopped gambling without any professional therapy or group support.

But what if we have tried to stop and have not done so yet? What if we have read all the self-help books yet continue to remain addicted and unable to break free? Then it may be time to seek some assistance, and there is absolutely no shame in this.

False pride and denial should not keep us from reaching out for help. When our future and perhaps even our life is at risk, taking that humble step is a small price to pay for recovery. Yet there can be no doubt that even with the very best therapy and the finest of support groups, the responsibility for recovery rests with the addict.

When recovering from addiction of any kind, it is usually best to avoid situations and locations where temptation might arise, at least until such time as recovery is well underway and the person has a substantial period of abstinence under their belt. Recovering addicts need to give themselves the very best chance of kicking the addiction, and being around others who are still using is just stacking the odds against recovery. Being in close proximity to the behavior or substance we once abused can trigger the old neural pathways in the brain that lead to craving. With enough time, new neural pathways can be established through our abstinent behavior, and we can become desensitized to the old stimuli, becoming more immune to activation of the old patterns, but we must always be vigilant.

Particularly when life takes a turn that disappoints or stresses us, the recovering addict can become surprisingly vulnerable to slipping into their former behavior pattern. It can happen subconsciously, and with even quite minor disappointments and stresses—hence the need to be vigilant in order to avoid cravings. When a craving does arise, it's important to determine the real cause of what we are feeling: Have we become overtired? Irritated? Sad? Bored? Fearful? Nervous? Have we been eating poorly, setting our neurotransmitters out of whack? Once we can identify what we're feeling, we listen to our chi; we know what we really need, and can take steps to fill this need instead of being driven by the craving.

All this will take real commitment and a conscious effort to change ingrained behavioral patterns, of course, but change is what ending an addiction is really all about. A person must *truly* want to change and be ready for change. When it comes to ending an addiction, 'ripeness is all'. No therapist and no amount of therapy can force anyone to stop making excuses, to stop justifying and rationalizing, and to stop lying and manipulating. The honesty needed to end an addiction has to come from within the individual. To recover, the addict needs to at last 'get real'.

Often, though, reality and the addicted person have a rather strange relationship. Many find it really difficult to 'let reality be reality', to again quote Lao Tzu. I have yet to meet an active addict who was not in some way kicking against the nature of life itself and trying to change the things that just cannot be changed. Indeed, it is this inability to accept life as it is, to honestly and openly embrace life's reality and to find meaning and a place within that reality, that has all too often produced the anxiety that helped goad the person into substance misuse or unwise behavioral patterns in the first place. Unfortunately, constant exposure to the addictive behavior brought about an even more confused and conflicted state of being. Perplexed and frightened, the addict often responds by assuming the role of the lost child.

Because of this, the great majority of addicts have a good deal of 'growing up' to do. If we are actively addicted and believe that we are not one of that great majority, there is a good chance we are simply in denial, and the sooner we end that denial the better off we will be. What this means, of course, is that though we are not to blame for our addiction, as adults we are responsible for it.

When presenting Julian's story earlier, it was clear that we were discussing dependence on a substance—alcohol, but I hope I have shown that it might just as easily have been any other substance: a drug such as cocaine or cannabis, or prescription drugs such as unnecessary painkillers, for example. In the field of addiction, there is little controversy about this. The exact chemistry might be different for different substances, the receptors and neurotransmitters may vary, but the similarity is there for us to see. It is easy to accept that a person can become addicted to a substance.

What is a bit more controversial, however, is the idea that a person can be addicted not to a substance but to a behavior. There are experts who disagree with this. They believe that assigning the term 'addiction' to any compulsive behavior a person feels unable to control, is an error. Their preference is to classify such behaviors as 'impulse behavior disorders'. While some behaviors may fall under such a heading—the compulsive urge to steal (kleptomania) and the compulsive urge to pull out hair (trichotillomania), for example—I believe a person is addicted when they have developed a tolerance to a substance *or* a behavior, when dependence has been established, and when they experience withdrawal symptoms while attempting to stop. There is an ever-increasing body of scientific evidence pointing to the fact that certain behaviors do indeed exhibit all of the characteristics needed to qualify them as addictions (Grant, 2010; Potenza, 2006; Albrecht, 2006; Marks, 1990; Bradley, 1990). And if this is not enough, try telling the loved one of a gambling addict that the person is not addicted.

Just as substances alter the brain's chemistry—changing the way we feel and respond and creating neural pathways that drive our impulses—so it is with behaviors (Baskerville & Douglas, 2010; Grant & Brewer, 2006). As with substance addictions, behavioral addictions produce consequences that can seriously harm. Behavioral addictions can fracture relationships, damage health, and wreck lives. When a behavior is repetitively and compulsively taken to an extreme, when we feel driven to automatically engage in it, we are out of control and have crossed the line that separates normal behavior from addiction (Goodman, 1990).

Although many of the actual behaviors people may become addicted to can, in and of themselves, be classified as harmless pastimes—shopping, exercise, or browsing the Internet, for example—addiction occurs when the behavior traverses the boundary between conscious choice and compulsion. When we put the behavior above all else and feel compelled to engage in it even though it is bringing negative consequences into our life or into the lives of others, or is threatening to do so, we need to admit we have a problem. It is the loss of control and the effect that the addictive behavior has on people's lives that qualifies it for the label of 'addiction'.

Compulsive gambling is certainly one such behavior, with more and more people consulting a therapist with a craving for gambling they just can't seem to control.

There's no denying that gambling is big business. In 2010, U.S. casinos, tracks and state lotteries generated 95 billion dollars in legal gaming revenue and this does not include illegal sports gambling and card playing. It is estimated that 6 to 8 million adults, and half a million teenagers meet the criteria for gambling addiction in the United States today (National Council on Problem Gambling, 2011).

In the U.K., gambling has now become so mainstream that one out of every two people now participates in some form of gambling at least once a month (Gambleaware, 2012), and this excludes such things as buying lottery tickets. Fixed-odds betting terminals, offering high stakes and high-speed play, have driven the growth of high-street betting shops, ensuring even bigger profits for the businesses—and big losses for a new breed of punter (Dispatches, 2012).

With the legalization and proliferation of online gambling these figures are certain to increase. In one way or another gambling is now a part of society, part of the national way of life. But it is an industry not without its share of victims. Problem gamblers are five times more likely to abuse drugs, eight times more likely to have bipolar disorder, and three times more likely to experience an anxiety disorder (Dispatches, 2012). There is no escaping the fact that gambling addiction can be a truly heart-breaking affair.

Johan was a well-paid and successful golf coach, much in demand with semi-professional and serious amateur golfers. His problem was that he had a gambling addiction. Over the years he had spent a fortune on a variety of gambling activities, from betting shops and racetracks to casinos and slot machines, gambling away his house, his car, and anything else that he could turn into the cash he needed to feed his addiction. Sometimes he would even call clients up, requesting them to pay weeks in advance for sessions, giving them all kinds of tall stories as to why this was necessary. No longer able to trust himself, he had been forced to turn over his earnings to his spouse, who now managed the finances and bills, giving him only the minimum amount of spending money on a daily basis, money that needed to be accounted for as he spent it—a fact he deeply resented.

He had come to me as a last resort. Completely defeated by his gambling addiction, Johan was ready to do anything to free himself, regain control, and turn his life around. He readily agreed to attend Gamblers Anonymous, the Twelve Step program for gamblers, even though it meant travelling to another city for meetings.

Deep in hypnosis, Johan returned to his childhood and to his very first experience with gambling. He was at a seaside resort in the off-season, it was raining, and he was bored. Turning off the main street, the boy had found himself in an amusement arcade full of bright lights and shiny fruit machines that glistened and flashed like something from a glamorous Hollywood movie. He had seen such machines before, but only on television. They were called 'one-armed bandits'. Now they were here, and so was he. The whole atmosphere seemed magical: The brightly colored lights, the singing of machines, and the sound of coins cascading down into the metal troughs were the perfect antidote to a boring, rain-swept day.

Soon the young Johan was feeding his holiday pocket money

into a machine, almost mesmerized as the pictures of lemons and cherries, bells, and sevens whirled by. Then it happened: First two, then all three reels lined up, and he had won! He had hit the jackpot! The lights flashed and the machine sang out as the deluge of coins cascaded down in an endless offering of jangling shiny treasure. What a reward! Johan's whole being was flooded with feelings of exhilaration and ecstasy. Never before had he known such a perfect high. Then the voice came, piercing the trance: 'Sorry, kid, you can't keep that money—you're too young!'

The boy recoiled in disbelief. Too young? First the shock and then the anger flushed like scalding blood through his system. He had won the money fair and square. It was his and now someone was trying to tell him that he couldn't keep it! 'Fuck off!' he yelled. 'That's my money! I won it!' But he argued in vain. Nothing he could say or do would change the man's mind. 'You're too young to be here, too young to gamble, and that's all there is to it, son. It'd be breaking the law, and I'd lose my license.'

With that, Johan was hustled to the door and sent back out onto the rain swept grey pavement, his pockets empty and his head reeling. From the dizzying heights of euphoria, he had been sent crashing back into the coldest reality. This was the initial sensitizing event, the experience that installed the program deep within his subconscious mind. From this moment on, Johan would be forever chasing that ecstatic feeling. Time and again he would attempt to reclaim that money, recapture that euphoric high he felt had been stolen from him.

As the boy grew, he found himself again and again in amusement arcades, sometimes skipping school in order to feed his pocket money or money that he had stolen from his mother's purse into the slots. Then when he was old enough, he discovered the betting shops, legal in the UK where he lived, and began hanging around them, putting every penny he could find—or sometimes steal—on horses, dogs, and football games.

When the bet was on, nothing else seemed to matter. All of his problems just faded away as the adrenaline and the dopamine and the endorphins swept through his system.

Sometimes he would win, and for a moment or two some of that elusive feeling returned, but it was always too brief and never enough, and Johan would quickly find himself feeding the money back until he had lost everything, endlessly searching for that missing feeling, that phenomenal rush.

The ecstatic feeling that young Johan felt when the reels lined up and the machine spewed out its reward is something common to almost all gambling addicts (Hewig et al. 2010). So many people I've treated experienced a euphoric high in the earliest stage of their gambling addiction, and they have been chasing that high ever since. When the bet is in play, nothing else seems to matter; time stands still and reality can wait.

Years ago, on a visit to South Korea, I found that I had booked myself into a hotel that boasted the largest gambling casino in Asia outside of Macao, where I struck up a conversation with the casino manager. I was curious to learn more about the mentality of his customers. 'We like them to win the first time they come in,' he told me with a smile. 'We usually have them after that—they keep right on coming back.' It's easy to understand why. The powerful cocktail of neurotransmitters rushing through the mind-body complex can easily kick-start a program of addiction which, left unchecked, can lead on to devastation and absolute ruin.

When allowed to continue, behavioral addictions have the potential to bring about complete destitution, a deterioration of life on all levels: psychological, social, physical, and spiritual. As with drug or alcohol addiction, a behavioral addiction is a progressive disorder that can lead to catastrophe, even death. Research shows that pathological gamblers are at greater risk of suicide than the average population (NHS Choices, 2013; Phillips & Welty, 1997), and it has been reported that gambling is linked to as many as one in five suicidal patients (Hagan, 2012; Volberg,

2002; National Council on Problem Gambling, 1997).

In my career as a therapist I have treated many people whose out-of-control gambling began in a similar way to Johan's. Slot machines (and fixed odds betting terminals) are known as the 'crack cocaine' of gambling addiction because of their fast action and ability to deliver those rapid blasts of dopamine, adrenaline, and other feel-good neurotransmitters at the touch of a screen, the push of a button, or the pull of a handle. With slots, the flashing lights and the ringing sound of those bright, shiny coins as they rain down lock into the person's visual and auditory centers, further exciting the system and accelerating the process of addiction.

With our sessions of intense therapy and his commitment to the support group program, Johan is now well into recovery from his addiction. Realizing there is no room for complacency, he lives one day at a time, back in control of his own finances, steering clear of gambling in all of its forms: proof that with the right approach and the correct attitude, it really is possible for even the biggest loser to become the greatest winner.

One of the fastest-rising addictions—and one that has no national borders—is that of Internet addiction, with more and more people hooked on sitting in front of their computer. Staring at that mesmerizing screen, we easily drift into the trance state where time becomes distorted, and in this trance, Internet addicts will often forgo sleep and proper meals to feed their dependence.

The Internet can, of course, offer a slippery slope into other forms of problem-causing behavior. Not only online gambling, but also online gaming addiction is now becoming a major problem for many, as is video-game addiction. Here the addicted person regularly enters into a fantasy world of virtual reality where they can role-play a character or adopt an alter ego that can become frighteningly real. Sometimes addicted players may even find themselves withdrawing from the real world and its needs, spending hour after hour in this 'virtual reality', becoming dissociated from actual reality.

Teens and preteens are thought to be most at risk, but gaming addiction can affect anyone at any age; in fact, the average age of a gaming addict is now believed to be around thirty-five years old. Like all addictions, this is a problem that is progressive in nature, having the potential to make the person gradually withdraw into a make-believe existence that impairs relationships, affects work, and negatively impacts on most other areas of normal, healthy living.

Often it is the relatives of the gamer who first see the problem and urge the increasingly withdrawn gaming addict to seek help. But as with any other addiction, effective treatment is not possible if the person does not recognize the problem and is not ready to halt the addiction. Once denial is ended and the addict commits to doing whatever is necessary to become free, hypnotherapy can greatly accelerate the process of recovery.

Another powerful form of Internet addiction involves the viewing of online pornography. This is another issue that, as a practicing hypnotherapist, I am called upon to treat with increasing frequency. A growing number of lives are being torn apart by this addiction with the easy accessibility of porn via laptops, tablets, and various mobile devices. Pornography is big business, with the online porn industry generating bigger revenues than Google, Microsoft, Apple, Yahoo!, Amazon, and eBay combined. Research reveals some truly staggering statistics in this area: Pornography accounts for 25 per cent of all search engine requests, and 12 per cent of all websites are porn sites (Ropelato, 2012). Every second, almost 30,000 Internet users view pornography, and 20 per cent of men admit to doing this at work (Ropelato, 2012).

Pornography addiction is, in fact, a form of sex addiction, and much of what we are discussing here also applies to sex addiction in any form (Carnes, 2001). Interestingly, a significant number of people with sexual addiction also have a substance addiction, and many have a history of sexual abuse, either in their childhood or adolescence (Book, 1997).

Sex addiction may be defined as a failure to control one's sexual behavior and a continuation of this behavior despite the possibility of significant harmful consequences. As with any addiction, it is compulsive. It's as if the sex addict can no longer simply decide not to engage in the behavior—they feel driven. Understandably, the sexual addict can go to extraordinary lengths to defend against their feelings of shame (Reid et al. 2009) and this, in common with other addictions, often involves some form of denial—not only to others, but to themselves.

Sexual addiction can take many different forms: compulsive and obsessive masturbation, frequent anonymous sexual encounters, regular extramarital affairs, unsafe sex, prostitution, obsessively cruising chat rooms, voyeurism, sexual harassment, as well as compulsive pornography viewing (Knauer, 2002). Though offering the illusion of intimacy, sex addiction is less about sex and more about trying to cope with feelings of inner estrangement. It's an attempt to satisfy a fundamental feeling of emptiness. Like all addictions, it has its roots in an absence of meaning.

Pornography addiction is an issue that is traditionally thought to afflict mainly men, but now an increasingly large number of women are also caught in its web. Perhaps because pornography carries with it moral stigma, and also because sex is by nature a private thing, this addiction most often begins when the person is alone, and it usually continues in this manner. It is an anonymous, solitary addiction. For these reasons, the addict tends towards a life of isolation.

What may have started as an infrequent and seemingly harmless activity, an erotic pastime or a bit of fun, can easily run away with a person. With repetition, pornography viewing can so easily become an overwhelming compulsion, bringing with it a multitude of problems, including mounting credit card debt, increasing subterfuge, and the anxiety that comes from having to live with an almost constant risk of discovery.

Paradoxically, though, as if to hasten discovery, the pornography addict may regularly view porn at the most inappropriate of times and in the riskiest of places, as if courting disaster. They may sneak onto the computer at night when a partner or other family member is near or access porn on work computers, for example. What is happening here is that the heightened sense of danger increases the flow of adrenaline, supercharging the luan chi even more. Such risky behavior may also be connected with an inner sense of shame and a subconscious desire to be punished.

Pornography addiction can also involve compulsive use of Internet chat rooms, and of course the addiction is not restricted to the Internet: Erotic magazines, videos, and DVDs can also prove addictive, as can telephone-sex chat lines and actual human contact, such as in 'massage' parlors. But the Internet differs from these in its rapid accessibility, which opens the gates to an instant and almost limitless selection and variety of pornography, one that even the largest adult video store cannot hope to compete with.

While compulsive masturbation may be an essential aspect of the porn addict's usual behavior, the addict often finds it increasingly difficult to reach orgasm, requiring more frequent exposure to porn and to more extreme forms of sexual stimulation in order to achieve the same result. This, of course, is simply part of the process all addicts undergo: Habituation means that more is required to produce the same effect. All addictions are progressive in nature—what once was enough to satisfy soon becomes insufficient—so the quantity or intensity will need to be increased to compensate, and eventually even this will not be enough. Sooner rather than later, porn addicts and other sex addicts arrive at the state where the brain's reward center no longer delivers the same intensity of pleasurable feeling. Too many of the receptor sites have closed down through overindulgence. Tolerance sets in, but the need for the thrill continues, more powerful than ever.

With the dopamine delivery system impaired and the pleasure circuit unable to operate effectively, the addict's ability to function normally in a real-life, intimate relationship can become seriously affected, causing a decline in sexual interest in, or intimacy with a partner, difficulty in reaching orgasm, erectile dysfunction, or premature ejaculation. Once we understand the nature of the addiction process, it's easy to see how the porn addict is forced to spend so much time viewing porn, and the person addicted to playing the numbers game of promiscuity so much energy chasing after sex, often casting caution to the winds and adopting a devil-may-care attitude that can place them and other people in jeopardy.

When the person has had enough of living life in this way, perhaps because of discovery or a crisis that the addiction has brought about or simply because they have awakened to the fact that they can no longer continue like this with impunity, then recovery can begin. Hypnotherapy can greatly aid and accelerate this process, and participation in support groups, with organizations like Sex Addicts Anonymous or Sex and Love Addicts Anonymous, will help provide the peer support that has proven helpful for so many on their journey of recovery.

Being hooked on shopping is another addiction that hypnotherapists are often called upon to treat. This condition has been given the rather amusing, vegetable-sounding name *oniomania*. In reality, though, it is anything but funny. We all have the need to sometimes shop. Items like food, clothing, and household and recreational items are all essential purchases, and we can derive a certain amount of harmless pleasure from shopping for them. But when we find ourselves shopping compulsively and in order to feel better on a regular basis, we need to examine whether we have a problem.

Research on shopping addiction has produced conflicting results, with some studies indicating that 80 to 90 per cent of those affected are women (Faber & O'Guinn, 1992; McElroy et al. 1994), while other studies report that the addiction affects men and women equally (Koran, 2006). According to PayPal's Managing Director Carl Scheible, 'The online revolution has turned men into shopaholics' (WalesOnline, 12th August 2006). As far as Internet shopping goes, men far outspend women (PayPal Online Retail Report, 2009; iProspect, 2012), which would suggest that men are just as in love with shopping as women—they just don't like going to the stores. Either way, there can be no doubt that this addiction is responsible for an enormous amount of misery and distress in people's lives and is a condition that needs to be recognized and addressed.

For the person addicted to shopping, store sales can be a nightmare, and with the proliferation of TV shopping channels pushing products twenty-four hours a day, massive credit-card debt can now be accumulated in the comfort of one's own living room. Often shopping addicts find themselves storing purchased items and never using them—sometimes leaving them in a drawer or closet with the price tag still on.

In addition to seeking out a qualified hypnotherapist to address the underlying drivers and emotional consequences of this addiction, shopping addicts are well advised to follow certain principles, including destroying credit cards, paying with cash, never shopping alone, and finding other ways to spend leisure time. It is also wise to avoid all TV shopping channels, to cultivate outside interests, and to move towards finding some kind of meaning in life other than shopping. Once more, we see the importance of *meaning*. For the shopping addict, the attitude of 'I shop, therefore I am' (Benson, 2000) needs to be replaced with a different kind of belief, one that is based on a higher sense of self and self-esteem and an appreciation of the individual's own inherent value.

Finally, we come to the subject of work addiction. The question here is: When does genuine commitment to one's job become an actual addiction? It is a matter of degree and of the person's ability to consciously choose. As we have seen, addiction occurs when a person loses control of a behavior or substance, develops a tolerance to it, then undergoes withdrawal symptoms when attempting to stop. Of course, a solid work ethic is essential to living a meaningful life, but when balance is lost and an obsessive approach to work supersedes everything else, we have a serious problem.

Just like other addicts, the work addict in denial attempts to justify and rationalize the excessive behavior. Denial is a stage the person must pass through as the condition worsens and becomes increasingly obvious. The quality of work tends to diminish and frustration mounts as stress accumulates. But no matter how hard or how long the person works, they can never seem to fill the need that exists within. The luan chi continues to deliver its disturbing message, allowing no respite.

Constant, excessive overwork can have devastating effects, not only on a person's relationships and quality of life, but also on one's health (Robinson, 1996). In Japan, where the problem was identified in the early 1970s, the word *karoshi* has been coined, literally meaning *death from work*. It is a condition legally recognized there, with the Ministry of Labor regularly making payments to families of workers who died from overwork. In the West, numerous studies show that overworking and high job strain correlate highly with our biggest killer—cardiovascular disease (Price, 2004; Landsbergis et al. 1993). There can be no doubt that constant work leads to chronic stress and can have serious, even fatal, consequences.

Balance needs to be brought back into the work addict's life, with time devoted to relaxation, activities involving family and friends, exercising, and eating properly. In addition to hypnotherapy, which can help the person deal with underlying emotional and psychological difficulties, support groups like Workaholics Anonymous can be very useful. There are also online groups that offer peer support for anyone with an addiction to work. Addiction knows no nationality, and the Internet makes international contact and communication easy.

Now let's talk about diet and nutrition. It is absolutely essential that the person recovering from any form of addiction eat a healthy and well-balanced diet. As we know, there really is no underestimating the effect of food on the mind-body complex and on our emotions and cognitive functioning. Very often the addicted person has neglected this vital aspect, taking too much sugar-laden junk food and caffeinated drinks into their system, eating irregularly, or eating very little or to excess. Recovering addicts need ample complex carbohydrates in order to maintain balanced blood sugar levels and stabilize mood.

Especially in the early phase of recovery, nutritional supplements—vitamins, minerals, and certain amino acids such as GABA (in the form of *Picamilon*) can be particularly helpful. The B vitamins, especially vitamin B12—so often seriously depleted through excess alcohol consumption—and the Omega-3 fatty acid EPA (which has been shown to be especially low in cocaine users) can also provide support. Because of the seriousness of addictions, such supplementation is best tailored to individual needs and taken on the advice of a competent health care practitioner or nutritionist who has specialized knowledge in the field *and* experience working with addictions.

The fact is, a person can become addicted to almost any substance and any behavior, and there are several common addictions that I have not had space to cover in this chapter. Whatever the addiction, they all share many similarities and can respond to a similar yet individually tailored and flexible approach. Treatment can be expensive, in many ways, but it is always less expensive than the price of on-going addiction.

No discussion of addiction would be complete without

mention of the role of family, friends, and loved ones. Often people are able to remain longer in their addiction through the misplaced love or kindness of a family member or friend who has supported them in some critical way. Love and compassion have made this person stand by and support the addict through the progressive addiction nightmare, and this has helped the behavior continue for far too long.

For an addict to recover, the kind of love needed is 'tough love'—the sort that finds the courage to say, 'I will no longer support you in your destructive addiction.' Understanding but firm confrontation may be necessary, and no idle threats should be made when arriving at this critical point. Words need to mean what they say, and there can be no going back once spoken.

Though the addict may try every kind of emotional blackmail and manipulation—appealing, promising, and threatening—steadfast tough love is indispensable if we are not to enable our loved one, making it easier for them to stay addicted. Painful though it is to watch, addicts must be allowed to hit their own personal bottom.

Addiction has a terrible effect not only on addicts but also on those who care about them. Family members, partners, and close friends often experience the same emotions as addicts (guilt, anxiety, fear and shame). Consciously or subconsciously, we may even believe we ourselves are responsible for the person's addiction, that we are somehow to blame. This is never true. Addicts are responsible for their own lives, and only they can make the decision to become free.

Family members may find counseling or therapy useful prior to and during the process of the addict's recovery. There are support groups such as Al-Anon that exist for family and friends of addicts. If no such group exists in your area, most Twelve Step programs have 'open meetings' that are attended not only by people in the process of recovery but also by families, partners, and friends. Such groups can provide invaluable assistance.

Contacts can be made with others who have been on a similar journey and now are willing to share their understanding and offer support. I even know of people who, unable to find any kind of group in their vicinity, have started their own. (Advice and materials for starting such a group can be obtained by contacting Al-Anon, AA, or other organizations.)

In this chapter I have told you of my firm conviction that complete abstinence is essential if recovery is to take place. It is a conviction shared by many, although not all, experts in the field. This does not mean the addict might not at some point in recovery slip and momentarily lapse back into the old way—recovery is not necessarily linear—but a lapse can be prevented from becoming a complete relapse by understanding what is happening.

Because of the weakened functioning of the frontal cortex part of the mesolimbic dopamine system, an addict's ability to choose wisely has been compromised, and this is exactly what a slip is—an unwise choice. Remember that the ability to choose wisely will be increasingly restored as we abstain from consuming the addictive substance or engaging in the addictive behavior. The longer we abstain, the more robust and better functioning our dopamine delivery system and all of our faculties become. (Remember, too, that an addict will always remain in some way 'in recovery' and so can never afford to become complacent.) Neither a lapse nor a relapse means failure. Nor are lapses and relapses inevitable. For many people, they never happen.

Addicts have tried to silence the messages their chi has been bringing for so long that they have lost touch with what their feelings are trying to tell them, which is another way of explaining why people may slip. An acronym used by Alcoholics Anonymous, but valuable for all who are in the process of recovering from addiction, is HALT: **H**ungry, **A**ngry, **L**onely, or **T**ired. Remembering this acronym helps alert a person to possible danger times—moments when we are more vulnerable. When people are aware they are more susceptible to a slip at such times, they can better prepare for such occasions and take appropriate action. The responsibility for this action rests, of course, with the recovering addict.

No one is going to tell the addict that recovery will be easy, but no one can say it is not possible. Hundreds of thousands of people all over the world have lost themselves to addiction and have recovered from it, and so have I. If we are to recover, we need to put at least as much energy and commitment into our recovery as we put into our addiction.

In order to remain clear, we need to find a renewed sense of meaning in our life, one that will change walls into windows and that will grant us the wisdom to know the difference between the things that we can and cannot change. But with an attitude of genuine willingness and an open heart, each and every one of us can make it.

Chapter Ten

Emotional Eating and Weight Management

'Let food be your medicine.'
~ Hippocrates

Like the air we breathe and the water we drink, in one way or another food surrounds us. Breathing may be the primary way we bring chi into our body, but equally important to our life on Earth is food. It contains its own life force, its own chi. When we eat, we absorb this and make it our own as it moves through us, fuelling our body, mind, and spirit.

Today, the Western world is reeling under the burden of plenitude. The U.S. is the most obese country in the world. Overweight yet paradoxically undernourished, at least 65 percent of the population is unhealthily heavy (WHO Country Comparison, 2013), and more than one third of all Americans over the age of twenty are clinically obese (Ogden & Carroll, 2012). In the U.K. the situation is little better, and Brits are among the fattest people in Europe (OECD Health Data, 'Obesity by Country', 2005). Figures show that almost 25 per cent of UK residents are clinically obese (Streib, 2007; BBC January 2008).

Being overweight can choke the life force, preventing us from enjoying life fully. Too much poundage affects our mobility and physical activities, making it hard to walk any distance, restricting our ability to play with children and grandchildren, and making it difficult even to find a comfortable seat in cinemas or on airplanes. It affects our leisure and our work; our physical, mental, and emotional health; our social and personal life—and our self-esteem.

Our children, too, suffer as we lead our youth into the perils of obesity at a younger and younger age. These young people often have more trouble making friends, are more likely to have behavioral problems and learning difficulties, and are more prone to low self-esteem. Overweight children are more likely to grow up to become overweight adults with an increased probability of serious health problems that will last throughout their lives. And there is every sign that things are getting worse, with some health experts now predicting that if current trends continue, we will soon see parents outliving their children (Chapman & Utton, 2013; Ontario Medical Association, 2012).

Moderate obesity shortens lives by about three years, while severe obesity shortens a person's life by ten years (University of Oxford, 2009). Obesity adds a staggering one hundred and ninety billion dollars to the annual healthcare costs of the United States (Cawley & Meyerhoefer, 2012). In the U.K. the figure is in excess of two billion pounds annually, with the National Health Service shouldering one billion pounds in treatment costs alone (National Audit Office, 2001).

And this obesity epidemic is now a worldwide problem (Popkin, 2009). Each year more and more people present with preventable disorders that are the direct consequence of unhealthy eating: heart disease; type-two diabetes; stroke, liver and gall bladder disease; high blood pressure; respiratory problems, and even cancer.

How on Earth did it come to this? What has gone wrong? These were the questions I asked years ago as I began working with people who came to me for help in controlling their weight and their overeating. Before accepting a hugely overweight client for therapy, I asked them to visit a medical doctor to determine that there were no physical reasons (such as endocrine malfunction, chronic disease or drug side effects) for the problem. I wanted to determine if the extra weight was a consequence of some such issue or entirely of how—and what— the person was eating. Once this had been cleared, we could begin to approach the problem from a psychological and behavioral perspective, with hypnotherapy.

Almost everyone had been on some kind of diet and most had tried several different kinds. They had worked their way through the meal replacement drinks and the slimming bars, the herbal remedies, teas, supplements, and slimming pills. You name it, they'd tried it, and though some of these things had seemed to work in the short term, sooner or later almost all of them had returned to their 'normal' way of eating, and the weight had gone right back on.

Most of the people who sought my help had read book after book on how to lose weight, and they'd scanned magazines for each new article that might give them the answer. Practically everyone knew just about everything a person could know about losing weight. Many of them knew more than the average doctor knows about nutrition—but still they overate.

Many had joined slimming groups, weight-watching programs, fitness centers, health spas, and gyms. Some had spent money on expensive exercise equipment or patented gadgets that now just cluttered up a room somewhere or sat in a closet collecting dust. They had bought the latest videos advertised on television and in glossy magazines, but despite all this, they were still overweight. Little wonder they felt like abject failures.

Could all of this 'failure' simply be ascribed to the power of habit and a lack of willpower? I thought not.

Of course habit plays a role, as does the unwise choice of the foods we eat. In our fast-paced modern world, it's easy to neglect healthy, balanced eating and opt for the easy option of fast food. Our children, too, have become accustomed to a diet rich in convenience food—full of fat, sugar, and empty calories.

When simple habit is the cause of overeating, then simple suggestion therapy can be of enormous help in breaking the pattern of habitual eating, and indeed for some people this is all that is really needed in order to reduce weight. (This involves repeating suggestions for positive change while the person is in hypnosis. Because hypnosis bypasses the critical factor, a person's subconscious receptivity to positive suggestion is greatly enhanced in this state.) But if we overeat for deeper emotional reasons, then in all probability this just won't be enough to bring about the powerful change that is needed. It could be that we have become food addicts and our dependence on food far exceeds our natural requirements. If this sounds like you and if you haven't already done so, I urge you to read the previous chapter on addictions before reading any further. That chapter explains the addiction process and how the body-mind system is altered by it.

If we have tried just about everything and still find ourselves turning to food to cope with life and feelings, we need to stop blaming habit, or our family, or our history, or our genetics, or the power of advertising, or even our own lack of willpower, and begin to accept responsibility for the part we ourselves play in our own lives and in our weight management—or the lack thereof.

When we use food in an attempt to assuage feelings like boredom, frustration, loneliness, anxiety, depression, and insecurity, or to recapture or prolong feelings of pleasure, it is obvious we are not eating in order to physically nourish ourselves. This is emotional eating, and we have become emotional eaters.

Quite a few of the people who came to me because of a weight problem seemed unwilling to admit this. But the fact is if you are overweight and the issue is not a glandular malfunction or other physical disorder, you are eating too much food for *you*. Your partner may eat as much as you do, and that may be all right for them, but you are a different person. You may very well eat no more than you did ten or twenty years ago, but since then your body and your metabolism have changed; if you're overweight, you're eating too much food for your present needs. And this is true no matter what your family or friends may say.

Research has shown that those who believe they have tried everything but cannot reduce their weight no matter what they eat or do not eat are simply underestimating the amount of food or number of calories they are consuming (Wansink & Chandon, 2006).

In order to reduce weight and regain a balanced way of eating, we need to banish two things: *denial* and *blame*. We may be overweight because of our overeating, but we are no more to blame for this than the shops and supermarkets that sold us the food, the restaurants that served it to us, or the celebrity chefs and advertisements that bombarded us with desire-provoking images. Before we can manage our eating in a positive way, we need to recognize that everyone sometimes gets out of balance and experiences difficult emotions, but that turning to food to distract ourselves is a dangerous strategy that provides no real solution. Food can never make difficult feelings go away for long, and it can never really help us cope with life. Food just cannot do any of these things—but *we* can.

The wonderful thing is that we really *can* change. We may have fallen into the trap of using food as a drug or a distraction or in an attempt to prolong feelings of pleasure, but just as surely, we can regain control, eat in a healthy way, and reduce our weight. Hypnotherapy can help us to do this.

Of course, if we really want to be at a healthy weight and feel good in our body and mind, we will need to eat those foods that nourish us and avoid those that harm us—even if this means having to sacrifice some of the habits that have been with us since childhood. We will need to end the blaming, accept responsibility, and then do something that solves the problem.

In my work with compulsive overeaters, I came to see it wasn't so much the food itself (although this did often play a part in it), as much as it was *their attitude* towards food that was responsible for their weight problems. This attitude was making them use food in a way it was never meant to be used. It was as if the emotional overeater was using food as a drug, something that could somehow modify reality and create a numbed-out state, where the uncomfortable and unwelcome feelings carried in their chi were cushioned and therefore temporarily less unsettling.

If we constantly overeat and continue to be overweight, it is our mind that needs fixing, our chi that needs to be attended to. Over the years I have worked with practically every kind of addiction and have found that what drives compulsive overeating is remarkably similar to what drives addictions in general.

Of course, some may say, 'Addictions are different. People can live without drugs and gambling and even without sex, but we can't live without food. We have to eat in order to live,' and they would be right. But here is the difference between healthy and compulsive overeating: When people constantly use food to distract themselves from feelings, that's not natural eating. It has little or nothing to do with nourishment and the natural enjoyment associated with the body's need to eat and a lot to do with addiction.

Not everyone who overeats is addicted to food, of course. As we have seen, some overweight people have simply fallen into faulty eating habits. Likewise, not everyone who is obsessed with food is overweight. I have worked with a good number of people who had enormous trouble with their eating and with their relationship with food who would never allow themselves to become overweight. Some of these people would go on eating binges and then purge themselves with laxatives or by inducing vomiting, while others would eat and eat and then go on a fast. Some, of course, were anorexic or bulimic, since no matter how thin they became, it was never thin enough, but not everyone could fit neatly into such diagnoses. There were those, too, who engaged in this kind of behavior but did not suffer from any form of body dysmorphia, or distortion of body image. They were neither anorexic nor bulimic, but they were obsessed with food and eating. Each one had the exact same problem: They were living their lives around food the way drug addicts live their lives around a substance.

If you are addicted to a drug, you are obsessed with it. You know first-hand about persistent, compulsive dependence. You crave a fix in order to feel all right. You make sure you get your fix when you need it, and you feel very uncomfortable when denied it. If you are addicted to overeating, the same thing is true with respect to food. Research has demonstrated a strong connection between the neural mechanisms underlying obesity and those of drug addiction (Volkow et al. 2008; Trinko et al. 2007; Gearhardt & Yokum, 2011).

As we saw in the previous chapter, addiction is not defined by the name of the substance involved—in fact there does not even need to be a substance—but by the *behavior*. Again, I am not suggesting that everyone overweight is a food addict. Some people who have difficulty managing their weight do so simply because of poor eating habits, poor food choices, or because of glandular or other difficulties. But in my work with people with weight issues, I found that the similarities between addiction and compulsive overeating were often too strong to ignore. I saw that every single addiction had the same underlying drivers: feelings of anxiety, anger, guilt, shame, emptiness, inadequacy, insecurity, and inner discomfort. Disturbed luan chi drove each addict—and it also governed those who regularly and obsessively overate.

My food-addicted clients just didn't know how to deal with these feelings other than to try to distract—or attempt to anesthetize—themselves with food. But what was also interesting was that many overeaters ate in response to not only uncomfortable feelings but to *happy* ones as well. When happy, enjoyable feelings came, they were using food in an attempt to heighten or prolong them.

Let me stress that it was *feelings of almost any kind* that caused these clients to eat and eat and eat some more. They just didn't know how to respond to the messages being carried in their chi other than to attempt to manipulate them with food.

All too often I saw that the more the person had tried to conquer overeating, the more out of control and powerless they felt. I also saw how almost every overweight client was unhappy with some aspect of who they were. In some way or another, their self-esteem had been damaged. Moreover, this was an aspect they felt powerless to change.

And this brings us to an essential understanding: *The single-most important factor in overeating and weight management is one's relationship with oneself.* It far outweighs calorie counting, diets, and even exercise, and has nothing to do with willpower or the lack of it. If our eating has become compulsive *over*eating, if we are having real trouble controlling our weight, then before we can ever eat in a permanently healthy way, our ability to personally deal with *feelings* must first be put back in order. We need to change our relationship with food *and with ourselves.*

As briefly mentioned earlier in this book, for many years I lived in the Far East. In China I learned that in olden days, before Western medicine made inroads, people paid their doctors to keep them well. If a person fell sick, the doctor was fired. Today most Chinese people, like most Westerners, visit the doctor only when they have symptoms of illness, when something is already going wrong. Almost universally, we visit the doctor because our symptoms tell us we must. We then expect the medical experts to make those symptoms go away and the problem disappear. The focus is almost always on the symptoms. But symptoms are not where the problem lies. As we have seen throughout this book, the problem lies in the reason why those symptoms exist; in why we feel the way we feel.

Before we eat food, we encounter it with all of our senses. We see it, smell it or touch it, and sometimes we can even hear it as it sizzles or steams—and then we taste it. As this happens, neurotransmitters are released, reactivating neural pathways, locking into the memories stored deep within the subconscious mind. Eating is a profound way of communing with the life that is all about us; in some ways it is more intimate even than sex. It is also one of the major ways we commune with our past, which produced all of our subconscious programming.

Do you remember the very first time you bit into a banana or tasted a piece of chocolate? How about the first spoonful of ice cream or mouthful of birthday cake? Perhaps you do and perhaps you don't consciously remember these things, but your subconscious, feeling mind certainly does. It has forgotten nothing. All these things are locked deep within its memory bank, inseparable from the feelings that went with them. And when we eat, we become reconnected with those memories, with our younger self—and with what that self *felt*.

Almost as soon as we are born, we are held close to our mother and we are fed. From the very beginning of our life, we form a deep emotional connection between being fed and being loved.

As children we cried, and for most of us, our crying was often answered by food along with human warmth that made us feel safe, valued and loved. Food served to reaffirm that we were indeed lovable. Sometimes, though, our crying—and our feelings—may have been ignored, or we might even have been chastised in some way for being so disruptive, and when this happened, the food we craved that could have brought us comfort might have been delayed or even denied. Either way, we *felt* it.

Sam was a busy salesman. He was also clinically obese. His job involved a lot of travelling and carried with it a good deal of pressure and stress. Results were what mattered to him and to his bosses in the head office who constantly demanded that targets be met. Everyone seemed to be on his back, from bosses and customers to his wife, with whom he never seemed to spend enough time, and she was always complaining about this.

When he came to see me, Sam had had enough of his compulsive overeating. He had tried just about everything possible short of radical surgery to control his food intake, yet still he was obese. He told me I was his last port of call before he opted to go under the knife.

In the safety of the therapy chair and in a deep state of hypnosis, Sam went back to his childhood, to the age of five, when he was in a children's home. There above him towered the strict and dour matron, telling him he must eat his food and may not leave the table until he did. But little Sam just didn't like that food. He hated cabbage, and the potatoes were hard and lumpy and covered with tasteless gravy, not at all like the lovely food his mother used to make for him when she was there and he was happy.

'Leave me alone!' he pleaded. 'I don't want to eat.' But the matron was not about to leave him alone; after all, it was her responsibility to make sure all the wards in her charge remained fed and healthy. 'I'll leave you alone when you eat,' she told him.

With tears streaming down his face, he had forced himself to eat, closing his eyes and swallowing bite after bite until his plate was empty. Only then did the matron leave him in peace.

This was the initial sensitizing event, the critical experience that led to Sam's overeating. At the age of five, a powerful belief had been implanted in his subconscious mind, as easily as a program might be installed in a computer: People will stop bothering you, stop pressuring you, if only you eat. Eat, and you can make the world go away. For Sam, eating food had become synonymous with an end to the feelings of being pushed and pressured and stressed.

As Sam grew, other experiences followed, and these subsequent sensitizing events reinforced the program, strengthening his inner belief that food could provide relief from the difficult feelings life so often seemed to produce. Now as an adult, he found himself automatically turning to food to deal with pressure and stress, to 'make them go away', just as eating had made the matron go away. Because of this, he had become dangerously overweight and unhealthy.

Only when we uncovered this program—embedded deep within Sam's subconscious—reprocessed the experience and repaired the mental programming that had been reinforced by various subsequent sensitizing events could Sam begin to eat in a balanced way. Working with various ego-states, or parts of Sam's psyche, we negotiated a better way of eating, one which would allow him to satisfy his needs without overeating. Once we did this, and the self-doubt fostered by his personal history was eased, Sam was able to stop using food as a way to cope with the pressures of his life.

Sam learned how to deal more effectively with the feelings that his chi delivered and how to choose those foods that would best nourish and satisfy his genuine hunger. He began to exercise regularly, too. These things are an essential part of any healthy eating and weight-reduction program, but now they became much less of an ordeal. His behavior could change because the *cause* of his old unhealthy overeating had been treated and properly processed. He no longer felt compelled to turn to food to distract himself from difficult feelings. Sam's behavior changed because his feelings had changed. At last he could listen to his chi.

Sam's case illustrates how food can be linked with emotion, although in his case negatively. As children, so many compulsive overeaters were rewarded with food for being good or for pleasing someone and this made their good feelings feel even better. When they hurt, they were consoled with food. They learned that food could rapidly distract them from unpleasant feelings and could intensify or prolong pleasure. Food was there when they loved and were loved, and it was there when they felt sad, unloved or rejected. Food became the loyal supporter, the constant friend.

In this way, food and emotion became somehow fused together. As they grew up, overeaters sometimes craved food when what they really wanted was love or genuine warmth and acceptance. Perhaps now we can see that when we find ourselves overeating, it is because food has become something more than food. It has become the way we again become connected to feelings we knew in our past. Even the thought of food can cause us to instantly re-access those neural pathways that transport us to previous states and bygone feelings. It is as if food itself is a subconscious portal leading to 'other voices, other rooms'; a time-tunnel, capable of whisking us back to former ways, previous perceptions and perceived states of being.

When the French writer Marcel Proust famously sat down to savor his madeleine cake, the taste automatically took him back to a previous time, to previous emotions and experiences. Seven volumes later it was still connecting him with his past. Food and the feelings and memories it triggered had led him to produce one of the twentieth century's greatest works of literature—*À la recherche du temps perdu*, or *Remembrance of Things Past* (More literally translated as *In Search of Lost Time*). Such is the power of our emotional connection with food.

Certain foods make us feel better more rapidly than others. High-fat foods alter the brain's chemistry, as do sugar-rich foods and refined, processed carbohydrates. These elevate blood sugar levels rapidly and stimulate the brain's reward centers, releasing the feel-good neurotransmitters dopamine and serotonin. In fact, brain-imagining scans have demonstrated that high-sugar and high-fat foods work almost exactly like morphine or heroin in the brain (Colantuoni & Schwenker, 2001; Hyman, 2011).

Chocolate, for example, can rapidly change the way we feel. When we eat it, not only are we reconnecting subconsciously with previous chocolate-eating experiences and the emotions that became fused with them, but research has actually shown that as chocolate melts in the mouth it increases both brain and heart activity to a level more intense than that brought about by passionate kissing (BBC News, 16th April 2007). Is it any wonder, then, that the overeater so often craves high-fat and sweet foods? They are a quick, easy, and legal way to get a socially acceptable 'fix'.

Once children learn to respond to and manipulate feelings by eating foods that produce a high, they stop learning more effective and balanced ways of coping with feelings. Eating to distract ourselves from unwanted feelings, we eventually put on weight, our bodies becoming distorted and as out of control as the emotions driving our eating. We weigh and measure, restrict and deny in an effort to right the imbalance. And with each failed attempt at permanent weight reduction, we find ourselves again overeating, feeling worse than ever.

If you have been nodding your head in recognition as you read this, it's because you have in some way lived this story yourself. You already know how terrible it has made you feel. The good news is that you are now in an excellent position to do something about it. New neural pathways can be established and old ones changed. You *can* end your emotional overeating and become slimmer and fitter. *You can change.*

But why did those diets and meal replacements and weight-watching groups fail? You were so determined and doing so well; they seemed to work to begin with, and you saw others lose weight and become slim. Why didn't they work for you? How come you couldn't stick to the routine? Are you really lacking in self-discipline? Is there something wrong with you? No wonder your self-esteem got pummeled and your self-confidence bruised.

Adeena came to see me after hearing me talk on the radio about overeating. Though it was the middle of summer, she wore a heavy, full-length coat that covered her entire body—a camouflage I am quite accustomed to seeing in people who consult me for severe skin conditions such as eczema and psoriasis. (Both of which, incidentally, usually respond well to the right kind of hypnotherapy.) Yet Adeena's problem was not her skin, but her weight.

Within minutes of taking her chair, Adeena burst out crying. It was obvious she was desperately unhappy. For years she had wrestled with her weight. Time and again she had gone on a diet, successfully shedding the pounds, only to quickly put them right back on when the diet inevitably ended.

Once she had been sylph-like and lithe and had received many compliments for her beauty, but then she started to binge-eat, and Adeena seemed to disappear behind layer upon layer of fat. The weight had crept on until she became clinically obese. Her size affected her self-confidence to such an extent that she even became hesitant to leave the house, and those close to her feared she was developing agoraphobia. She tried various diets and even found the courage to leave her home and accompany her sister to the slimming groups with their weigh-ins and pep talks. She had done well, worked hard, and over time she again became slim.

For a while it really had worked for her. In fact, she had even been named 'Slimmer of the Year'. A local newspaper had written an article about her, complete with pictures documenting her success, showing her slim, smiling, and happy. But then inexplicably, she began to overeat again, more compulsively than before, as if making up for lost time. Once more the weight went back on, the layers of fat making her feel like a complete failure, a disappointment to herself, and a mystery to her family and friends.

Adeena was filled with feelings of guilt and shame because she thought she had let down not only herself and those close to her, but also all the people at her slimming club to whom she had been held up as a shining example of what could be achieved. The red days and green days, the calorie counting and the weigh-ins all had helped her to reduce her weight, but then she seemed to lose her way: Her resolve had slipped, none of it seemed to work anymore, and the weight had gone right back on.

In hypnosis, Adeena returned to her earlier years and to the experiences that had caused her to use food as both distraction and reward. Being the oldest child in her large, extended family, she was expected to act as an example to her younger siblings. Often she got blamed when they misbehaved, and she sometimes felt left out when her younger brothers were receiving the attention she herself craved. Food was given as rewards and as bribes. It was withheld when she had been naughty—and sometimes when a younger brother or sister had been naughty—and she was sent to her room with no supper. Soon food had become a way of feeling better, of validating herself and being validated. Food and eating told Adeena she was doing all right, that she was loved and that she really did matter. Its absence meant that she was bad.

In working through these underlying issues during hypnosis, Adeena's subconscious mind came to see that food was not the solution. Step by step, her subconscious realigned and reprogrammed itself to current reality. Food was there to nourish, and it could indeed be enjoyed, but it could never solve the problem of difficult feelings, uncomfortable chi. Gradually those parts of Adeena that were responsible for feelings of inadequacy were addressed and brought back into greater balance and harmony. Self-hypnosis would help her to better handle whatever stresses life might bring. It would also enable her to relax and maintain a state of on-going stability that would not be dependent on food or overeating. There was no longer any need for diets or for calorie counting; Adeena ate what her more even feelings now told her to eat, not in a compulsive way, but in a natural and healthy way that allowed her to become and remain the slimmer, trimmer person she longed to be. Food was no longer a drug—it was food.

In many ways, Adeena's story is all too familiar. The overeater goes on and off diets, on and off meal replacements, and on and off forced regimens. Many people who struggle with their weight do not fully realize the reason why the diets, the regimens, and the meal replacements don't go on working. It is because nothing has been done about the *cause* of the overeating. Food plans and regimens work only on the level of the symptoms, focusing on quantities and calories. Moreover, they do this through a systematic deprivation-discipline-and-denial approach. They are based on the principal of *no*, and the subconscious mind—in its simple, almost child-like way—doesn't like 'no'. It likes 'yes'.

The understanding that the human mind dislikes no and likes yes has been used to great effect in advertising. Those clever marketing people at Coca-Cola harnessed this insight when they came up with the winning slogan: 'Yes, Coke, Yes!' This advertising catchphrase was responsible for selling more Coca-Cola than just about any other marketing ploy in the history of the company. It is the *nature* of the subconscious mind to reject the negative and welcome the positive.

The conscious mind, as we have seen, uses willpower to get things done, and willpower is a wonderful thing. It can indeed work marvels—for a time. But it wasn't really made for the long haul. After the short or even medium term, the job that conscious willpower has begun—eating less food, for example—gets handed over to the subconscious, to habit, and to our old friend: feelings. It's their responsibility to continue the work that the conscious mind began, attempting to implement the no.

But if the subconscious is working on different programs, as it so often does, programs that tell it that food will make it *feel* better and that food is a useful solution to life's difficulties and discomforts, this is what will happen: Sooner or later we will compulsively eat, no matter how much we consciously don't want to.

Willpower can certainly help in the beginning. In fact, a degree of willpower is necessary to get things underway and to keep them moving, but unless the subconscious mind agrees with what the conscious mind is trying to achieve, willpower may eventually be overwhelmed by feelings. Because of this, no long-term weight-management approach will prove lastingly effective until the subconscious mind's programming has been aligned with what we consciously want. When this happens, we don't really need to *try* to eat in a healthy manner—it just *feels* natural to do so. We are in harmony with our free-flowing chi and the feelings that it brings.

Be aware, though, that even after a person's subconscious has been realigned with the conscious mind and its desires through hypnotherapy, there may be occasions when the old compulsion to eat returns momentarily.

The idea won't be overwhelming as it was before you altered your subconscious and created new neural pathways that support a healthy relationship with food. But at times like this, you will have to exercise your power of choice. Remind yourself that this is the luan chi speaking, responding to the uncomfortable stress (tiredness, fear, irritation, anger, whatever), and that it will pass.

It is essential that you find another way to relax and comfort yourself when stressed or upset—without resorting to the 'food solution'. This is why I teach rapid self-hypnosis techniques to all of my weight-management clients. Self-hypnosis is a wonderful way to 'chill out' and relax; a really effective way to manage stress. If you do go down that old route of emotional eating, you will reactivate the old pleasure-reward pathway inside the brain, and it will—surprisingly quickly—snap back into usable shape. This can result in days or even weeks of struggle in returning to a state of balance.

Even though fixing the psyche is a major part of the solution, we need to be aware that addictions involve physical as well as psychological elements. The physical components are the old neural pathways, the overused pleasure-reward circuit, that triggers the physical cravings, as well as the body's biochemistry, which is heavily dependent on receiving a constant supply of the right nutrients for healthy functioning.

Get past the emotional need the stress engenders by taking care of yourself in a healthy way, and that initial impulse to 'eat to deal' will quickly fade. Powerful cravings won't be triggered, and you will remain in balance. You can choose to eat or choose not to eat: Choose the new neural pathways or the old, overgrown, but quick-to-be-activated old pathways. *Realizing you do have a choice is essential in these situations.*

For a person who has not realigned their subconscious, the behavior of overeating can serve multiple psychological functions. As with every form of destructive behavior, overeating begins with a positive intent. Sometimes, for example, food and eating can be used by the subconscious in an attempt to protect us from harm. The layers of unattractive fat can act as a suit of armor, designed to keep people from coming too close and hurting us.

Such was the case with Cheryl, an attractive but seriously overweight woman in her early thirties who was already experiencing type two diabetes because of her overeating. In hypnosis, Cheryl went back to a time when she was a young exchange student in Europe. She was walking back to her lodging early one evening when she was attacked and raped by a man who repeatedly called out: 'Tu es belle! Tu es belle!'—'You are beautiful! You are beautiful!' Filled with horror, Cheryl entered the trance state known as *shock*, the words 'You are beautiful!' becoming instantly linked with her feelings of repulsion and fear. For Cheryl's subconscious mind, being beautiful was now something to be feared, something that could attract dire consequences: She was guilty of being beautiful. Perhaps it was she herself, with her beauty, that had provoked the rape; maybe she was responsible.

Filled with shame and unexpressed feelings of guilt and rage, Cheryl had told no one of the terrible experience, doing her best to bury those feelings deep within. But no matter how deeply she tried, they found a way to surface. From that day on, Cheryl found herself eating in a compulsive manner, piling on the fat that a part of her subconscious mind told her she needed to protect herself. If she had been raped for being beautiful, her deeper mind would ensure that this could never happen again. She would remain safe by becoming fat and unattractive. Though Cheryl knew that things had changed following the rape, she had never really understood how that experience had affected her weight. She just found herself craving food, especially high-fat and sweet things, and she couldn't really understand why.

By the time she reached me, she had already worked her way through the diets, the books, and the weight-loss experts. Nothing seemed to work; she might take weight off for a time, but then the armor went right back on. It was only when the protective part of Cheryl came to realize that its strategy was harming and not keeping her safe that she was able to regain her natural eating patterns and resume her natural state and healthy weight. This we accomplished with hypnosis.

Of course, a person does not need to have been raped or abused in order to don a suit of armor. Indeed fat, and the size that comes with it, is a mask many people wear, a strategy adopted by a less-obvious part of themselves, often for reasons known only to that subconscious aspect of the psyche, but usually revealed in the process of hypnotherapy.

The subconscious mind may also prevent a person from maintaining a healthy weight in an attempt to punish. After all, carrying a great deal of extra weight can be an excellent way of punishing not only ourselves, but also others. This can manifest itself in attitudes such as: 'I don't really deserve to be slim and healthy and attractive, so I don't care if I overeat...' or 'After what you've done, I'll be damned if I'll change and become slimmer just to keep you happy!' and so on.

Our attitudes can work in a very powerful way to affect our weight. In my professional experience, the person who comes for help with weight management usually also needs help working through unprocessed anger and guilt, and any comprehensive weight-reduction program designed to last must be equipped to deal with both of these powerful emotions.

We need to be fully aware of that part of us that, despite all of our understanding and good intentions, might still insist we continue to overeat. It is a part that exists in many of us, operating much in the same way as a member of the wartime resistance might operate, covertly and under deep cover. I call this part 'the self-saboteur'.

As we discussed in Chapter 1, each of us has several different aspects to our personality—several personas that make up this thing that we call 'the self'. Sometimes these parts—or *ego states*—jostle for control and so are in conflict. The less conflict, the more balanced and harmonious our life is. The 'self-saboteur' is just such an ego state, and when it steps forward, and gains the executive position, our other more sensible parts can be pushed to the side. The logic of our conscious mind can quickly be bypassed, and good intention can find itself flying out of the window, along with our willpower.

The important thing to realize about the self-saboteur aspect is that it doesn't really want to hurt us. In fact, quite the reverse: It believes it is helping us. The problem is that it so often gets it wrong, defeating the very best efforts of our willpower and rational conscious mind and conflicting with other, more balanced aspects of the subconscious. (Self-sabotage can have other causes, of course. It may be used by the subconscious in order to punish, to compensate for feelings of guilt or shame, and it may more commonly come into play as a function of low self-esteem.)

We can see, then, that in order to change our relationship with food it is essential to first change our relationship with our inner self, especially with any part or ego state that might have been holding us back—be it the self-saboteur or any other part. Any weight-reduction therapy or healthy-eating program that fails to take this into account will be failing the person who seeks help.

Something more needs to be clear before we begin any really effective weight-management program, and that is our expectations. Sometimes people think they can drop a massive amount of weight in a few weeks or a couple of months and then automatically keep it off. Unfortunately, the chances of this happening are quite slim. The body has an inner 'fat thermostat', so to speak, that monitors our weight and works with other elements in the body to keep it in a state of equilibrium called *homeostasis*. When we lose weight too quickly, this shocks the body, triggering an alarm that tells the brain we're starving (even though we aren't). While it may not go off immediately, sooner or later this alarm sounds. Then everything in the body cries out for food, food, and more food. We *feel* like we are starving, on a food program that previously felt comfortable and fine. Yet again, it is our *feelings* that take precedence over everything else. This is the mechanism behind statements such as: 'I maintained my ideal weight for about ten minutes. Then I started going right back up.' It's as if the weight is a yo-yo, and when a certain low point is reached, the body snaps back to its former state of equilibrium, the fatter version of ourselves.

If a person can reduce their excess weight gradually and stay slim for long enough, the body's 'fat thermostat' will automatically reset to the new weight, making that weight the 'new normal'. The body will then not react against being slimmer, trying to restore the sense of equilibrium felt at the higher weight by getting us to overeat. The best way to make this adjustment is to get there gradually, so that the body can adjust in gentle increments. This avoids the shock that ultimately propels the body back up the scale.

If you are overweight, you gained your weight by degrees, and the wisest way is to reduce it little by little. Reducing it by more than a few pounds a month is too fast and probably won't result in sustained weight reduction.

It's heart-breaking for anyone to drop a massive amount of weight and immediately yo-yo up again. Spare yourself that deflating disappointment by gently easing, not racing down the scale. Make gradual modifications to your diet (such as eliminating between-meal snacking, giving up sweetened soft drinks, desserts, and sugar), and when one new routine becomes a habit, move on to the next modification, reducing portion size, for example, and eating more fresh vegetables. You will start to feel better almost immediately, and this will more than compensate for the 'slowness' of progress on the bathroom scales, which, incidentally, I urge you to dump because scale weight is a notoriously inefficient indication of actual weight reduction. Better by far to trust the way you feel as you fit into your clothes. Let your clothing, not the scales, tell you how you're doing.

The truth is that *the very best diet is no diet.* Achieving a healthy weight and maintaining that weight is a long-term lifestyle choice. It is not something that can be realistically achieved and then maintained by some new miracle diet or breakthrough slimming pill. In order for you to become slimmer, trimmer, and healthier for life, you have to do your bit, play your part. *This means making the right life-style choices.*

Pay attention to the amount of sleep you get. When we do not get sufficient sleep, the body's *leptin* levels automatically drop. Leptin is the neurotransmitter that informs the brain when we have eaten enough food. It relays the feeling that we are now full. For this reason, being tired can feel like being hungry, so make sure you get enough sleep!

Another expectation that derails many people in their weight-reduction program is the idea that getting thin will solve all problems. If we think losing weight will automatically make us smarter, free us of self-doubt and deep-seated fears, make us feel less shy, or bring us the prince or princess of our childhood dreams, we're headed for enormous disappointment. It's just not going to happen solely because of weight reduction. All of these things are possible, of course, and hypnotherapy can powerfully assist in much of this, but they will not come about simply because our body has become slimmer.

Quite the contrary, in fact: Growing slim can bring on a host of new difficulties for a shy or insecure person if they have not addressed their issues and corrected the subconscious programming responsible for their low self-confidence or low self-esteem. Good hypnotherapy aims to do just that. If, for example, the subconscious reason we are fat is to insulate ourselves from being hurt, then when we get thin, we will feel dangerously exposed and vulnerable unless we have taken care of the misguided programming.

If we have taken off weight because we believe that will magically transform our life only to find it doesn't bring us that new job, new partner, or fabulous lifestyle, then the self-saboteur is fully capable of saying something like: 'There you are, you see—I told you it was pointless. You've denied yourself the comfort and pleasures, abandoned the armor, reduced your weight, and now look: it's still the same. Better go back to eating like before. At least that makes you feel good while you're doing it…'

Realistic expectations are essential if we are to master our overeating and become slimmer and trimmer. They are a prerequisite if we want to remain healthy eaters for the rest of our lives.

Now that we understand quite a bit more about the psychological causes and drivers of emotional overeating and weight gain, it's time to briefly turn our attention to the actual food itself. Though this is not a book about nutrition, in addition to being a hypnotherapist I am a nutritionist and no chapter about weight management would be complete without some form of discussion on the type of food we eat. Thomas Edison once said, 'The doctor of the future will give no medicine, but will interest his patient in the care of the human frame, in diet, and in the cause and prevention of disease.' Sadly, that future has yet to arrive, but increasing our knowledge of food and nutrition is of real value if we wish to live a balanced life and maintain a healthy weight.

What role does the *kind* of food we eat have in making us overweight? So far we've been talking a lot about *healthy eating*, but what exactly does this mean?

The popular media is awash with confusing and confused nutritional information. Visit any bookshop and you will find row after row of books proclaiming that they can help you to rapidly shed the pounds by eating this and not eating that. The majority of the best-selling diet books have been sold during the last decade, testimony to our modern society's burning desire to lose weight.

If you are like the majority of people who come to me for help with their weight, you have already tried some of those diets, read some of those books. But the true science has been submerged beneath a tidal wave of incorrect information, nonsensical theories, fad diets, and the vested interests of the food industry and its powerful lobbying and propaganda machine.

If we are to eat in a healthy manner, we need a clear definition of healthy eating. Well, let me offer this:

> Healthy eating means eating a reasonable amount of foods that contribute to good health while eliminating foods that are harmful to health.

At the very top of the list of nutrients so often accused of being responsible for our weight problems, and therefore of having a harmful effect on our health, are carbohydrates and fats. So let's begin with carbohydrates. Are they really something that should be avoided at all costs?

In spite of what those popular diet books say, the answer is NO. Of course, if we eliminate or greatly reduce our carbohydrate intake, then we will reduce our weight, especially in the short-term, but this is simply because we will be reducing the number of calories we eat (Sacks et al. 2009; Anderson & Chen, 1980). Reduction of food means a reduction in weight, whether that food is protein, fat or carbohydrate rich.

Far from avoiding carbohydrates, we should in fact be eating an abundance of them—provided they are the right kind of *complex* carbohydrates (Campbell & Campbell, 2006). Complex carbs are found in foods such as whole grains, cereals, brown rice, and vegetables. These foods are healthy, and we need to include them in our daily diet. Eliminating or seriously restricting complex carbohydrates can bring about an imbalance in body and mind. The American Heart Association, the American Dietetic Association, the American Kidney Fund, and the U.K. Food Standards Agency, amongst others, have all published statements warning about the dangers associated with low-carbohydrate, high-protein diets (St Jeor et al. 2001; Physician's Committee for Responsible Medicine, Atkins Diet Alert).

The human brain uses a form of glucose called glycogen for fuel. Protein, fat, vitamins, and minerals cannot provide the fuel the brain needs. Glycogen is to the brain what gasoline or petrol is to your car. It is produced through the breakdown of the carbohydrates we eat.

Lack of carbohydrates can easily alter the way we feel, bringing on mood swings, lethargy, despondency, and irritability because in addition to its glycogen-lowering effect, a lack of carbohydrates rapidly causes serotonin levels to slump (Wurtman & Wurtman, 1995). Carbohydrates also increase the availability of the amino acid tryptophan, the serotonin precursor (Herrera et al. 2011). Not only this, but when we do not eat sufficient carbs, the body cannot burn fat in an efficient way (Martz, 2002; Vander et al. 1998).

The fact is that we need carbohydrates, so forget those no-carb and low-carb diets. No properly conducted long-term study has demonstrated success with a low-carb diet (Campbell & Campbell, 2006; Larsen et al. 2004; Astrup et al. 2003). Odd then, that the biggest-selling books in the history of publishing—books about the Atkins Diet—so vehemently maintain the opposite. The founder of this dieting regimen, Dr Robert Atkins, was a brilliant marketer and exceptionally astute businessman. He was not a nutritionist but a cardiologist with serious heart problems, who suffered from high blood pressure. He died an extremely wealthy yet obese man—at the age of 73, having suffered a major heart attack the previous year—still promoting his scientifically unsound low-carb, high-fat, high-protein nutritional theories (Bone, 2004).

Equally as questionable are the latter-day spin-offs of the Atkins Diet, such as the South Beach and the French Dukan diets. All such diets share another major flaw: When we eliminate carbohydrates from our diet then fiber, naturally occurring vitamins, minerals, trace elements, and perhaps yet to be identified nutrients are also removed. Research has clearly shown that weight loss on these diets is due not to carbohydrate restriction, but depends on the number of calories consumed and the length of time on the restricted calorie diet (Sacks et al. 2009; Bravata et al. 2003).

But what about fat?

Well, it *is* important that we eat meals low in fat—especially saturated fat, the kind that comes from animal produce. In addition to being high in calories, animal fat also contains enormous amounts of cholesterol, which accumulates in the arteries, posing a real danger to health. Foods containing trans fats are also best avoided completely. (Trans fats are formed when oil is 'hydrogenated', a process that hardens the oil, so it's best to reject any food that mentions hydrogenated as part of its product contents.)

There is a popular but misguided view that says: 'We've been focusing on low-fat eating for years now and we're becoming even more overweight, and that proves that fat is not the problem.' Ask yourself how this can be true, when research shows that today we are in fact consuming *more* fat per person than we did a few decades ago when the low-fat message first began to be disseminated (Rajen & Basiotis, 1998; Campbell & Campbell, 2006).

Even if we were taking in a smaller percentage of our calories from fat today, it would simply be because the number of calories we consume by bingeing on high sugar and processed carbohydrate junk foods and drinks has simply outpaced our fat consumption. The fact is that, as a collective, we have by no means adopted a low-fat way of eating (Drewenski & Popkin, 1997; WHO Global & Regional Food Consumption Patterns).

And, by the way, one gram of fat contains nine calories, while one gram of carbohydrate provides only 4 calories, so gram for gram, ounce for ounce, fat is more than twice as calorific as carbs. If we wish to be healthy, it is recommended that we get a *maximum* 30 per cent of our total daily calories from fat (The George Mateljan Foundation). Personally, I think this figure far too high, and I am not alone in this. Expert cardiologist Dr Caldwell Esselstyn (2008) believes that we should not only eliminate fats from our diet, but also avoid *all* forms of oil—be it olive, corn, coconut, or any other kind. Oil is 100 per cent saturated fat calories, which damages the innermost lining of the arteries, the endothelium, when ingested. If we are wise then we will obtain the little oil that we do need naturally from the foods we eat (Barnard, 2003), not from fats and oils they are cooked in or by adding it in the meal preparation or cooking process. Eating a varied diet that includes the occasional and sparing use of nuts and seeds is the healthiest thing to do (Esseltsyn, 2008).

So what about a high-protein diet, which is advised by so many weight-loss gurus? Well, far from eating a high-protein diet, if we really do want to be healthy, we will get no more than 8 to 10 per cent of our calories from protein—and we will get more than this simply by eating a varied, whole-foods plant-based diet (Campbell & Campbell, 2006). It is not even necessary to eat meat, fish, eggs or dairy in order to get this small amount of protein. Even if we are athletes, engaged in rigorous physical exercise, we need no more than ten to twelve per cent of our calories from protein (Anderson et al. 2010; Tarnopolsky, 2004), and this is easily achieved by eating from a varied menu of plant-based whole foods.

Then what about supplements?

There are no specific supplements, amino acids, vitamins, minerals, pills, potions or sachets needed to accelerate your weight reduction and eat healthily. However, some nutritional supplementation may be beneficial in the beginning of a weight-reduction program for people whose irregular eating habits and unbalanced food choices have created a deficiency. When a person regularly eats a varied range of fresh foods, especially from a whole foods plant-based menu (fresh vegetables, whole grains, legumes, beans, and fruits), supplements are no longer required. They have all that is necessary for good health.

As we have seen, if we want to become healthier and lighter, we will make sure that our subconscious has re-processed its underlying difficulties and is aligned with our conscious desire to reach and maintain a balanced, healthy weight. We will keep our fat intake to a minimum; eat a variety of whole foods—including complex carbohydrates, an abundance of fresh vegetables, and a reasonable amount of fresh fruit—while reducing or eliminating our consumption of animal produce. Processed foods are best avoided altogether, since they are denatured, lifeless, and consequently weak in vibrant chi. In addition, they are usually high in salt, hidden sugars and fats. The closer foods are to their natural, unadulterated state the better they are for us. We will also restrict our alcohol intake (since alcohol is very calorie dense), while drinking plenty of water, which hydrates and helps with feelings of satiety. If we are wise, we will exercise on a regular basis, too.

Regular exercise is something that cannot be neglected by anyone who wants to reduce weight and feel good. If you have not exercised for some time, be sure to check with your doctor before beginning any exercise program, then start slowly and gradually build up the intensity. There's no denying that exercise requires a certain amount of self-discipline, but it is well worth it for the results it brings. Regular exercise not only burns up excess calories, but it produces positive changes in our entire nervous system and in our mood. When our mood is high, we are less likely to turn to food in order to feel better.

By the way—and you will have heard this before, but it bears repeating—never skip breakfast. Studies have repeatedly demonstrated that eating a balanced, healthy breakfast helps to maintain reduced weight and stabilize mood. Start the day with a piece of raw fruit, since this will alkalize the body, which tends towards acidity. Disease flourishes in an acidic environment.

In making our food choices, it's always best to focus on what it's best to have rather than on what we shouldn't have. When we stop concentrating on what isn't there and begin to focus on what is there—the wonderful symphony of flavors and wide variety of different, tasty foods that nourish and support our good health—making the right food choices becomes much easier. It won't seem like depriving yourself if you substitute the things you are eliminating from your eating regimen with new delicious foods that also are good for you. Learning to delay instant gratification brings with it an even greater reward: the freedom to choose. When we are free to choose, we are free from addiction. The way to a healthier, slimmer you lies in a modification of old eating habits and in an alteration of your *relationship* with food and with yourself—not in dieting.

Hypnotherapy can put you back in touch with your authentic self, helping you to re-draw those outmoded maps, delete the faulty programs and re-write the scripts that have been forcing you to eat compulsively and to put on so much unhealthy weight. As a human being you are the result of hundreds of thousands of years of research and development. Everything you need in order to be healthy is right there, built into you, waiting for you to access and to return you to a lighter, more balanced weight, but you need to play your part, too. The choice between being healthy or unhealthy is yours and yours alone, and each time you put food into your mouth you make that choice.

When we stop using food as a way of distracting ourselves from those feelings and emotions that we find too powerful or inconvenient to handle, our balance is restored and we can eat in a healthy manner, the way nature intended us to eat.

When food at last becomes food and resumes its correct role as the provider of healthy chi—the pleasant, enjoyable and life-sustaining nourishment that it is meant to be—then we regain control not only over our weight, but also in so many areas of our life. As this happens, the chi that food contains flows through us, becoming our own vital energy, providing us with all we need in order to live a balanced, healthy life.

Chapter Eleven

Self-Confidence and Self-Esteem

'If I have lost confidence in myself, I have the universe against me.'
~ Ralph Waldo Emerson

Few things affect the way in which we live our life more than self-confidence. With it we can achieve inner balance, material stability, and perhaps even greatness. Without it, each day can be a struggle. The level of confidence we hold within ourselves affects our happiness, our relationships, our creativity, and our success. In a circle of increasing returns, the more confidence we have, the more we can accomplish. The more we accomplish, the better we feel about ourselves. And the better we feel about ourselves, the more self-confidence we generate.

Lack of self-confidence, on the other hand, adversely affects our relationships, our education, our career prospects, and even our health. It dampens down our chi, holding us back and making life much harder than it otherwise would be.

Take a moment now and look back over the years. How different might your life have been if you had all the confidence you needed exactly when you needed it? What opportunities did you pass up because you lacked the confidence to grab them? What might you have accomplished if you had found enough self-confidence to step beyond your doubt?

You can't bring back those lost opportunities, but you can use them now to motivate yourself into action, to decide that history will not go on repeating itself. Remember that nothing is ever wasted if we learn from it. If those experiences show you what you lost, they can also show what you can gain when you have the confidence to reach out and embrace life.

No matter how little self-confidence you may have or how much confidence you may have lost, you *can* become more self-confident. No one needs to continue performing to old, self-defeating scripts that are holding them back. It will take some work, but with a little effort, anyone can develop self-confidence.

Becoming self-confident is more than learning a few simple tricks. It just cannot be reduced to just a handful of techniques or efforts at positive thinking. I know all about the bestselling authors who have made money promising instant confidence in a week by resorting to a few easy tactics. Perhaps you've bought a couple of those books, tried some of those techniques. Maybe they even looked like they might be helping for a while, but all too soon you found that the basic problem didn't go away: You still lacked the confidence you needed.

Those superficial strategies are unlikely to make much of a dent in the deeply entrenched programming that has been holding you back for so many years. It is this subconscious programming that has been affecting your chi, forcing you to doubt yourself, stealing away your natural confidence.

In order to become really confident, you will need to leave the surface and delve deeper down. Hypnotherapy provides a wonderfully effective way to journey into your personal history, uncover those experiences that taught you to doubt yourself and your abilities, and then reinterpret or reprocess the *meaning* you have given to those experiences. Remember that it is the meaning we give to our experiences that defines our inner landscape. This is what shapes our beliefs—and what creates our lack of self-belief.

If you find yourself struggling with self-doubt, understand that these feelings are not based on fact, although they have tried to fool you into believing otherwise. They are the product of luan chi, the distorted energy that has been flowing through you, energetically feeding you information—or misinformation. *Feelings* of inadequacy are not the same as inadequacy. Because we *feel* inadequate does not mean that we *are* inadequate. Lack of confidence and low self-esteem has everything to do with conditioning. As with so many of our difficulties, these have their roots in the subconscious mind and how it has been programmed. In previous chapters, we saw how subconscious programs can be rewritten and more helpful ones installed. This can be done with self-confidence and self-esteem programs, too.

When we are confident we can almost feel our vigorous, healthy chi flowing through us, energizing and informing us that we can reach out, that no matter what happens, we will somehow be able to deal with it. With confidence comes the understanding that we will remain safe, that we can cope, and that we are capable of living and allowing others—even those whose opinions and beliefs we do not necessarily share—to do the same. Real confidence means we can give ourselves permission to take risks, to be assertive without being aggressive, to be open without being unnecessarily defensive. Above all, confidence means that we can live our own, authentic life, not someone else's version of what our life should be.

A mistake many people make, however, is in thinking that self-confidence means that we are always 100 per cent sure of ourselves, that we never experience any anxiety or hesitation and are certain we will always do well in any undertaking. This is not at all what self-confidence is. *Real* self-confidence means we can push on regardless of uncertainty, anxiety, or even in the presence of fear. It is an inner understanding that despite apprehension and challenges, we will move forward, that we can step into the unknown and depend on ourselves to somehow handle it.

In other words, self-confidence means we trust ourselves. That is the meaning inherent in the Latin root of the word: *confidentia*, which translates as 'having trust or reliance'. When we are self-confident, we know we are indeed capable, that we can tackle whatever we need or choose to, and that we can probably do it well. We also know that even if we fail, it is not the end of the world, nor the end of us.

Self-confidence can present itself in numerous different forms, according to the role or situation we find ourselves in—personal independence, workplace confidence, social confidence, or peer confidence, for example. It can even assume an almost physical quality that is commonly known as 'charisma' or 'stage presence'.

Yet self-confidence is not a thing some people automatically have and other people automatically don't. It is something fluid and malleable and it has a lot to do with habit. If being confident meant having to wait until we actually had the feeling, we might have to wait quite a while before doing anything. The great thing is that the feeling will come as we cultivate the habit.

So how do we cultivate the habit of self-confidence? If you've read the chapter on habits, you know all habits are acquired through repeated *action*. In order for confidence to manifest and work in our life, it has to be activated; it is something that we have to *do*. The more we do it, the more habitual it becomes. In this sense, confidence is just as much a verb as it is a noun—something we do as much as something we feel.

Think about it: If confidence had nothing to do with action, it would be of very little consequence, like some recreational drug that self-indulgently triggers the release of endorphins, encouraging us to sit back and feel good about ourselves as the world passed us by. Without action, confidence would be pretty meaningless. What if we felt supremely confident but simply left it at that, allowing everything else to remain the same? We would never reach out and connect with others, never ask someone out, never pass an exam, never go for a promotion, never change careers, never give a performance, never complete a project, never move forward.

If faith without action is useless then so too is self-confidence.

The real power of self-confidence lies in the doing. And fortunately, with practice, we humans can learn to do just about anything. In fact, we are very good at learning how to do things.

But for people who lack self-confidence, it can seem as if practically everyone else has it in spades while they have little or none. This, of course, can never be true. Even the most unconfident person feels confident in some things, whether it is talking to a close friend, practicing a hobby, surfing the Internet, doing a familiar job, or riding a bicycle. In one sphere or another, everyone knows how to be—or more correctly, how to do—confidence.

In fact it's not at all unusual for a person to feel confident in some areas of life while feeling completely unconfident in others. The experienced professional or skilled worker, for example, may feel completely confident while working in a familiar setting, handling even the most demanding tasks, but ask that same person to stand up and make a presentation or give a talk in front of a group of people, and the free-flowing chi instantly becomes luan chi, conveying the feelings that make confidence simply drain away. A person might feel entirely comfortable mixing socially with friends, family, and work colleagues, but introduce that same person to strangers, and they may freeze into an awkward silence, becoming completely tongue-tied and surprisingly shy.

I have worked with celebrities who told me they have all the confidence they need when standing on stage in front of an audience or before the camera, yet they have absolutely no confidence in their social or personal life. Others visited me because the more famous they became, the more they felt their professional confidence slipping.

I cannot help wishing the celebrities I helped, some of whom have talked openly to the media about their difficulty with confidence, would also mention *how hypnotherapy assisted in overcoming it* because this would perhaps inspire and help so many other people who struggle in a similar manner. Yet very few are willing to talk about how their difficulty has been resolved. It is as if seeking professional help through hypnosis is seen by these individuals as a weakness that must always be kept hidden from the eyes of others. Some never talk about the difficulties they have had with confidence, an aspect of their life that they choose to keep hidden in order to protect an image.

Of course, it's not only celebrities who keep their self-confidence issues hidden. So often I hear those who consult me because of low confidence say things like: 'People might think I'm confident, but I'm really not. It's a front, an act I put on to get by, but on the inside I'm always struggling.'

What is to blame for such lack of self-confidence? You probably already know from what you've read in this book: The culprit is *the past*. While difficult occurrences such as the end of an important relationship, a divorce, or the loss of a job can send us into a tailspin, such experiences are more likely to be symptom-producing events, not the origin of our problem. Of themselves, they are unlikely to keep us unbalanced for very long were we not already insecure within ourselves to begin with. Once again, it is our childhood experiences that largely dictate our emotional resiliency and the level of self-confidence we feel as adults.

Adara was a young lawyer with aspirations to become a high court barrister. The problem was that she lacked self-confidence. Though well educated and qualified, the thought of standing in court and arguing a case in front of a judge and jury made her legs go weak and her face red. Though she knew it was irrational, she just didn't feel the judge and jury would listen to or respect her. At the same time, she also knew that she would have to let go of this crippling, fearful feeling if she wanted to move ahead, fulfill her potential, and accomplish her dreams.

Deeply relaxed and in hypnosis, Adara easily drifted back to her childhood and to the initial sensitizing event that had kicked off her deep-seated lack of confidence. She was five years old. It was a warm summer day; she was wearing a pair of pretty yellow and red shorts and had skipped into the cul-de-sac in front of her house to play with the neighboring children. Adara had been observing them from the window of the front room as they played with a lovely new scooter. Seeing her, they had motioned to Adara to come outside and play. She hadn't thought twice, rushing out of her front door and happily joining in the fun. Suddenly her mother's voice rang out, piercing the laughter, 'Adara, come here now!' The little girl knew she was in trouble. Immediately she left the other children and scurried back inside, her heart pounding, not knowing what she had done wrong.

As soon as the door closed, her mother was screaming at her. 'You have brought shame on yourself and on the family! How could you do this to us?' The little girl received a big, hard slap on her bare legs. Adara's family was strict Muslim, and for a girl to expose her legs and her body in front of others, as this little girl had done, was shameful in their eyes. 'You should be ashamed of yourself!' her mother yelled, and Adara was sent to her room, tears streaming down her reddened face.

In the trance-like state that is early childhood, Adara had heard her mother's words, and powerful messages instantly transformed themselves into beliefs, becoming embedded in the bio-computer of the child's subconscious mind. For the mature, adult mind, the experience would seem almost trivial, something to be forgotten and left behind in the mists of childhood, but the powerful emotion it had produced was enough to disrupt the little girl's chi and plant the tiny seed of self-doubt. This ostensibly harmless experience was all that it took to install a program that would be reinforced time and again by a string of subsequent sensitizing events as Adara grew into adulthood.

So many times she was told she would never go very far, that she wasn't the brightest of girls, and that she should work towards being the kind of woman a successful man might want to take for a wife. This was the distorted information that would infiltrate her chi. Little wonder, then, that the grown-up Adara lacked the self-confidence to stand up in court and argue her case.

Once the origins of her confidence difficulties were understood, Adara was helped in reprocessing the meaning that her subconscious mind had assigned to those earlier experiences. Deep in trance, the grown-up Adara was guided to talk with the child Adara, helping her to see how the past external invalidations were faulty and unhelpful and could therefore now be replaced with a more realistic self-image. The doubting ego states that had been so preoccupied with protecting her from embarrassment and shame could now loosen their restrictive grip and allow more assertive parts of her personality to play their role. As a result, confidence could be restored, and Adara could move forward in a positive and much more self-assured manner. (If you picked up this book and turned immediately to this chapter, I suggest you read Chapter 1 in which I explain *ego-states*.)

She would have to practice, of course, as we humans need to make a habit of anything we want to become really good at, but that was her choice—she chose to practice law, to stand up and talk in front of others, and to make a habit of it. Adara understood that feelings of uncertainty would still sometimes be there; after all, there could be no absolute certainty that she or anyone else would ever win a case, but now she could handle that uncertainty. Her chi unblocked, she could push through those feelings of apprehension and move forward with her professional life.

Adara's story demonstrates an important fact: Nobody is born with a lack of self-confidence or with low self-esteem. Even if we can't remember a time when we felt truly confident, the fact is that each baby enters the world with all the trust necessary for self-confidence to grow. Each of us is born with a natural capacity to acquire an abundance of self-confidence and self-esteem. No one has more of this capacity than anyone else. Confidence is everyone's birth right. We each have the right and the ability to earn the respect of ourselves and of others.

Everyone has the capacity to become more confident. But before we can do this, we must first acknowledge what has been standing in our way. What stops us from being totally self-confident?

Take a moment right now, and think back to a particular situation in which you lacked self-confidence. Go ahead and search your memory bank; I'm sure you can remember one. Now close your eyes and go through it in your mind. Imagine it as vividly as you can. See what you saw, hear what you heard, and notice what you're thinking and feeling as you do this. Notice your energy level as your chi changes. See if you can pinpoint what it is that has caused these feelings of uncertainty. It won't take long—just go ahead and do it now.

Was the feeling you connected with in this exercise uncomfortable? You might even be able to give it a name, such as tension or anxiety. If you followed that feeling deeper, to what was *behind* your self-doubt, you probably found the emotion of *fear*. When we doubt ourselves, we fear we are not good enough, or cannot trust ourselves to do what needs to be done. Often there is also the fear that other people will witness or come to know about our ineptness. We fear being exposed, appearing inadequate, foolish, or fake—and embarrassed, humiliated or rejected because of this.

People who are not confident in social situations, or when meeting others, for example, fear they will be scrutinized and found wanting, uninteresting, or uninformed, or that they might slip up and say or do something embarrassing or humiliating. Because of this fear, they try their best to remain in the background and under the radar.

Likewise, people who lack self-confidence at work or when entering a room full of people, speaking in front of others, or giving a presentation, for example, not only do not trust themselves, they also fear they will be placed under the microscope where their incompetence or inferiority will be revealed for all to see, causing them deep humiliation. It is the same for any situation where we lack self-confidence—completing a project, passing an exam, speaking to a stranger, or asking a colleague out for a drink, to give a few examples. Fear of what the other person may think causes the person with low self-confidence to pass by golden opportunities that could ensure their success and even change their life. The fear of embarrassment, humiliation, or rejection lurks somewhere inside every single person who lacks self-confidence.

Is the confident person someone who knows no fear and no anxiety, while the person who lacks confidence knows nothing but fear and anxiety? Not at all. The real difference is that confident people have learned how to push through the fear so it does not paralyze them. Even the most confident people sometimes feel fear and anxiety, but they do not let this stop them from taking action. In repeatedly taking action, the fear is calmed and conquered.

Let's look at a couple of people who had the confidence to accomplish what they wanted and who have even become famous because of it. The erudite Stephen Fry, celebrated British actor and author, once wrestled with an intense lack of self-confidence and self-esteem, yet he pushed through this successfully. His lack of confidence has not stopped him from appearing on stage, on television, in films, and in print.

Likewise, Angelina Jolie, the popular movie actor, has publicly admitted her struggles with low self-confidence and self-esteem, yet this has not prevented her from getting up in front of the public and allowing herself to be scrutinized. The Canadian poet and singer Leonard Cohen, who has performed in front of hundreds of thousands of people, suffers at times from severe 'stage fright' before giving live performances. Woody Allen admits he sometimes vomits before going on stage.

Can it be true that even people as much in the public eye as celebrities might lack confidence? Certainly, but they have learned to push through their fear. They know that *confidence lies in action.*

The point is that we do not need to wait until we feel flushed with confidence in order to move into confidence. If we wait until we feel absolutely sure of ourselves, we might wait a very long time indeed—so long, in fact, that we may act too late or never act at all. While waiting for the good ship Confidence to come in, we might very well miss the boat of Opportunity. Really confident people are not people who never know fear; they are people who do not allow their fear to stop them. They are people who have changed the word *risk* into the word *challenge*, and in doing this they have developed the right attitude. They have become willing to take that little leap into the unknown and to trust that they will somehow come out of it all right.

Here then is an important understanding: Self-confidence is not the absence of fear, but the ability to move forward and take action in spite of fear. This ability increases with repetition, becoming a habit. The more we do it, the more we trust we can do it, and the more we trust, the more confident we become. Action is the foundation of self-confidence. Repeated action is the cement that strengthens self-confidence.

Hypnotherapy can help with this process—it identifies the root beliefs about ourselves that cause us self-doubt and works towards changing those beliefs to something much more helpful and healthy. But we still need to continually push ourselves beyond our comfort zone. All of the therapy in the world is useless if we do not place ourselves into situations where we can develop the *habit* of self-confidence. If we remember to regard 'confidence' as a verb, as an action, we won't go far wrong.

In previous chapters I mentioned my own personal experience with depression and addiction, so it might not come as a surprise when I tell you that I have also wrestled with low self-confidence and self-esteem. Like so many of the people who now come to consult with me, I, too, had lost golden opportunities, let wonderful chances slip through my fingers simply because I lacked the confidence to reach out, to do what was needed in order to grasp life's gifts and really live.

Today I confidently talk before large groups, speaking frequently on stage, on the radio, and in front of the camera. I can socialize without the need of alcohol or drugs to anesthetize or embolden me. I teach, lecture, conduct seminars and corporate training, and enjoy my work as a busy therapist, but this does not mean I never feel anxious or afraid. I still sometimes feel these emotions, but I have learned to act in spite of those feelings, to push forward and simply to *do*. I have developed the *habit* of self-confidence and know from personal experience that it can indeed be built.

So far we've been talking about self-confidence, but we have said little about its close relative: self-esteem. Though not identical to self-confidence, self-esteem is closely allied with it. The word is taken from the Latin *aestimare,* which means 'to value or appraise'. When we have high self-esteem, we value and appraise ourselves favorably. When we have low self-esteem, the opposite is the case. Low self-esteem causes us to devalue and denigrate ourselves. It turns us into our own worst critic.

Whereas self-confidence is all about self-trust and self-reliance, self-esteem is our sense of self-worth. It is our *perception* of ourselves. This perception influences our self-acceptance and ultimately our ability to accept other people. This is why individuals with low self-esteem may experience strong emotions for another person but often find it difficult to actually love. Love requires opening oneself up, dropping one's defense mechanisms, and inviting another person to see, share, and accept even the most fragile and vulnerable parts of ourselves.

Not only this, but it means being secure enough to fully reciprocate in kind. If we are unable to accept and value ourselves, to see our own self-worth, it is very difficult to really share ourselves with another. While we may develop an emotional dependence that we *call* 'love', we may well remain strangers to the real thing.

When we lack self-esteem, we are unable to validate ourselves from within. As a result, our sense of security depends largely on other people. We are constantly seeking to be validated from without, so people and events beyond our control determine how we feel about who we are and therefore about life in general. In psychology, this is called having an 'external locus of control'. (We will be talking more about this shortly.)

We can see now how self-confidence and self-esteem are interrelated. Lack of self-esteem undermines a person, stopping them from embracing the challenges that being confident requires. Living in this essentially fear-driven way can easily turn us into people-pleasers who spend so much of our time worrying about other people's opinion of us while ignoring our own. Not only this, but low self-esteem can easily trigger feelings of habitual anxiety and mood swings. When our self-esteem is low, it's as if there is nothing to support us. If we fail, there is nothing to fall back on, so we cannot afford to fail. And if we cannot afford to fail, we are inclined to shy away from putting ourselves out there and transforming *risk* into *challenge*—we simply lack the confidence to do so.

With high self-esteem, we are more grounded in ourselves. We have a clearer idea of who we are. Because of this, we can allow ourselves to embrace challenges, and risks do not seem so risky. The mistakes we make do not stand in the way of our progress. They cannot keep us down for the count because we are resilient enough to learn from them and to use this learning to accomplish our own self-determined goals. This in turn motivates us, providing the kind of energy that leads on to a fuller, more meaningful life. Little wonder that people who have high self-esteem report being happier within themselves (Mruk, 2006).

In the past, the idea that high self-esteem is a positive

attribute has taken some battering. The influential American psychologist Albert Ellis thought the concept of self-esteem unrealistic and self-defeating (Ellis, 1997). He argued that it is perfectionistic and grandiose. For him, a better quality to strive for would be *self-acceptance*. As if to support this view, research conducted in the mid-1990s appeared to demonstrate that violent criminals tend to have high levels of self-esteem (Baumester et al. 1996). This has added strength to the argument that self-esteem correlates with arrogance, prejudice, self-deception, and egotism. The conclusion that many have drawn is that we should have nothing to do with it.

It would be difficult for me to disagree more. Of course, self-acceptance is key to feeling good about ourselves, but to say that high self-esteem is a bad thing simply because some criminals have it is about the same as saying that we should not keep dogs or be vegetarian because Hitler kept German shepherds and didn't eat meat. (Incidentally, the idea that Hitler was vegetarian is a myth 'cooked up' in collusion with Joseph Goebbels, his minister of propaganda. According to Albert Speer and other informed biographers, Hitler would occasionally go on 'vegetarian binges' because of gastric upset, but his main diet contained such things as liver dumplings, pork sausage, sliced ham, and a special favorite, squab—young fledgling pigeon.) The fault is not with self-esteem itself but with the way its detractors view it, unfairly equating it with negative qualities. Ellis thought it to be based on 'perfectionistic and grandiose thinking', while research has confused it with arrogance and narcissism. In fact, arrogance, perfectionism, egotism, and so forth are as far away from genuine self-esteem as one can possibly get.

The reality is that arrogance is a compensation for deep-seated feelings of inferiority—the very opposite of high self-esteem. Perfectionism is usually linked to a fear of criticism—the person with genuine self-esteem is able to accept criticism and use it as feedback. Grandiose thinking and egotism are products of a distorted self-image—again, the opposite of authentic self-esteem.

Narcissists (the term psychologists give to arrogant, egotistical people) very often have a perverted self-image. They usually believe they have some kind of special entitlement, and they organize their 'self-knowledge' in an overly egocentric and childishly self-serving manner. Narcissists often attempt to manipulate people for their own ends and, in extreme cases, may even resort to violence to achieve their desires. American serial killer Ted Bundy, and Britain's Kray twins are classic examples of the narcissistic personality taken to extremes.

The person with high self-esteem, however, tends to have a balanced self-awareness. They often exhibit the tendency not of aggressively manipulating others, but of openly pursuing positive goals, and leading others towards positive outcomes. This reinforces their self-respect and earns them the respect of others.

When self-esteem is high, we more easily accept our own strengths and limitations as well as those of others, and we tend to maintain a forward-looking and optimistic attitude towards life in general. Self-acceptance and self-esteem go hand in hand.

High self-esteem also performs a protective function: It helps us cope with stress, making us more resilient and deterring feelings of anxiety. Chi flows freely in people with high self-esteem. They effectively handle situations that arise and step up to whatever challenges life may present, knowing they have what it takes to discover the solution and to come out safely on the other side.

Low self-esteem, on the other hand, produces feelings of insecurity, leading to personal or social withdrawal and unrealistic expectations. Low self-esteem generates oversensitivity to criticism, fear of making mistakes, and chronic indecision. People with low self-esteem also tend to be far less forgiving in their personal relationships than other people. Perhaps unsurprisingly then, low self-esteem plays a major role in a variety of psychological difficulties, such as addictions, depression, and eating disorders.

Like so many other problems, the origins of low self-esteem can almost always be traced back to the formative years of infancy and early childhood and to the way we were treated back then. It is here that parents, caregivers, and teachers plant the seeds of self-doubt—usually unintentionally. As we have seen, all sorts of childhood experiences can have powerful negative effects, embedding the kernels of low self-esteem that easily sprout and mature as the person grows.

All children, like all adults, need and deserve to have their natural emotional needs met. We humans need to feel we are worthwhile and lovable. The more often a baby is held, appropriately touched, and lovingly caressed, the safer and more valued the infant will feel. Responding to children's emotional states when they are reacting to the birth of a sibling or the death of a pet, or when they are having problems in school or moving from one school to another, for example, are all part of the nurturing of a child's sense of security and self-worth. Talking about children as if they aren't there, not including them in decisions that affect them, exposing them to constant parental arguing or inappropriate sexualization—these sorts of behaviors usually translate into major problems as that child grows into an adult.

The sense of security and self-worth we have as children depends not only on our immediate family but also on the larger social context. In school, teachers who consistently find fault in a child can damage that person and change the course of their life. Coming from a social or ethnic minority and experiencing prejudice or being ridiculed for looking, behaving, or speaking differently can negatively influence how children view themselves well into adulthood. And it isn't always the adults who damage children. Kids can damage other kids with their taunting, rejection, and bullying. Sometimes children with very supportive families and teachers develop low self-esteem, anxiety, and other emotional problems because of their treatment by other children.

Our self-esteem can also be damaged when we have left our childhood and become adults. If a partner or family member constantly criticizes us, or if a boss or colleague regularly questions our performance or makes derogatory remarks, we can come to doubt ourselves and question our own abilities. If our self-esteem was not high to begin with, this additional pressure can corrode it even more, creating feelings of great anxiety and despondency.

Some experts believe self-esteem to be a fixed personality trait, but I certainly do not share that view. My work as a therapist and my own life experience have shown me that self-esteem is malleable. It can indeed be eroded or dramatically enhanced. But here is the thing: If we want to improve our self-esteem, we need to *earn* it. If self-esteem is to be strong and authentic, it needs to be rooted in our personal experience of successful outcomes. As Thomas Carlyle pointed out, 'Nothing builds self-esteem and self-confidence like accomplishment.'

Just as self-confidence needs to be *built*, self-esteem needs to be *earned*. In building self-confidence, we learn to deal affirmatively with situations life brings our way. In earning self-esteem, we learn to actually like and respect ourselves.

People with low self-esteem do the opposite. They usually treat themselves harshly, engaging in endless self-criticism. In my therapeutic practice, time and again I have asked people with low self-esteem to reflect and tell me if there is anyone in their life they treat as badly as they treat themselves. No one has ever said yes.

Relentless self-criticism hardly improves things. If it helped, perfection would have been acquired long ago. Constant criticism serves only to damage, never to build—a fact that all parents should be taught before the birth of their first child and all teachers should have underscored at the outset of their training. Constant criticism is a self-defeating, downward spiral: The more we are criticized, the worse we feel, and the worse we feel, the more we beat ourselves up. As the humanist psychologist Carl Rogers pointed out, so many of people's problems exist because they despise themselves.

People with self-loathing are forced to look outside themselves for positive validation. In doing this, they turn over control of their feelings and destiny to external forces, which brings us to something I mentioned earlier: having an 'external locus of control'. People who function in this manner tend to be negative about life and their place in it, while people with an internal locus of control, being more self-reliant, believe they are the primary authors of their destiny and have a greater chance of succeeding in their endeavors and so of feeling good about themselves.

When we depend on other people's opinion of us, it is easy to put our own needs and wants to one side and become 'people-pleasers'. People-pleasing brings with it a host of negative consequences, such as an inability to form healthy boundaries in relationships, difficulty in managing or supervising others, problems accepting positive feedback, and—because people-pleasers find it hard to say 'no' to others—problems managing time. Moreover, because of the constant need to prove one's worth to others and the energy expended in the effort, people-pleasing can lead to chronic fatigue and eventual burnout.

If our sense of self-worth depends on pleasing others, it is not true self-esteem: it is 'other-esteem'. By attempting to endlessly please and placate other people, we find ourselves renouncing our own rights, turning our back on our own needs, and simply wearing ourselves out.

Brendan was a bespectacled man in his mid-forties who worked in a large accountancy firm. He came to see me because he was suffering from chronic stress and what he described as 'total burnout'. In our pre-hypnosis chat, Brendan lost little time telling me about his lack of self-confidence and feelings of low self-worth. 'I had a bit of a difficult start in life, so that probably has something to do with it,' he said. 'I've worked hard all my life, but I still don't know how I've managed to last this long. I'm at my desk before anyone else but always end up taking work back home. No matter how much I do, it never seems enough. I don't really feel appreciated—just taken for granted. People keep putting things on my desk because they know I won't say no. I can't seem to help it; I just don't want to let them down.'

Reclining in the therapy chair, Brendan soon entered a state of deep trance where he quickly went back to experiences in his childhood. He had been born in the 1950s, a time when ideas of morality were quite different from today, and his teenage mother had not been married when she became pregnant with him. She had wanted an abortion but was unable to find someone who could perform it, so she had been forced to give birth to the boy. For the first three or four years of Brendan's life, his mother struggled to make ends meet, receiving scant support from her family who treated her as a disgrace. Eventually she met and married a man whose wife had died, leaving him with two young children to bring up. It seemed an ideal solution to everyone's problem.

Though the boy Brendan was treated quite well by his stepfather, he did not fare so well with his mother, who saw him as the embodiment of the shame that had been forced upon her. Sometimes she told him of the sacrifices she had been forced to make because of him and of how much it had cost her to do her duty by him. Although Brendan was the youngest person in the household, by the age of seven he was made to rise early each morning and prepare breakfast for everyone else, including his older stepbrother and stepsister who seemed to delight in lording it over him. When things weren't done just right, Brendan got the blame. His mother hardly ever praised him or even bothered to thank him for all of his effort and hard work. No matter how earnestly he tried, he just couldn't seem to please her.

Once, when making tea, the boy had badly scalded himself with boiling water and had to be taken to the hospital for his burns. There was anger in his mother's voice as she chided, 'Tell them you were playing in the kitchen—that you shouldn't have reached up for the kettle!' More than anything, he longed for his mother's love and approval, but because this wasn't forthcoming, he was willing to settle for a quiet life, and in order to get this, he constantly bent over backwards to keep his mother and everyone else as happy as possible.

All these experiences were revisited in hypnosis, and Brendan's subconscious mind was helped to reinterpret them so that their meaning changed, his negative interpretations becoming replaced with ones more helpful. Later we worked with those aspects of Brendan's psyche, or ego states, that were still holding him back and causing him self-doubt. As his therapy progressed, he learned that this new, affirmative way of being did not lead to rejection but brought about a greater degree of respect from others, and as he earned this, he also earned a heightened respect for himself. In applying the self-hypnosis techniques he had been taught, Brendan could now manage and release stress as it appeared. He no longer needed to use all of his energy in some futile attempt to please others.

While Brendan's mother does not appear to have been a people-pleaser—at least as far as her son was concerned—she does seem to have played the martyr, constantly reminding her son of how much she had been forced to sacrifice because of him. The role of martyr, sometimes called *the martyr complex,* is most often a guise adopted by people who usually have serious problems with their own self-esteem. In this role, a person can go to great lengths to show they have placed someone else's needs—often a dependent relative's—before their own, and that they have made great sacrifices because of it. Martyrs believe they have been called upon to suffer in the name of duty or love and often let others know how difficult their life is because of it. Underlying such a role, there is most often a great sense of resentment.

People suffering from the martyr complex are usually very willing to take on responsibility for other people's lives—and may find themselves drawn to careers where they can do this professionally—yet they usually find themselves evading full responsibility for aspects of their own life. This is part of the reason why I believe anyone entering the helping professions—be it psychiatrist, psychologist, psychotherapist, counselor, or hypnotherapist—is well advised to go through their own course of therapy, and also participate in ongoing supervision.

In many ways, the martyr complex is similar to an addiction in that it usually tells the sufferer that *they* do not have it. When confronted with their martyr-like behavior, such people will often display a knee-jerk reaction, feeling offended and retreating behind a veil of righteous indignation. If challenged, they resort to defense mechanisms, blaming the person (friend, family member, or therapist) who has shone the light of truth upon the role they have been playing.

Uncomfortable though it may be, only through rigorous self-honesty will martyrs ever free themselves from the inauthentic role they play and move on to a life lived with high self-esteem. Sadly, many find it just too convenient to luxuriate in this state. They refuse to recognize the role they are playing or to do what is necessary to emerge from it.

Like other psychological issues, the martyr complex is most often initiated in the childhood years and generally involves a parent. We know that as babies we are completely dependent on our parents and caregivers; without them we could not survive. We have an instinctual need to be accepted, liked, and loved by them so that they will continue to nurture and take care of us. If a parent or caregiver is overly demanding, critical, or distant, or if they manifest neurotic tendencies such as the martyr complex, we will naturally become anxious and insecure.

Instinct tells us that if our mother or primary caregiver stops loving us, they may also stop taking care of us and we could be in danger of abandonment, so there is real survival value in pleasing and, if necessary, placating the adult who holds such power. For the young child, avoiding disapproval and pleasing the mother or other primary caregiver is in many ways tantamount to survival.

Many people-pleasers learned early in infancy that through placating an overly demanding parent or caregiver—even if this meant sacrificing their own needs and abandoning their own desires, as a martyr must—they could sustain that person's emotional interest and perhaps also maintain or win that person's love, or at least a facsimile of it.

The solution to the martyr complex, as well as to the people-pleasing syndrome, lies in changing our locus of control from external to internal—not in some silly, self-indulgent manner, but in a mature way that fosters our own independence. When we stop making other people our means of validation and cease turning over control of who we are to them, we take our life back and earn our own self-esteem. This is accomplished in steps, and that means taking action. We have to earn our progress.

Only when we recognize on all levels, conscious and subconscious, that we are inherently love-worthy, that we are worthwhile, and that our excessive people-pleasing responses are outdated and unnecessary, will we be able to let those childish behavior patterns go and move forward into an adult life of true self-care and robust self-esteem.

Advanced hypnotherapy can rapidly accelerate this process. When we at last learn to please ourselves—not in a childish, selfish way, but in an honest, nurturing, and loving way—we are freed from our past conditioning and can become the authentic, independent person we were born to be.

As we have seen then, self-esteem has to be earned, and it is earned through the actions that lead us to accomplish. When we push ourselves to go beyond our limiting self-beliefs, challenging ourselves again and again, our self-esteem is automatically enhanced and our self-confidence strengthened.

An excellent way to systematically accomplish anything, from personal inner change to life achievements, is to set goals, both short and long-term, so that our action has clear direction. The SMART mnemonic, often taught in management and self-development classes, is useful here, reminding us to keep our goals:

Specific
Measurable
Attainable
Realistic and
Time-Bound

There are other variants of SMART, but this is the one I have found useful.

When a person first comes to me for help in changing the way they have been feeling or behaving, I ask precisely what it is that they hope to gain from therapy. Many simply say, 'to be happy' or 'to feel better'. But these are very vague goals.

In order to effectively move forward, it is far better to be specific. How would you know if you were happy? What would change? How would you feel if you felt better? What would you be able to do that you can't do now? These are the kind of questions that lead to a more *specific* and *measurable* goal. The more specific we can be with our goals and the more we know how to measure our progress, the more successful we'll be in reaching those goals.

Our goals also need to be *realistic* and *attainable*. We may think we'd like to be a famous singer, for instance, but if we can't carry a tune in a bushel basket, that may be an unrealistic goal to pursue. On the other hand, many unrealistic goals can be drawn into the realm of realistic by setting smaller goals that lead to the big goal. For example, perhaps the person who can't carry a tune could create a goal of taking singing lessons and developing their voice. If they did this and succeeded at learning to sing beautifully, then setting a goal to become a famous singer might no longer be unrealistic. Of course, if we really are tone-deaf, or if all objective feedback tells us our singing grates, then we need to be realistic and perhaps pursue some other goal.

A goal is unrealistic if it is too big a stretch to achieve based on where you are now. If your intended goal is of this nature, it is better to either replace it with another goal, or put it on the back burner and replace it with a stepping-stone goal, and then perhaps other stepping-stone goals—taking on the bigger goal when you've accomplished the smaller ones that lead to it. If you start out with an unrealistic goal, you only discourage yourself and sabotage your efforts. So begin with something doable, and work your way up to great things.

We can—and should—aim for the stars. We need great dreams to live great lives. Mediocre dreams result in mediocre lives. The sky really is the limit, and it is achievable: Each one of us has the potential to become our own Neil Armstrong or our own Richard Branson. Our dreams need to be grand, or we sell ourselves short. But to attain great dreams we must set small goals that build on one another. If we do this, we will climb, step by step, up the ladder of our dreams. It is folly to set only mediocre goals that don't include a map to achieving our most cherished dreams. We must push beyond our limiting beliefs of what we are capable of and strive to become the greatest version of ourselves. Only then will life be lived in joy and fulfillment.

It's wise to give ourselves a *time frame* for any goal so that we stay on track. Having a realistic time frame for accomplishment helps maintain focus and avoid procrastination. Having a deadline keeps things moving forward, but if you need to adjust the deadline, be flexible.

In fact, flexibility is part of the achievement. You may find that, en route to your goal, you must revise your strategies. Rather than feeling discouraged when this happens, realize this is a natural part of the process. We create plans and strategies to achieve our goals based on what we know now, but as we move towards the goal, our knowledge increases, and we typically must revise our plan and strategies to make them practical. Some people don't understand this and equate a strategy that does not work smoothly with failure. Then they give up on their goal and on themselves. Don't let that happen to you. *Expect* that revisions to your plan will periodically be needed (especially if your goal is long-term). Flexibly revisit your plan for achievement, and alter it as needed to make it fit your lifestyle and your needs. If you do this, you will keep on moving forward.

It's important to structure rewards and celebrations into your game plan. These help you keep going after the initial excitement of starting on the path to a new goal wears off. Sometimes the actions you're taking to reach your goal may start to feel boring and routine, like drudgery. When this happens, think of different actions (strategies) that will be more enjoyable and still move you forward. Keep it fresh, and you will stick with it. Part of staying motivated is creating milestones along the way to a long-term goal and celebrating those small achievements. Looking forward to the reward you have promised yourself when you reach the next milestone will help you persevere in moments when you may feel less inspired.

Becoming our true, authentic self—with all the confidence and self-esteem needed to live a good, productive, and fulfilling life—takes work. Sometimes the people who knew the 'old' us find it a little uncomfortable adjusting to this 'new', more confident, more assertive person we are becoming. They may even try to hold us back, hoping to maintain the old familiar status quo. But when we press on with our own inner development, most people will eventually see that the new you, though less easy to manipulate and control, is a better, more secure, and more joyful human being, and probably even more likeable, too. If they really have our best interests at heart, they will learn to welcome and even celebrate the more authentic person they see unfolding before them.

But some of the people in our lives may not have our best interests at heart. Sometimes friends or family members are jealous of the changes they see us making and try to sabotage us, consciously or subconsciously. If you suspect this is happening, protect yourself from that person. If they are someone you cannot eliminate from your life, at least reduce your exposure to their influence. Don't allow insecure, jealous people from your past to keep you stuck in old self-defeating patterns. Dare to be great in spite of them. When you do, you will meet new people, and make new friends who better match the positive, self-confident person you are becoming. Be willing to let old associations dwindle or even fall away if they tug you back from becoming all you wish to be and achieving your great dreams.

Working meaningfully on achieving greater confidence and self-esteem means being committed to change, and change always comes at a cost. Human beings are creatures of habit, so it's not unusual to encounter some degree of resistance to change as the old internal status quo is unsettled and adjusted. When our chi brings such new information, it can feel a bit strange to begin with.

As we progress with our journey, building our self-confidence and earning our self-esteem, we need to understand that feelings of apprehension, nervousness, and sometimes even guilt may manifest themselves, especially when we are asked to act in a self-interested way. Limiting beliefs may surface, placed there long ago—perhaps by parents or teachers—that tell us such things as it's immoral to succeed in a material way, unethical to make a good profit from our labor, or wrong to try to reach beyond 'our station in life'. It is important to understand that these limiting beliefs and the emotions they generate come from our child-like or confused ego states and don't belong to the adult we now are and that we need not be held back by such things. Fortunately, hypnotherapy can help to process and rapidly clear these feelings and the faulty programming that drives them.

With the proper therapy and just a little time, those confused states will become calmer as they learn that asserting yourself and acting in a self-affirming way does not necessarily lead to the rejection or negative consequences that they fear. Eventually all parts of you will come to see that you are safe now, so you really can move forward in confidence.

Self-confidence tells us to go ahead, accept the challenge, and push through any fear that might try to block us. Self-esteem tells us that even if we do fail, we ourselves are not a failure—we will still be all right, and we have what it takes to handle the blow and move on with our life. With continued action and perseverance—and by reaching out beyond the usual, the comfortable, and the familiar—we can accomplish our goals and earn the self-respect that is the foundation of healthy self-esteem.

Remember that a reasonable amount of regular, healthy exercise is also essential for us to feel good in our body and mind. Exercise strengthens our chi, and study after study demonstrates the beneficial effects that exercise has on the way we feel about ourselves. Research has shown beyond any doubt that regular exercise has a positive impact on self-perception and self-esteem, improving mental well-being and life quality in general (Galper et al. 2006; Hassmen et al. 2000; Chaouloff, 1997).

Having high self-esteem and real self-confidence does not mean we will become some kind of Superman or Superwoman, superior to the rest of humanity. It does not mean we will become little buddhas or bodhisattvas, levitating above it all, as we remain blissfully aloof and completely free from anxieties.

We know even confident people sometimes experience feelings of trepidation and fear, and everyone occasionally feels overwhelmed. But self-confidence and high self-esteem permit us to push through those periods.

Self-confidence and self-esteem allow us to act from a place of genuine self-deserving where we are our own best friend. In this authentic state, we are able to accomplish our goals and build on our achievements, growing our self-respect and feeling good about ourselves.

Feeling good about ourselves—regardless of past programming and what we have or have not been taught about ourselves—is the birth right of all of us. The essence of each of us is valid, valuable, and worthwhile. The profound truth is that we come into this world lovable and deserving of love, and all this is part of our unique human heritage, precious and priceless as the chi that flows through us.

As we continue to build our self-confidence and earn our self-esteem, we become free at last to be the person we were born to be, the person we really were all along. And as the Dalai Lama observed, 'With the realization of one's own potential and self-confidence in one's own ability, one can build a better world.'

Chapter Twelve

Balanced Living

'It takes courage to grow up and become who you really are.'
~ e.e. cummings

At the beginning of *The Chi of Change*, I explained that it is not a treatise on Oriental philosophy, or a self-help book, but a guide to the wonderful therapeutic approach called hypnotherapy. In writing, my aim has been to bring clarity to many of the emotional and psychological problems we humans can encounter, and to show how hypnosis combined with good therapy can help in overcoming them.

Throughout the book we have seen how so many of our difficulties are the result of out-dated beliefs and faulty programming, of confused ego states that function in unhelpful ways, and we have seen how hypnotherapy can greatly help in re-processing, realigning, and setting things right.

In this closing chapter, I want to discuss some things that my work as a therapist and my journey as a person have taught me about living a good, balanced, and healthy life because I have found that when we get these things clear, our chi and our lives flow a lot more freely.

Perhaps the most basic understanding that we make as we grow from little babies to full-grown adult human beings is that life is all about relationships. In the beginning, it is about our relationship with our parents and family, and later it is about our relationship with the people we meet as we move out into the world. And, of course, it is about the relationship we have with ourselves.

Let's begin by looking at our relationship with others. Can you imagine a world where you were the last person alive?

Where you would never again hear a voice other than your own, never again look into eyes other than the ones that look back at you from the mirror? It might be a welcome relief for a little while, with no one making demands on your time, energy, or resources, but how long would it be before you longed for other people to share the world with you? When we think about this scenario, it's easy to see how important other people are to us, even though we often take them for granted.

Not all the people we meet on our life's journey are kind, accepting, and easy to get along with, of course. Some care about us, and some are careless, knowingly or unknowingly causing us harm. This is the way it has always been. The person who has never been hurt by another, just as the person who has never hurt another, has yet to be born.

If we are fortunate, we know genuine friendship. If we are very fortunate, we know genuine love. These things make life worthwhile, giving it warmth and depth. Friendship and love sustain us and contribute so much to life's meaning.

As social animals, we are meant to mix with others, to cultivate friendships based on trust and respect. Genuine friendship helps us to develop as people, adding a degree of objectivity to our subjectivity, aiding clarity and balance, and offering support and feedback unavailable elsewhere. With friendship we can join forces with others, sharing the joy and the difficulties, celebrating the seasons of plenty and better enduring the times when hardship comes calling. As the French paleontologist and philosopher Teilhard de Chardin wrote, 'The world is made round so that friendship can encircle it.' And when friendship encircles our world, it's a better, nicer place to be.

The word *friend* can cover a range of different relationships, of course, from the close and intimate friendship with a partner to the friendship based mainly on things such as common interests or shared history. The one thing that all real friendships share, though, is the desire to remain in and to cultivate that friendship.

How many friends does a person need? Well, thoughts differ, and there is really no scientific answer to this question. It depends on what works best for us as individuals. Some people believe two close friends are enough and others believe five or six is the right number. The average number of close friends most people have appears to be around five, but there is a limit to the number of really close friends a person can have before friendship becomes diluted. Our closest friends form the nucleus of our 'friendship network', with others, perhaps ten or so, forming an additional layer. Some of these are family members, and others are people we like and with whom we share common values or interests. Then there are additional layers that include people we talk with on the telephone occasionally or meet up with from time to time and who add to our social world.

Research conducted by Dr Peter DeScioli and Kurzman (2009) at the University of Pennsylvania shows that our feelings about our friends are often based on how our friends feel about us, something called *the alliance hypothesis* of friendship—more evidence of the power feelings have to influence our lives.

While the closest and most enduring friendships may have their roots in a platonic love, friendship is not what we generally think of when we say 'love'. Love can come in so many different forms. It can be the familial love between parent and child, for example, or the platonic love that builds real and lasting friendship. It can be romantic love, or the love involving Eros, the sexual principle that feeds physical desire, and it can also be something higher, something called *agape,* a kind of spiritual love that is completely unconditional and selfless.

Many of us take the love between parent and child for granted. This love seems built into our genes. It is profound and unique, and no one will ever be able to replicate it. We ourselves may have experienced such love, but not every person has been so fortunate. We are born helpless and dependent into this world, relying on the love and kindness of our parents or those who care for us in order to survive, grow, and become independent. This early love, or the lack of it, stays with us in one form or another throughout our lives.

Later in life, we may become the parent to our parent as age takes its toll, perhaps reversing the role of dependence. The slow decline of an aging parent can be one of the hardest things to witness and go through. To see the person who means so much to us, who has been there from the beginning, diminish and fade before our eyes can be absolutely heart breaking. Not only this, but it can make us angry.

At such times—and such times may last for years—it is important to remember the lessons life has taught us. We and those for whom we must now care are passing through a process that inconveniences, annoys, and upsets both them and us. Now is the time for perspective and above all, a time for patience. It is not our mother or father we really are angry at, although they may be the target of such emotion, but rather it is the apparent unfairness of the aging process, the fragility of human life itself.

If we feel anger, it is because life is taking away someone who matters to us, who has always been there and who now is leaving. Though the journey may be long and grueling, wearing down even the strongest, patience and still more patience must be found if we are to do what needs to be done as we are called upon to do it. It is at such times that our love and our spirit are tested.

So many people who consult with me arrive carrying the burden of remorse, an enormous sense of guilt about a parent or loved one they believe they have failed at the very end. All too often they feel they acted selfishly, impatiently, irresponsibly, or childishly—the way they acted so many times in their lives when with Mom or Dad.

The sad language of regret falls from the tongue: 'If only I'd had more patience ...,' 'I could have been kinder ...,' 'I should have done so much more ...,' 'I just wish I'd told her I love her ...,'

'I wish I'd been there for him at the end ...' Though therapy can greatly help with these feelings, it is so much better to have mustered the courage and found the patience necessary to help the person when they were alive—the person who has helped us so much (or who has hurt us); the person without whom we would not be here. No matter what our relationship with our parents has been, it is we who must live with ourselves after they are gone. To know we have done all we could to help them when they needed us frees us from regret. That is truly priceless.

If you or someone you care about is going through this kind of process with an aging relative, do not be afraid to ask for help. Because the emotions you are experiencing are being generated largely in the present, it may well be wise to seek counseling rather than hypnotherapy. Good counseling can offer the emotional support that eases your burden. Your doctor's office should have contact details of a support group, or you can access one online. Most doctors are also able to refer you for one-on-one counseling, often with little or no charge, that will help you to cope better with your situation.

Now let's talk about the kind of love called 'erotic' or 'sexual'. Our love life often begins with physical attraction, and we naturally may feel sexual urges towards someone we find attractive. Although sex is an important aspect of a loving relationship, especially in the beginning where it ignites the fires of passion, any relationship based solely on sex has only a slim chance of staying the course. Eros may well be the first god to enter the arena of love, but he is also the first to leave. With the passage of time, the flame of sexual desire can lose its brilliance, eclipsed by familiarity and routine, and if sexual attraction has not been replaced by something more enduring, it can fade away, taking with it what we mistook for love.

To confuse the passion of sexual attraction with love is to open oneself up to real disappointment, yet this is a confusion so many unhappy people have fallen into. The solution is to awaken from this illusion and then to do something about it—to develop shared values, strengthen the relationship, and find areas of mutual interest and respect where each partner is nurtured. But this is only accomplished through patience and a willingness on both sides to finally say goodbye to childhood and to commit.

Perhaps the form of love we are most familiar with is romantic love. In many ways, this kind of love is the backdrop of our culture. It's the love that singers sing about and that drives the sales of bestselling novels. It's the love featured in Hollywood and Bollywood movies and in sad French films—the kind of love we grew up wholeheartedly believing in or brokenheartedly doubting. Most of us were looking for this kind of love when we married or entered into a relationship. If we 'married for love', chances are that in the beginning Eros fanned the flame. Our partner, triggering the flow of endorphins and hormones such as oxytocin (which plays a huge role in pair bonding), physically attracted us and this fed into our romantic vision of love, filling us with all the heart-fluttering passion that convinced us 'this is the one'.

The difficulty is that this kind of love can also lose its intensity and fade with the passage of time. What once was the raging sea of high romance can eventually dwindle down to the tame backwater of familiarity as the logistics of life—the demands of making a living, paying the bills, raising children, and growing older—begin to take their inexorable toll. When this happens communication can slowly begin to break down as one or both partners find themselves thinking: 'This isn't what I signed up for' or 'This isn't the person I married.'... 'He/she has changed...' And in some ways, they are right. As the writer Lillian Hellman observed: 'People change and forget to tell each other.'

What happens when the honeymoon ends? For so many people, the fading of the rose that is romantic love and its replacement by a predictable sense of the mundane leads sadly on to the gradual demise of the relationship. Feelings of being stuck in a situation where 'love has flown out of the window' can turn what once was a rose garden into a thorny cage. For others, the continual quest to recapture those powerful, endorphin-fuelled feelings of high romance becomes a form of addiction that can lead to failed relationship after failed relationship, and for still others, to marriage after broken marriage.

When we learn to transform romantic love into a deeper love that is built on shared values, consideration, respect, and on genuine partnership and friendship, we can enter into a love that really sustains and endures. The rose of real romance is preserved, not in its original dewy form, but in a form that will last. But this is grown-up love, and it takes effort, humility, and copious amounts of give-and-take. It is love as action, something we do rather than allow—not simply a collection of feelings, but a series of decisions. And this kind of love takes that most human of qualities: the ability to forgive.

In fact, if there is one single element that brings sanity and balance into all of our relationships, be they with a partner or spouse, a mother or father, a brother or sister, our children, family, or friends—or indeed with ourselves—it is simple forgiveness. People make mistakes. Some of these hurt us and some hurt others. Some mistakes are accidental, and some are intentional—after all, it is a real mistake to hurt someone intentionally. When this happens, we can choose to hold onto that hurt and to harbor resentments, but then we condemn ourselves to the life of a victim. Grudges are toxic and resentment can exact the heaviest of tolls. Our anger and resentment permeate our chi and keep us in chains, with a big part of us stuck in the past—stopping us from living the life we were born to live, the freer life we deserve to live.

There is an ancient Chinese saying: 'Hatred corrodes the vessel in which it is stored.' And so, too, does anger. Forgiveness ends the corrosion, erasing hatred and anger, restoring the vessel—our body-mind—and helping us to heal. Perhaps that great Swedish statesman Dag Hammarskjöld put it best when he said: 'Forgiveness is the answer to the child's dream of a miracle by which what is broken is made whole again, and what is soiled is made clean again.' When we approach life with an open heart and an attitude of forgiveness, our relationship with other people, and with ourselves, will be on the surest of footings.

Throughout this book we have seen how the mind can be compared to a powerful biological computer and that mind and body are, in fact, one. Of course, if human beings were nothing more than software and hardware, a sophisticated combination of electro-chemical responses triggered by past programming and biology, we really would be little more than bio-machines. But we are not machines and never will be. The reason has to do with an important aspect of our humanity that machines cannot explain or contain: namely, our spiritual nature.

We may be as fit as an Olympic athlete, eating all the right foods, respecting our body, and treading lightly on the earth. We may have sorted out our past and its faulty programming. We may be getting along with friends, family, and colleagues. But when the light goes off at night, we are left with the person who lives behind our eyes and who must somehow journey on, a person whose identity and needs are not only physical, personal, and social, but also spiritual.

If we ignore this important aspect of ourselves, we ignore the thing that makes us intrinsically human. When we do this, we deny ourselves the balance, fulfillment, and harmony we humans so desire and deserve.

Life is filled with joy and beauty and the most wonderful gifts of friendship and love. But life also has its challenges, and there's no denying it can be hard. Sooner or later we all encounter experiences that shake us to the core. In everyone's life, there are moments of doubt and even sometimes of despair. This has been called 'the dark night of the soul'. At such times—and they can last far longer than a few moments, extending for some people into weeks, months, or even years—we feel alone indeed. It's as if we've reached some kind of ending and have nowhere left to go. The life force within us, our chi, feels completely stalled, our energy almost totally drained. Lost in the increasing darkness of our existence, we begin to lose hope and drift further into what appears to be the meaninglessness of it all.

Does this mean that we have become mentally ill? I think not, and if you have read the book this far, you will know this conviction is part of my philosophy. In fact, not only are such experiences normal at some time in our lives—they are actually essential if we are to become our true and authentic selves. Here, amidst all the chaos, is the opportunity to emerge from our illusion, to free ourselves from whatever myths we have bought into (put there by our culture or our history) and to finally be who we are. It is at moments like these that we begin to separate what we have been taught or programmed to believe (our 'knowledge') from what we ourselves believe (our 'knowing'). In so doing, we discover our genuine selves. And with this discovery comes real change.

Today the medicalization of human behavior, of distress, and of difference, is becoming more pervasive and complete. Medicine is big business. As we saw with depression, many things once regarded as life difficulties are now diagnosed as illnesses. The list of these so-called illnesses grows each time a new manual of mental disorders is published. This approach to human psychology would have us believe there are medical solutions to social, emotional, and even spiritual difficulties, and that solutions can be prescribed and found in pill or capsule form. Not only does this medicalized model completely ignore social causes of distress (such as inequality, poverty, trauma, or abuse) and the individual's unique background of experiences—it completely ignores our spirituality, as if it didn't exist. This means ignoring the most intimate and significant part of who we are.

Far from being an illness, our times of distress—painful, confusing, and unwelcome though they may be—contain within them a wonderful, hidden gift: the gift of transformation. In a lonely, broken state, we can at last hear what our quiet inner voice has been trying so hard to tell us: We simply cannot continue as we have been. We must change. And the change cannot be on the physical or mental level alone. For change to be real, it also has to take place on the spiritual level.

The word 'spiritual' is confusing, if not threatening to many people. Confounding it with religion, we may tell ourselves that we have been running with it all our lives and that we are already believers—or that we have been running as fast as we can in the opposite direction, and we intend to keep right on doing so. Either way, what we miss seeing is that all this restlessness, this running, serves to exhaust us. The fact is that while religion may contain aspects of spirituality, religion does not equate with spirituality.

What then *is* spirituality? It is something personal to each one of us, something that seems to defy definition but that underlies our existence, permeating it at the deepest, subtlest level. Some equate it with consciousness. Some call it the soul.

Strangely enough, our spirituality is something that is often hidden from or denied by the logical mind, which is usually focused outward into the world of activity, away from our quiet, inner self. But no matter how caught up we may become in our outer lives—how we may forget there is more to us than our body, our likes and dislikes, our temperament, and our opinions—our spiritual aspect can be ignored or denied for only so long.

Sometimes our spirituality can catch us unawares, as if we glimpsed ourselves in a mirror, not knowing the mirror was there, thinking that it was someone else. Perhaps we've sensed it in the stillness before dawn, in the colors of the setting sun, or in the quiet grandeur of a forest. It may have been reflected back to us in the eyes of another: a child, a loved one, or an animal. Perhaps we felt it inside a house of worship or listening to a piece of music that transported us to a place we had forgotten existed. We might have sensed it in the movement of the ocean, or as we meditated, pulsing with the rhythm of our breath or heartbeat—that power within the life force, the mysterious chi that permeates all that lives.

At such times we may have been given a hint of what Teilhard de Chardin meant when he said: 'We are not human beings having a spiritual experience. We are spiritual beings having a human experience.' We may have *sensed* our spirituality in any number of places, but we can only really *find* it within our self.

In those long, dark nights of the questioning self, we feel ourselves grind to a halt, our chi urging us to be still, to look beyond the chaos, hear beyond the cacophony. In this enforced inner quiet, we may suddenly encounter what we have been fleeing and desiring at the same time: our spiritual self.

This is the experience that changes endings into beginnings and that starts to make sense of it all. In the inner quiet, we find the self that had been buried in the dust of our own mad rush, our own particular busyness. This self can steer us through fear, unhappiness and confusion and guide us into clarity, vision, and calmness. It is this self—written perhaps with a capital 'S' because it is the deepest, most profound level of our personhood—that seeks meaning in life. And it is this self that can help reveal that meaning.

Many of us come to this self broken and in pain. We may be on antidepressants, sleeping pills, or painkillers; we might be self-medicating through alcohol, drugs, or other behaviors meant to distract us from our discomfort. We might be having anxiety attacks or be haunted by regret. Events, people or relationships might have traumatized us. Perhaps we are full of inexpressible sadness that seems never to lift, or maybe we feel close to breaking because of the weight of a past we have carried for far too long and just cannot seem to set down and leave behind. Whatever has brought us to this point, this crossroads, it will not have been easy and we will have done our best to resist and fight it through whatever means we could find. But still our luan chi runs through us, bringing with it such disturbed energy, such unsettling information—such distressed feelings. We remain confused and lost. We still hurt.

Whatever difficulties bring us to this place of encounter with our inmost self, when that moment happens and the door opens, we never again are the same.

Many people turn to hypnotherapists when they are suffering through such difficult experiences, before they reach the place of self-knowing. And a good, experienced hypnotherapist can bring tremendous relief. As we have seen throughout this book, hypnotherapy can reprocess and re-program the subconscious; it can realign ego states, helping the person become closer to their authentic self or selves. Professional hypnotherapy can greatly assist in helping people become freer, calmer, and clearer within themselves. It can do all of these wonderful things, but it cannot awaken a person to their spirituality or give a person meaning and purpose in life. It is meaning that we truly crave. This is what really kindles the flame in the darkness of mere existence.

As Teilhard de Chardin observed, life is a very special experience—or perhaps more correctly—it is an endless procession of special experiences. Each experience intertwines and interacts with every other experience. And this we have also seen throughout *The Chi of Change*: The meaning people give to their experiences determines the effect those experiences have upon them. Likewise, it is the meaning we give to the experience of life itself that determines the effect our life has—not only on us, but on other people and even on the planet.

How do we have a spiritual experience and how do we find meaning and purpose? A spiritual experience may spontaneously descend upon a person who has suffered greatly or endured great shock. In the First World War, it was reported that soldiers would often drop into a profound state of transcendence when a grenade would land at their feet, lie there, and fail to go off. The shock of the experience suddenly opened to them a level of their being that transcended space and time. Some say people who crave intensely adventuresome experiences, like skydiving or race car driving, rock climbing or surfing waves as high as mountains, are drawn to these activities because they jolt the psyche into that same transcendental state, described by some as 'feeling intensely alive'. In the same way, people who have undergone unbearable suffering often spontaneously drop into this state, and it feels as if the sun has just come out in the sky, after months of storm and hurricane. Many people seek an experience of their inmost self through meditation, self-hypnosis or through hours spent in the presence of nature. Others of course experiment with drugs in an attempt to open 'the doors of perception', to short-circuit the process through exogenous substances such as peyote, mescaline, magic mushrooms, LSD, and ibogaine.

But how does a person find meaning? The trick is to change the word *find* to the word *choose*. We don't actually *find* meaning in life—we choose it; we assign it. Life's meaning is different for different people. For some, it is making a lot of money or perhaps acquiring fame or power. For others, it is being a good citizen or doing one's duty. For others, it is joyful expression, creativity, or learning and wisdom. For others, it is adventure; or helping people, animals or the planet; being a good mother, father or friend, and for still others, it lies in assisting people to find greater clarity so that they can discover their own meaning in life.

There is no one single meaning to existence. There are many to choose from. I know there are religions and philosophies that disagree with this statement. If the meaning these belief systems assign to life works for you—if it doesn't hold you back and harm you or anyone else—then that's okay. Why not choose their meaning?

Yet externally acquired meanings can never be every person's meaning, just as my meaning may not be your meaning, and your meaning does not have to be something you read in a book—this one included—or that someone else told you about, no matter how recently or how long ago. Meaning really isn't a 'one size fits all' kind of thing.

Existence is too vast and life's experience too rich and diverse to settle on one catch-all meaning for everyone who lives. Life does not need one single meaning, nor can it be restricted to that. Perhaps there are as many meanings as there are people. Once we let go of the idea that there has to be 'a' meaning, we free ourselves to live in a different way; we become more flexible, more spontaneous. We listen to what *we* feel and think about living and become more ourselves. When we come to understand that life has the meaning we *choose* to give it and the meaning we give to our life does not have to be static but something that can change and evolve as *we* change and evolve, then we begin at last to live more authentically.

The same is true for our life's purpose. It is *you* who decide your life's purpose. Honoring the values you hold precious—the things that really matter to you—you *decide* the purpose that is uniquely yours. Who do you want to become? What do you want to achieve or express or experience? Do you want to be a well-rounded person? Someone you yourself would like to be friends with? Someone others can look up to and respect? Someone who achieves things of substance? Someone who does good in the world? Someone who contributes to our understanding of the world and of the life with which we have been gifted? A respected teacher? A great dancer, artist, or scientist? Perhaps you'll choose a quiet but profound purpose, like helping others, spreading more hope or joy in the world.

The point is that *we* get to decide our purpose and create our personal vision. When these are authentic and based on our genuine inmost feelings and desires, we will hold to our life's purpose through thick and thin, even when life experiences challenge us. It is *we* who choose who we will be and what we are going to do with our all too brief time on Earth.

In his book *Man's Search for Meaning,* Auschwitz survivor and psychiatrist Viktor Frankl writes: 'Man does not simply exist, but always decides what his existence will be, what he will become in the next moment.' With purpose and meaning in our lives, and with a sense of our own spiritual nature, we are capable of greatness.

Perhaps you will think me an idealist, and I am content to be called that. I have even been called 'one of life's enthusiasts', and I am happy about that label, too. After all, I *am* enthusiastic about life, and I believe people have a *need* to be idealists. We need to aim for the stars and see what we are capable of at our best. We will never aim for the stars if we think the achievement of dreams and greatness are impossible.

If we treat people with respect and can see past their surface quirks to their inner potential, we help them to draw out that inner greatness. The German philosopher Goethe made this point when he said, 'If you treat an individual as he is, he will remain how he is. But if you treat him as if he were what he ought to be and could be, he will become what he ought to be and could be.' When we recognize this, it alters our perspective on other people, as well as on ourselves. We change for the better, and our sense of life's purpose and meaning expands and deepens.

Living peacefully—with respect, purpose, and meaning—enables us to exist in harmony with our chi—in balance with ourselves, with our fellow creatures, and with the earth on which we miraculously walk. In this harmony, we may come to recognize and express our inmost potential, our spiritual nature, that which was waiting for us all the time, somewhere deep within.

I hope this book has helped to bring more clarity and an even greater sense of hope to your life and that it has shown you how hypnotherapy can play a continuing part in this. We humans really *are* capable of greatness. You are human, so *you* are capable of being great, of living a good life—one that has meaning and purpose for you. Make it a life as special and wonderful as you are—your own carved out, self-created, personal destiny. You really are unique.

And now, finally, I want to ask you to do something for me. It's what Christopher Robin asked that loveable bear Winnie the Pooh to do in the story that is part of so many people's childhood memories: 'Promise me you'll always remember: You're braver than you believe, stronger than you seem, and smarter than you think.'

May your chi flow and guide you safely home to yourself.

References and Relevant Reading

Chapter One

A.A. The Big Book (1939) New York: Alcoholics Anonymous Services

Berdanier C.D. (2000) *Advanced Nutrition: Macronutrients, Micronutrients, 2nd edition.* CRC Press

Boyne G. (1989) *Transforming Therapy.* Westwood Publishing

Coward H. (1996) *Taoism and Jung: Synchronicity and the Self.* Philosophy

Elman D. (1964) *Hypnotherapy.* Westwood Publishing

Emmerson G. (2003) *Ego State Therapy.* Crown House Publishing

Flew A. (1979) *A Dictionary of Philosophy.* London: Pan Books

Freud S. (1920) *Beyond the Pleasure Principle (ed. 2003).* Penguin Modern Classics

François de la Rochefoucauld (1613-1680) *Maxims.* Oxford University Press

Frith C. (2007) *Making Up the Mind: How the Brain Creates Our Mental World.* Blackwell Publishing

Gropper SS, Smith JL. (2009) *Advanced Nutrition and Human Metabolism, 5th edition.* Wadsworth Gengage Learning

Jung C. (1961) *Memories, Dreams, Reflections.* Random House

Jung C. (1951) *Foreword to the English Version of The I-Ching,* trans. Richard Wilhelm, Routledge

Kipling R. 'IF' (1910) *Rewards and Fairies*

Kozorovitsky Y, Gross G, Kopil C, et al. (2005) Experience induces structural and biochemical changes in the adult primate brain, *Proceedings of the National Academy of Sciences, 102*:17478-17482

Lao Tsu (100 BC) *The Tao Te Ching (ed. 2011).* Vintage Books

Moncrieff J. (2008) *The myth of the chemical cure: A critique of psychiatric drug treatment.* Palgrave Macmillan

Neibuhr R. (1937) First publication of what was to become

known as *'The Serenity Prayer'* in US Christian student publication

Nin A. (1932) *D.H. Lawrence: An Unprofessional Study*. Paris: Edward Titus

Proust M. (1913-27) *À la recherche du temps perdu ('Remembrance of Things Past', or 'In Search of Lost Time')*. Eng. Wordsworth Editions, 1960

Star J. (2001) *Tao Te Ching: Definitive Edition. Translation and Commentary of Lao Tsu*. Tarcher/Penguin Books

Wilhelm R. (1951) *I Ching or Book of Changes*. English Edition, Routledge

Chapter Two

Banyan C. (2003) *The Secret Language of Feelings*. Banyan Publishing, Inc.

Bear MF, Connors BW, Paradiso MA. (2007) *Neuroscience: Exploring the Brain*. Lippincott Williams & Wilkins

Borysenko J. (1988) *Minding the Body, Mending the Mind*. Bantam Books

Cohen KS. (1997) *The Way of Qiqong*. Ballantine Books

Conrad P. (2007) *The Medicalization of Society: On the transformation of human conditions into treatable disorders*. Johns Hopkins Press

Cornelius R. (1996) *The Science of Emotion*. New Jersey: Prentice Hall

Dalgleish T. (2004) *The emotional brain*. Nature: Perspectives, 5, 582–89

Damasio AR. (2000) *The Feeling of What Happens: Body and emotion in the making of consciousness*. New York: Harcourt Brace

Davis PJ. (1999) Gender differences in autobiographical memory for childhood emotional experiences. *Personal Social Psychology 6, 3*: 498-5107

DSM-IV, Diagnostic and Statistical Manual of Mental Disorders. (2000) American Psychiatric Association

Denton DA. (2006) *The Primordial Emotions: The Dawning Of Consciousness*. Oxford University Press

Ellsworth PC, Scherer KR. (2003) Appraisal processes in emotion. *Handbook of Affective Sciences*. Oxford University Press

English A, Stengel B. (2010) Exploring fear: Rousseau, Dewey, and Freire on fear and learning, *Educational Theory, 60, 5*:521-542

Fiori M. (2009) A new look at emotional intelligence: a duel process framework. *Personality and Social Psychology Review February 2009 13:* 21-44

Frith CD. (2007) *Making Up the Mind: How the Brain Creates Our Mental World*. Blackwell Publishing

Guilia G, Noham W, Leun JO. (2011) Sex differences in the use of anticipatory brain activity to encode emotional events. *Journal of Neuroscience, 31, 34*:12364 –12370

Gerhardt S. (2004) *Why Love Matters: How affection shapes a baby's brain*. Brunner-Routledge

Gershon M. (1998) *The Second Brain*. HarperCollins

Glatzer ed. (1974) *I Am a Memory Come Alive: Autobiographical Writings by Franz Kafka*. Schocken

Gray J. (1993) *Men Are From Mars, Women Are From Venus*. Harper Collins

Horwitz A. (2003) *Creating Mental Illness*. University of Chicago Press

Jung C. (2010) *Four Archetypes*. Princeton University Press

Kaptchuk TD. (1983) *The Web that Has No Weaver*. Congdon & Wead Inc.

Kaltenmark M. (1969) *Lao Tzu and Taoism*. Stanford University Press

Le Doux JE. (1996) *The Emotional Brain: The Mysterious Underpinnings of Emotional Life*. New York: Simon & Schuster

Le Doux JE. (1998) Fear and the brain, *Biological Psychiatry, 44,* 1229-1238

Lipton BH. (2005) *The Biology of Belief*. Hay House

Nussbaum MC. (2001) *Upheavals of Thought: The Intelligence of Emotions*. Cambridge University Press

Myers DG. (2004) *Theories of Emotion, Psychology: 7th Edition*. New York: Worth Publishing

Oatley K, Jenkins JM. (1996) *Understanding Emotions*. Oxford: Blackwell.

Ohman A. (2000). Fear and anxiety: Evolutionary, cognitive, and clinical perspectives. In M. Lewis & J. M. Haviland-Jones (Eds.), *Handbook of Emotions*. Guilford Press

Ohman A, Soanes JJF. (1998) Emotional conditioning to masked stimuli: expectancies for aversive outcomes following non-recognized fear-relevant stimuli. *Journal of Experimental Psychology, General, vol 127*, 69-82

Pert C. (1997) *Molecules of Emotion: The Science Behind Mind-Body Medicine*. New York: Scribner

Pessoa L. (2008) On the Relationship between emotion and cognition. *Nature Review Neuroscience* 9:148–158

Phelps EA. (2004) Human Emotion and Memory: interactions of the amygdala and hippocampal complex. *Current Opinion in Neurobiology, 14*, 196-202

Plutchik R. (2002) *Emotions and Life: Perspectives from Psychology, Biology, and Evolution*. Washington, DC: American Psychological Association

Rolls ET. (1999) *The Brain and Emotion*. Oxford University Press

Sarno JE. (2006) *The Divided Mind*. Regan Books

Scarantino A. (2010) Insights and blind spots of the cognitivist theory of emotions. *British Journal for the Philosophy of Science, vol 61, issue 4*, 729-768

Seigal DJ. (1999) *The Developing Mind: How Relationships and the Brain Interact to Shape Who We Are*. Guilford Press

Solomon R. (1993) *The Passions: Emotions and the Meaning of Life*. Indianapolis: Hackett Publishing

Thoreau HD. (1854) *Walden (ed. 2004)*. Bantam

Waley A. (1958) *The Way and its Power: A Study of the Tao Te Ching and its Place in Chinese Thought.* Grove Press

Chapter Three

Adler A. (1927) *Understanding Human Nature*. Oneworld

Boyne G. (1989) *Transforming Hypnotherapy.* Westwood Publishing

Cameron OG. (2007) Understanding comorbid depression and anxiety. *Psychiatric Times, 24, 14.*

Dai-Ja Jang, Myeong Soo Lee, Byung-Cheul Shin, et al. (2008) Red ginseng for treating erectile dysfunction: a systematic review. *British Journal of Clinical Pharmacology, 66,* 4:444–450

De Andrade, E, De Mesquita, AA, De Almeida C, et al. (2007) Study of the efficacy of Korean Red Ginseng in the treatment of erectile dysfunction. *Asian Journal of Andrology, 9, 2*:241–244

Ellman D. (1964) *Hypnotherapy*. Westwood Publishing

Frith CD. (2007) *Making Up the Mind: How the Brain Creates Our Mental World*. Blackwell Publishing

Helmy MM, Senbel AM. (2012) Evaluation of vitamin E in the treatment of erectile dysfunction in aged rats. *Life Sciences, 9, 90 (13-14)*:489-94

Hughes RN. (June 1996) Drugs which induce anxiety: caffeine. *New Zealand Journal of Psychology, 25 (1)*: 36–42

Lao Tsu. *The Tao Te Ching* (ed. 2011). Vintage Books

Mahajan SK, Prasa, AS, McDonald FD. (1984) Sexual dysfunction in uremic male: Improvement following oral zinc supplementation. *PubMed, Contributions to Nephrology, 38:*103-11

Merry T. (2002) *Learning and Being in Person-Centered Counselling.* PCCS Books

Moncrieff J. (2008) *The Myth of the Chemical Cure: A critique of psychiatric drug treatment*. Palgrave Macmillan

Ng CF, Lee CP, Ho AL, Lee VW. (2011) Effect of niacin on erectile function in men suffering erectile dysfunction and dyslipidemia. *Journal of Sexual Medicine, 8, 10*:2883-93

Spector G. (2012) *Identically Different: Why You Can Change Your*

Genes. Weidenfeld & Nicolson

Seigal DJ. (1999) *The Developing Mind: How Relationships and the Brain Interact to Shape Who We Are*. Guilford Press

Sprenger KB, Schmitz J, Hetzel D, Bundschu D, Franz HE. (1984) Zinc and sexual dysfunction. *PubMed, Contributions to Nephrology. 38*:119-28.

van Deurzen E. (2002) *Existential Counselling and Psychotherapy in Practice*. Sage Publications

Zhang CG, Kim SJ. (2007) Taurine induces anti-anxiety by activating strychnine-sensitive glycine receptor in vivo. *Annals of Nutrition and Metabolism*

Chapters Four and Five

Abdou AM, Higashiguchi S, Horie K, et al. (2006) Relaxation and immunity enhancement effects of Gamma-Aminobutyric Acid (GABA) administration in humans. *Biofactors. 26,* 3:201-8

Angst J, Davidson J, Keller M, et al. (1998) *Social Phobia - A Comprehensive Course for Medical Practitioners*. World Psychiatric Association

Anxiety and Depression Society of America (2012) from http://www.adaa.org/about-adaa/press-room/facts-statistics

Australian Institute of Health and Welfare (1998) *National Health Priority Areas Mental Health: A Report Focusing on Depression*. 'Depression statistics in Australia are comparable to those of the United States.'

Ayers S. (2007) Weinman, A., et al. eds. *Cambridge Handbook of Psychology, Health and Medicine, 2nd edition*. Cambridge University Press

Barlow DH. (2004) *Anxiety and Its Disorders, 2nd edition*. Guilford Press

British Journal of Psychiatry (2006) *May, 188*: 432-8.

Broman-Fulks JJ, Berman ME, et al. (2004) Effects of exercise on anxiety sensitivity. *Behavior Research and Therapy*

Bruce TJ, Sayeed SA. (1999) Social anxiety disorder: A common, under-recognized mental disorder. *American Family Physician, Nov 15; 60(8):*2311-2320

Bruce M, Lader M. (1989) Caffeine abstention and the management of anxiety disorders. *Psychol Med, 19*: 211-14

Cowely D.S., & Roy-Byrne, P.P (1991) The biology of GAD and chronic anxiety. In R. Rapee & D.H.Barlow, *Chronic anxiety: Generalized anxiety disorder and mixed aniety-depression*: 52-75. New York: Guilford Press

Darwin C. (1872) *The Expression of the Emotions in Man and Animals. 3rd Edition. 1998.* Harper Collins

El Idrissi A, et al. (2009) Effects of Taurine on Anxiety-like and Locomotor Behavior of Mice. *Advances in Experimental Medicine and Biology, 643:* 207-215

Graeff FG. (2002) On Serotonin and Experimental Anxiety. *Psychopharmacology, 163, 3-4*: 467-476

Howard K, Kopta S, et al. (1986) The dose-effect relationship in psychotherapy, special issue: Psychotherapy research. *American Psychologist, 41 (2)* 159-164

Hughes RN. (1996) Drugs which induce anxiety: caffeine. *New Zealand Journal of Psychology 25 (1):* 36–42

ICD-10: The ICD-10 Classification of Mental and Behavioral Disorders: Clinical Descriptions and Diagnostic Guidelines. *World Health Organization*

Kessler RC, McGonagle KA, Zhao S, et al. (1994) Lifetime and 12 Month Prevalence of DSM-3-R Psychiatric Disorders in the USA. In a survey of 8,098 people, the National Comorbidity Survey found that 6.6% of respondents noted that they experienced a fear of using the toilet away from home.

Kinsey AC. (1948) *Sexual Behavior in the Human Male.* Indiana University Press

Kessler CR, Demier O, Frank RG, et al. (2005) Prevalence and treatment of mental disorders. *The New England Journal of Medicine*

Kessler R, Stein MB, Berglund P. (1998) Social phobia subtypes in the national comorbidity survey. *American Journal of Psychiatry, 155*: 613-619

Kimura K, Ozeki M, Juneja LR, Ohira H. (2007) L-Theanine reduces psychological and physiological stress responses. *Biological Psychology 74,* 1:39-45

Kong WX, Chen SW, et al. (2006) Effects of taurine on rat behaviors in three anxiety models. *Pharmacology Biochemistry and Behavior, Volume 83,* 2:271-276

Lang PJ. Davis M, Ohman A. (2000) Fear and anxiety: Animal models and human cognitive psychophysiology. *Journal of Affective Disorders*

Lépine JP. (2006) The epidemiology of anxiety disorders: Prevalence and societal costs. *Journal of Clinical Psychiatry, 63 Suppl* 14:4-8

Lickey JA, Gordon B. (1991) 'Anxiety is a mental disorder when it is more intense than is justified by the actual threat.' *Medicine and Mental Illness.* Freeman

Lindenbaum J, et al. (1998) Neuropsychiatric disorders caused by cobalamin deficiency in the absence of anemia or macrocytois. *New England Journal of Medicine 318:*1720-1728

Lindsay SJE, Powell GE. eds. (1998) *The Handbook of Clinical Adult Psychology. 2nd edition.* Routledge

Lydiard RB. (2003) The Role of GABA in anxiety disorders. *Journal of Clinical Psychiatry, 64 Suppl 3*:21-27

Nagaswa H. (2011) 'Among humans, the ability to accurately recognize other people's expressions and judge their emotions is a vital social skill. This study has shown that dogs that live closely with humans are also able to recognize positive facial expressions, indicating that these dogs have acquired the social skills helpful to survive.' 26 February, 2011, Animal Cognition (As reported in *World Science, retrieved March 2013.*) from www.world-science.net/exclusives/110302_dogs.htm

National Comorbidity Survey (NCS) and National Comorbidity Survey Replication (NCS-R) (2005). Harvard School of

Medicine

National Institute for Health and Clinical Excellence (2011) Clinical guideline on the diagnosis and treatment of social phobia (social anxiety disorder)

USA National Institute of Mental Health from http://www.nimh.nih.gov/statistics/1anyanx_adult.shtml

Nazareth I, Boynton P, King M. (2003) Problems with sexual function in people attending London general practitioners: cross sectional study. *British Medical Journal, 23; 327(7412)423*

NHS Choices. (2010) 'PTSD affects up to 30% of people who experience a traumatic event. It affects around 5% of men and 10% of women at some point during their life.' Retrieved February, 2012, from http://www.nhs.uk/conditions/post-traumatic-stress-disorder/pages/introduction.aspx

Mason R. (2001) L-theanine boosts alpha waves, promotes alert relaxation. *Alternative and Complimentary Therapies, 7*:91-95

Murray M, Pizzzorno J. (1998) *Encyclopedia of Natural Medicine, Revised 2nd edition*. Rocklin, CA: Prima Publishing

Rogers C. (1961) *On Becoming a Person*. Boston: Houghton Mifflin

Salmon P. (2001) Effects of physical exercise on anxiety, depression and sensitivity to stress: a unifying theory. *Clinical Psychology Reviews, 21*, 36-61

Sareen J, Cox BJ, Tracie OA, et al. (2005) Anxiety disorders and risks for suicide ideation and suicide attempts: a population-based longitudinal study of adults. *Archives of General Psychiatry. 2005;62(11)*:1249-1257

Shorter E. (2008) *The Troubled History of Mood Disorders in Psychiatry*. Oxford University Press

Smith ML. (1977) Meta-analysis of psychotherapy outcome studies. *American Psychologist, 32 (9)* 752-760

Smith ML. (1982) What research says about the effectiveness of psychotherapy. *Hospital and Community Psychiatry, 33 (6)* 457-461

Smits AJ, Otto M.W. (2000) *Exercise for mood and anxiety disorders.*

Oxford University Press

Smits JAJ, Zvolensky MJ. (2006) Emotional vulnerability as a function of physical activity among individuals with panic disorder. *Depression and Anxiety, 23*, 102-106

Somers JM, Goldner EM, Waraich P, Hsu L. (February 2006) prevalence and incidence studies of anxiety disorders: a systematic review of the literature. *Canadian Journal of Psychiatry, 51 (21):* 100-13

Standal S. (1954) *The Need for Positive Regard: A contribution to client-centered theory*. University of Chicago

Stein MB, Gorman, JM. (2001) Unmasking social anxiety disorder. *Journal of Psychiatric Neuroscience, May; 26(3):* 185–189

Symons J, Carey MP. (2001) Prevalence of sexual dysfunction: Results from a decade of research. *Archives of Sexual Behaviors, 30, 2:* 177-219

Tsuang MT, Bar JL, Stone WS, Faraone SV. (2004) Gene-environment interactions in mental disorders. *World Psychiatry, June; 3 (2);* 73-83

Waldinger MC, et al. (2005) A multinational population survey on intravaginal ejaculation latency time. *Journal of Sexual Medicine* 2: 492-497

Weisberg RB. (2009) Overview of generalized anxiety disorder: epidemiology, presentation, and course. *Journal of Clinical Psychiatry*

World Health Organization (2009) Global Perspectives on Mental-Physical Comorbidity in the WHO World Mental Health Surveys

Zhang CG, Kim SJ. (2007) Taurine induces anti-anxiety by activating strychnine-sensitive glycine receptor in vivo. *Annals of Nutrition and Metabolism*

Chapters Six and Seven

Ayers S. Weinman A, et al. eds. (2007) *Cambridge Handbook of Psychology, Health and Medicine. 2nd edition.* Cambridge

University Press

Austen. (2006) *The Owner's Manual for the Brain: Everyday Applications from Mind-Brain Research, 3rd edition.* Bard Press

Beezhold BL, Johnston CS, Daigle DR. (2010) Department of Nutrition, Arizona State University. Vegetarian diets are associated with healthy mood states: A cross-sectional study in Seventh Day Adventist adults. *Nutritional Journal. 1, 9*:26

Bentall RP. (2009) *Doctoring the Mind: Why psychiatric treatments fail; Allen Lane edition, 2010.* Penguin Books

Blumenthal JA, et al. (2007) Exercise and pharmacotherapy in the treatment of major depressive disorder. *Psychosom Med. 69*

Bosely S, Evans R. (2008) *Drug Giants Accused over Doctor's Perks.* The Guardian Saturday 23 August 2008

Bourre JM. (2005) Dietary Omega-3 fatty acids and psychiatry: mood, behavior, stress, depression, dementia and aging. *The Journal of Nutrition Health Aging. Vol. 9*: 31-8

Brady K. (2001) *Clinical challenges: Anxiety and substance abuse.* Program and abstracts of the 154th Annual Meeting of the American Psychiatric Association; May 5-10, 2001

Breggin PR. (2008, 2nd Edition) *Brain Disabling Treatments in Psychiatry: Drugs, electroshock and the role of the FDA.* New York: *Springer Publishing Co.*

Breen G, Todd Webb B, Butler AW, et al. (2011) A genome-wide significant linkage for severe depression on chromosome 3: the depression network study. *American Journal of Psychiatry*

British Journal of Psychiatry, (2006) *May; 188;*432-8

Chouinard G, et al. (1990) A pilot study of magnesium hydrochloride (magnesiocard) as a mood stabilizer for rapid cycling bipolar affective disorder patients. *Progress Neuro-Psychopharmacology & Biological Psychiatry, vol 14;* 2, 171-80

Conrad P. (2007) *The Medicalization of Society: On the transformation of human conditions into treatable disorders.* Johns Hopkins Press

Coppen A, Bolander-Gouaille C. (2005) Treatment of depression:

Time to consider folic acid and vitamin B12. *Journal of Psychopharmacology,19,1*:59-65

Craft L. (2004) Benefits of exercise for the clinically depressed. *Journal of Clinical Psychiatry, Primary Care Companion, Vol 6*: 104-111

Department for Work and Pensions/Department of Health (2009). *Working Our Way to Better Mental Health: A framework for action.* London

Depression Alliance, www.depressionalliance.org

Devane CL, Chiao E, Franklin M, Kruep EJ. (2005) Anxiety disorders in the 21st century: status, challenges, opportunities, and comorbidity with depression. *American Journal of Managed Care, 11 (12):* S344-353

Doe-Young K, Camilleri M. (2000) *Serotonin: A Mediator of the Brain-Gut Connection.* Gastroenterology Research Unit, Mayo Clinic and Mayo Foundation. Rochester, Minnesota

Giannini AJ. (2002) Magnesium oxide augmentation of verapamil maintenance therapy in Mania. *Psychiatry Research.14*;9391:83-7

Gunnel D, Saperia J, Ashby D. (2005) Selective serotonin reuptake inhibitors (SSRIs) and suicide in adults: A meta analysis of drug company data from placebo controlled trials submitted to the MHRA's safety review. *British Medical Journal, 330* (7488), 385

DSM-IV, Diagnostic and statistical manual of mental disorders (2000) *American Psychiatric Association*

Harrington A. (1999) *The Placebo Effect: An interdisciplinary exploration.* Harvard University Press

Högberg G, Gustafsson SA, Hällström T, et al. (2012) Depressed adolescents in a case-series were low in vitamin D and depression was ameliorated by vitamin D supplementation. *Acta Paediatrica, 101, 7*:779-783

Hoang MT, Defina LF, Willis BL, Leonard DS, Weiner MF, Brown ES. (2011) Association between low serum 25-hydroxyvitamin

D and depression in a large sample of healthy adults. *The Cooper Center longitudinal study, 86, 11*:1050-5

Hotchner AE. (1955) *Papa Hemingway: A Personal Memoir*. De Capo Press

Glenmullen J. (2005) *The Antidepressant Solution: A Step-by-Step Guide to Safely Overcoming Antidepressant Withdrawal, Dependence, and Addiction*. Free Press

Gutzler A. (2006) *Perinatal Depression Focus Group Report*. Perinatal Connections

ICD-10: The ICD-10 Classification of Mental and Behavioral Disorders: *Clinical Descriptions and Diagnostic Guidelines*. World Health Organization

Illinois Department of Public Health, *Facts about Postpartum Depression*

Janis IL, Astrachan M. (1951) The Effect of electroconvulsive treatment on memory efficiency. *Joural of Abnormal Psychology 46*, 501-11

Jasper, A. (2009) *Exercise for Mood & Anxiety Disorders*. Oxford University Press

Jones JE. (1974) 'Non-ECT', *World Medicine, Sept. 1974, 24*

Johnstone L. (2000, 2nd ed) *Users and Abusers of Psychiatry*. Routledge

Johnstone L. (1999) Adverse Psychological Effects of ECT. *Journal of Mental Health 8*, 69-85

Jureidini JN, McHenry LB, Mansfield PR. (2008) Clinical trials and drug promotion: selective reporting of study 329. *International Journal of Risk and Safety in Medicine, 20*(1-2), 73-81

Kahn A, Levanthal RM, et al. (2002) Severity of depression and response to antidepressants and placebo: An analysis of the food and drug administration database. *Journal of Clinical Psychopharmacology, 22(1)*, 40-5

Kendler KS, Gallagher TJ, Abelson JM, Kessler RC. (1996) Lifetime prevalence, demographic risk factors, and diagnostic validity of nonaffective psychosis as assessed in a us community sample. the national comorbidity survey. *Archive of Genenal Psychiatry, 53*:1022-1031

Khan A, Khan S, Kolts R, Brown WA. (2003) Suicide rates in clinical trials of SSRIs, other antidepressants and placebo: Analysis of FDA reports. *American Journal of Psychiatry 160(4)*, 790-2

Kendell RE. (1998) 'What are Royal Colleges for?' *Psychiatric Bulletin 22;* 721-3.

Kessler CR, Demier O, Frank RG, et al. (2005) Prevalence and treatment of mental disorders. *The New England Journal of Medicine*

Kirsch I, Deacon BJ, Huendo-Medina TB, et al. (2008) Initial severity and antidepressant benefits: A meta-analysis of data submitted to the food and drug administration

Kirsch I. (2009) *The Emperor's New Drugs: Exploding the Antidepressant Myth*. New York: Basic Books

Lacasse JR, Leo J. (2005) Serotonin and depression: A disconnect between the advertisements and the scientific literature. *PLOS Medicine 2(12)*, e392

Lancet (2012) Living with grief. *The Lancet, 379* (9816)

Lasagna L, Masteller F, et al. (1954) A study of the placebo response, *American Journal of Medicine 16*, 770-9

Lester H. (2005) Shared care for people with mental illness: a gp's perspective, advances for psychiatric treatment. *The Royal College of Psychiatrists*

Lindenbaum J, et.al. (1998) Neuropsychiatric disorders caused by cobalamin deficiency in the absence of anemia or macrocytois. *New England Journal of Medicine 318:*1720-1728

Luby JL. (2010) Preschool depression: The importance of identification of depression early in development. *Current Trends in Psychological Science, August 2010; 19*(4)

Maes M. (1994) *Journal of Affective Disorders 42*(5):349-358. 5-140

Maes M, et al. (1997) 'Lower serum zinc in major depression is a sensitive marker of treatment resistance and of the immune/inflammatory response in that illness' *Bioogical Psychiatry: 31*(2):13

Maes M, et al. (1998) Fatty acids, cytokines, and major depression. *Biological Psychiatry, 43*:313-14

Martins JG. (2009) 'EPA but not DHA Appears to be Responsible for the Efficacy of Omega-3 Long Chain Polyunsaturated Fatty Acid Supplementation in Depression: Evidence from a Meta-Analysis of Randomized Controlled Trials'. *Journal of American College of Nutrition, 28, 5*:525-42

McLean B. (2001) A Bitter Pill. *Fortune.* 13 August, 2001

Melander H, Ahlqvist-Rastad J, Meijer G, Beerman B. (2003) Evidence b(i)ased medicine – selective reporting from studies sponsored by pharmaceutical industry: review of studies in new drug applications. *British Medical Journal, 326(7400)*, 1171-3

Mind, Executive Report (May 2007) *Ecotherapy: The Green Agenda for Mental Health*

Mischoulon D, Fava M. (2002) Role of S-adenosyl-L-methionine (SAMe) in the treatment of depression: a review of the evidence. Harvard Medical School, Depression Clinical and Research Program. *American Journal of Clinical Nutrition, 76, 5*:1158S-61S

Mischoulon D, Raab MF. (2007) The role of folate in depression and dementia. *Journal of Clinical Psychiatry, 68(Suppl 10)*:28–33

Moncrieff J. (2006) *The Myth of the Chemical Cure: A critique of psychiatric drug treatment*. Palgrave Macmillan

Moncrieff J. (2008) The creation of the concept of the antidepressant : An historical analysis. *Social Science and Medicine*

Munk-Olsen T, Laursen T, Videbech P, et al. (2007) All cause mortality among recipients of electroconvulsive therapy. *British Journal of Psychiatry, 190*, 435-439

Murray M, Pizzzorno J. (1998) *Encyclopedia of Natural Medicine, Revised 2nd edition* Rocklin, CA: Prima Publishing

National Institute for Health and Clinical Excellence (UK) (2004) *Depression: Management of Depression in Primary and Secondary Care*

National Institute of Mental Health (USA): The Numbers Count: Mental Illness in America. *Science on Our Minds Fact Sheet Series*

National Sleep Foundation, USA. (2012) Retrieved February 2012, from http://www.sleepfoundation.org/article/sleep-related-problems/sleep-aids-and-insomnia

Nestler EJ, et al. (2002) Neurobiology of depression. *Neuron 34*:13–25.

O'Hara MW, Swain AM. (1996). Rates and risk of postpartum depression – a meta-analysis. *International Review of Psychiatry 8*: 37–54

Olofson M, Blanco C, et al. (2006) National trends in the outpatient treatment of children and adolescents with antipsychotic drugs. *Archives of General Psychiatry*

Parker G. et al. (2006) Omega-3 fatty acids and mood disorders. *American Journal of Psychiatry 163 (10):*184

Parker G, Brotchie H. (2011) 'D' for depression: Any role for vitamin D? Food for Thought II. *Acta Psychiatry Scand 124, 4*:243-249

Paulson JA. (2010) Focusing on depression in expectant and new fathers: prenatal and postpartum depression not limited to mothers. *Psychiatry Times, 27* (2)

Peet M, Horrobin DF. (2002) A dose-ranging study of the effects of ethyl-eicosapentaenoate (EPA) in patients with ongoing depression despite apparently adequate treatment with standard drugs. *Archives of General Psychiatry 59, 10*:913-9

Pratt L, Brody DJ, Gu Q. Antidepressant use in persons aged 12 and over: United States, 2005-2008. *NCHS Data Brief No 76*. October 2011

Reeves GM, Nijjar GV, Langenberg P, et al. (2012) 'Improvement in depression scores after 1 hour of light therapy treatment in patients with seasonal affective disorder.' *Journal of Nervous and Mental Disease 200,* 1:51-5.J

Roberts M. (2010) Post-natal depression in men 'often undiagnosed', BBC News, 18 May, 2010, retrieved March 2013 from http://news.bbc.co.uk/1/hi/health/8687189.stm

Rose D, Fleischmann P, Wykes T, et al. (2003) Patients' perspectives on electroconvulsive therapy: Systematic review. *British Medical Journal, 326,* 1363–1367

Ross C. (2006) The sham ECT literature: Implications for consent to ECT. *Ethical Human Psychology and Psychiatry*

Sackheim H, Prudic J, Devanand J., et al. (1993) Effects of stimulus intensity and electrode placement on the efficacy and cognitive effects of electroconvulsive therapy. *New England Journal of Medicine, 328,* 839-846

Sackheim H, Prudic J, Fuller R, et al. (2007) The cognitive effects of electroconvulsive therapy in community settings. *Neuropharmacology*

Salmon P. (2001) Effects of physical exercise on anxiety, depression and sensitivity to stress: A unifying theory. *Clinical Psychology Reviews, 21,* 36-61

Satz T. (1970*) Ideology and Insanity: Essays on the Psychiatric Dehumanization of Man*. New York: Anchor Books

Scott AIF. (2005) College guidelines on electroconvulsive therapy: An update for prescribers. *Advances in Psychiatric Treatment, 11,* 150–156

Service User Research Enterprise (2002) review of consumers' perspectives on electroconvulsive therapy. *Institute of Psychiatry,* London

Shear MK, Simon N, Wall M, Zisook S, et al. (2011) Complicated grief and related bereavement issues for DSM-IV. *Depression and Anxiety, 28,* 2, 103-17

Shorter E. (2008) *Before Prozac: The Troubled History of Mood Disorders in Psychiatry*. Oxford University Press

Sinha JK, *et al.* (2011) 8th IBRO World Congress, Florence, Italy

Spillmann MK, et.al. ((2001) Tryptophan depletion in SSRI recovered depressed outpatients. *Psychopharmacology (Berl) 155, (2)*:123-127

Stagnitti M. (2005) Antidepressant use in the US non-institutionalized population 2002, Statistical Brief 77, Rockville, MD: Medical Expenditure Panel. *Agency for Healthcare Research and Quality*

Stompe T, et al. (2001) Guilt and depression: a cross-cultural comparative study. *Psychopathology, 2001, 34(6)*:289-98

Sublette ME, Ellis SP, Geant AL, Mann JJ. (2011) Meta-analysis of the effects of Eicosapentaenoic Acid (EPA) in clinical trials in depression. *Journal of Clinical Psychiatry*, 72, 12:1577-84

Squire L, Slatter P. (1983) Electroconvulsive therapy and complaints of memory dysfunction: A prospective three year follow-up study. *British Journal of Psychiatry*

Tariq MM, Streeten EA, Smith HA, et al. (2011) *Vitamin D: A potential role in reducing suicide risk?* Mood and Anxiety Program, Department of Psychiatry, University of Maryland School of Medicine

Teicher MH, Glod C, Cole C. (1990) Emergence of intense suicidal preoccupation during fluoxetine treatment. *American Journal of Psychiatry 147*(2), 207-10

Teimer H, et al. (2002) Vit B12, folate and homocysteine in depression: The Rotterdam study. *Americal Journal of Psychiatry*

TIME magazine, August. 26, 2002, *Inside the Anxious Brain*

Turner EH, et al. (2007) Selective publication of antidepressant trials and its influence on apparent efficacy. *New England Journal of Medicine. 358*: 252-260

UK ECT Review Group (2003) Efficacy and safety of electroconvulsive therapy in depressive disorders: A systematic review and meta-analysis. *Lancet, 361*:799-808

Wood J. (2011). 'Antidepressant use up 400 percent in U.S.' *Psych Central*. Retrieved on January 14, 2013, from http://psychcentral.com/news/2011/10/25/antidepressant-use-up-400-percent-in-us/30677.html

World Health Organization 2008, *The Global Burden of Disease 2004 update.* http://www.who.int/healthinfo/global_burden_disease/GBD_report_2004update_full.pdf

Zhao G, Ford ES, Li C, Greenlund KJ, Croft JB, Balluz LS. (2011) Use of folic acid and vitamin supplementation among adults with depression and anxiety: a cross-sectional, population-based survey. *Nutritional Journal Sep 30;10*:102

Chapter Eight

Bennet H. (2005) *Waking Up Dry: A Guide to Help Children Overcome Bedwetting.* American Academy of Pediatrics

Beyond frequency: Habit as mental construct (2006) *British Journal of Social Psychology, 45, 3*:639-656.

CDC – Centers for Disease Control and Prevention, USA. (2012) Smoking and Tobacco Use

Centers for Disease Control and Prevention. (2004—2005) Smoking-Attributable Mortality, Years of Potential Life Lost, and Productivity Losses—United States, 2000—2004. *Morbidity and Mortality Weekly Report 2008; 57* (45): 1226-8

Elman D. (1964) *Hypnotherapy*. Westwood Publishing

Glasser OC. (1910) The formation of habits at high speed. *Journal of Comparative Neurology and Psychology, 20, 3*:165-184

Lally P, van Jaarsveld CHM, Potts H, Wardle J. (2009) How are habits formed: modeling habit formation in the real world. *European Journal of Social Psychology*

Mathews R. (1992) How one in five has given up smoking. *New Scientist Magazine, Issue 1845.* (Reporting on research conducted by Schmidt and Viswesvaran, University of Iowa)

Office for National Statistics. (2011) General lifestyle survey 2009 report: *Smoking and drinking among adults*

Office for National Statistics. (2012) General lifestyle survey overview: *A report on the 2010 general lifestyle survey*

Substance Abuse and Mental Health Administration. (2010) Results from the 2010 National Survey on Drug Use and Health: *National Findings*. Rockville (MD): Office of Applied Studies

Wood W, Neal DT. (2007) A new look at habits and the habit-goal interface. *Psychological Review, 114*:843–863.

Chapter Nine

Albrecht U, Kirschner NE, Grüsser SM. (2007). Diagnostic instruments for behavioral addiction: An overview. *Psychosocial Medicine 4*: Doc11

Baskerville TA, Douglas AJ. (2010) Dopamine and oxytocin interactions underlying behaviors: Potential contributions to behavioral disorders. *CNS Neuroscience & Therapeutics, 16, 3*:e92-e123

Beasley JD. (1992) *Diagnosing and Managing Chemical Dependency*. New York: Amityville

Berridge KC, Robinson TE. (1998) What is the role of dopamine in reward: Hedonic impact, reward learning, or incentive salience? *Brain Research Review 1998;28*:309–69

Blaszczynski A, Nower L. (2002) A pathways model of problem and pathological gambling. *Addiction, 97, 5:487-499*

Blum K, (1991) *Alcohol and The Addictive Brain*. New York: The Free Press.

Boisvert RA, Martin LM, Grosek M, Clarie AJ. (2008) Effectiveness of a peer-support community in addiction recovery: Participation as intervention. *Occ Ther International, 15,* 4:205-220

Book P. (1997) *Sex & Love Addiction, Treatment & Recovery*. New York: Lucerne Publishing

Benson AL. ed. (2000) *I Shop Therefore I Am: Compulsive Buying and the Search for Self*. Northvale, NJ: Jason Aronson

Bradley BP. (1990) Behavioral addictions: Common features and treatment implications. *British Journal of Addiction, 85, 11*:1417-

1419

Carnes P. (2001) *Out of the Shadows: Understanding Sexual Addiction 3rd edition.* Hazelden

Faber RJ, O'Guinn TC. (1992) A clinical screener for compulsive buying. *Journal of Consumer Research, 19*:459–469

Grant JE, Brewer JA, Potenza MN. (2006) *The Neurobiology of Substance and Behavioral Addictions.* University of Minnesota Medical School

Grant JE, Potenza MN, Weinstein A, Gorelick DA. (2010) *Introduction to Behavioral Addictions.* University of Minnesota Medical School

Hagan K. (21 April, 2010) *Gambling Linked to One in Five Suicidal Patients.* Melbourne: The Age

Hagedorn WB, Juhnke GA. (2005) Treating the sexually addicted client: establishing a need for increased counselor awareness. *Journal of Addictions & Offender Counseling 25,* 2:66-86

Hassay DN. Smith CL. (1996) Compulsive buying: An examination of consumption motive. *Psychol Marketing. 13*:741–752

Hewig J, Kretschmer N, Trippe R, et al. (April 2010) Hypersensitivity to Reward in Problem Gamblers. *Biological Psychiatry, 67* (8) 781-783

Hornbacher M. (2011) *Waiting, A Non-Believer's Higher Power.* Hazelden Press

Hughes K. (2007) Migrating identities: The relational constitution of drug use and addiction. *Sociology of Health and Fitness, 29, 5*:673-691

iProspect (2012) *Survey of online buying habits.* Retrieved February 2013, from USA Today.com

Kim J, Haridakis PM. (2009) The role of internet user characteristics and motives in explaining three dimensions of internet addiction. *Journal of Computer-Mediated Communication, 14*:988-1015

Knauer S. (2002) *Recovering from Sexual Abuse, Addictions, & Compulsive Behaviors.* New York: Haworth Press

Koran LM, Faber RJ, Aboujaoude E, Large MD, Serpe RT. (2006) Estimated prevalence of compulsive buying behavior in the United States. *American Journal of Psychiatry, Oct; 163(10)*:1806-12

Kuzma J, Black DW. (2006) Compulsive shopping—when spending begins to consume the consumer. *Current Psychiatry. 7*:27–40

Landsbergis PA, Schurman SJ, et al. (1993) Job stress and heart disease: evidence and strategies for prevention. *New Solutions 3, 4*: 42-58

Li C-Y, Mao X, Wei L. (2008) Genes and (common) pathways underlying drug addiction. *PLOS Computational Biology 4(1):* e2.10.1371

Marks I. (1990) Behavioral (non-chemical) addictions. *British Journal of Addiction, 85, 11*:1389-1394

McElroy SL, Keck PE Jr, Pope HG Jr, Smith JM, Strakowski SM. (1994) Compulsive buying: A report of 20 cases. *Journal of Clinical Psychiatry, 1994 Jun; 55(6)*:242-8

Milton AL, Everitt BJ. (2009) The psychological and neurochemical mechanisms of drug memory reconsolidation: Implications for the treatment of addiction. *European Journal of Neuroscience, 31, 12*:2308-2319

National Council on Problem Gambling (2011) 'Statement of Keith S. Whyte, Executive Director, National Council on Problem Gambling. 'Internet Gaming: Is There a Safe Bet?' United States House of Representatives Energy & Commerce Committee, October 25, 2011'

National Council on Problem Gambling, Problem and Pathological Gambling in America: *The National Picture* (Report) January 1997

Nestler EJ. (2000) Genes and addiction. *Nature Genetics, vol 26*. Department of Psychiatry and Center for Neuroscience, University of Texas Southwestern Medical Center, Dallas, Texas, USA

PayPal Online Retail Report. (2009) Survey of online spending habits of 1000 adults. Reported in Guardian.co.uk Retrieved February 2013

Phillips D, Welty W, Smith M. (1997) Elevated suicide levels associated with legalized gambling. *Suicide and Life-Threatening Behavior 27 (4)*: 373–378

Potenza MN. (2006) Should addictive disorders include non-substance-related conditions? *Addiction, September, 101*: 142-51

Price AE. (2004) Heart disease and work. *Heart. September; 90(9):* 1077–1084.

Reid RC, Harper JM, Anderson EH. (2009) Coping strategies used by hypersexual patients to defend against the painful effects of shame. *Clinical Psychology & Psychotherapy, 16,* 2:125-138

Reith G. (2004) Consumption and its discontents: Addiction, identity and the problems of freedom. *The British Journal of Sociology, 55,* 2:283-300

Robinson BE. (1996) The psychosocial and familial dimensions of work addiction: Preliminary perspective and hypotheses. *Journal of Counseling & Development, 74,* 5:447-452

Ropelato J. (2012) *Internet Pornography Statistics.* From TopTenReviews.com

Shaffer HJ. (2004) Understanding the means and objects of addiction: Technology, the Internet, and gambling. *Journal of Gambling Studies, 12 (4):* 461-469

Sellman D. (2010) The ten most important things known about addiction. *Addiction, 105, 1*:6-13

Seo D, Sinha R. (2011) Neural mechanisms of stress and addiction. *Neuroimaging in Addiction*

Trimble MR, George MS. (2010) The addictions and disorders of motivation. *Bio Psychiatry, 3rd Edition,* 215-229

Volberg R. (2002) The Epidemiology of Pathological Gambling. *Psychiatric Annnals 32(3):* 171-178

Volkow ND. (2004) The reality of comorbidity: Depression and drug abuse. *Biological Psychiatry*

Wardle H. (2007) *British Gambling Prevalence Survey 2007*. National Centre for Social Research, Gambling Commission

West R. (2001) Theories of Addiction. *Addiction, 96, 1*:3-13

Wise RA. (1998) Drug-activation of brain reward pathways. *Drug Alcohol Depend. 51*, 13-22

Chapter Ten

AKF, American Kidney Fund Web site, retrieved February, 2013, from http://216.248.130.102/AboutAKF/Newsroom_020425 .htm

Anderson JW, Randles KM, Kendall CW, et al. (2004) Carbohydrate and fiber recommendations for individuals with diabetes:A quantitative assessment and meta-analysis of the evidence. *Journal of American College of Nutrition 2004 Feb;23(1)*:5-17

Anderson JW, Chen WL, Sieling B. (1980) Hypolipidemic effects of high-carbohydrate, high fiber diets. *Metabolism 29*: 551-558

Anderson J, Young L, Prior S. (2010) Nutrition for the Athlete, Colorado State University Extension. Retrieved February 2013 from http://www.ext.colostate.edu/pubs/foodnut/09362.html

Astrup A, Larsen TM, Harper A. (2004) Atkins and other low-carbohydrate diets: A hoax or an effective tool for weight loss? *The Lancet, 364, 9437*: 897–899

BBC News, 16 April 2007. *Chocolate better than kissing*. Reporting research conducted by Dr David Lewis, University of Sussex

Beezhold BL, Johnston CS. (2012) Restriction of meat, fish, and poultry in omnivores improves mood: A pilot randomized controlled trial. *Nutritional Journal, Feb 14,11*:9

Bone J. (2004) 'Diet doctor Atkins "obese", had heart problems: coroner. Widow angrily denies opponents' claims that heart condition caused by controversial diet.' *Ottawa Citizen, 11 February, 2004*:A11

Bravata DM, Sanders L, Huang J, et al. (2003) Efficacy and safety of low-carbohydrate diets: a systematic review. *JAMA, 289*:1837-1850. ('This review of 107 research studies on various low-carbohydrate, high-protein weight-reduction diets found that weight loss on these diets is due not to any special effect of carbohydrate restriction, but on the extent to which the dieters' caloric intake fell and how long they continued on the lower calorie diet.')

Brehm BJ, Seeley RJ, Daniels SR, D'Alessio DA. (2003) A randomized trial comparing a very low carbohydrate diet and a calorie-restricted low fat diet on body weight and cardiovascular risk factors in healthy women. *Journal of Clinical Endocrinology & Metabolism, 88*:1617-1623

Cameron M. (2002) *Carbohydrate's Role in Fat Loss*

Campbell, TC. (1979) Influence of nutrition on the metabolism of carcinogens (Martha Maso Honor's Thesis). *Advanced Nutrition Research 2*

Campbell TC, Campbell TM II. (2006) *The China Study*. ('The Most Comprehensive Study of Nutrition Ever Conducted and the Startling Implications for Diet, Weight Loss and Long-term Health.') BenBella Books

Cawley J, Meyerhoefer C. (2012) The medical care costs of obesity: An instrumental variables approach. *The Journal of Health Economics, 31*:219-30.

Chadwick DJ, Krahn DD. (2007) The epidemiology of obesity. *The Origins and Consequences of Obesity,*1-16. CIBA foundation symposium

Chapman C, Utton T. (2013) *Parents May Soon Outlive Obese Children*. Retrieved on Sunday 17 January, 2013 from MailOnline.

Chao A, Thun MJ, Connell CJ, et al. (2005) Meat consumption and risk of colorectal cancer. *JAMA. 12;293(2)*:172-82

Ciliska D. (1990) *Beyond Dieting*. New York: Brunner/Mazel

Colantuoni C, Schwenker J, McCarthy P, et al. (2001) Excessive sugar intake alters binding to dopamine and mu-opioid receptors in the brain. *Neuroreport. 12(16):* 3549–3552

Drewnowski DS, Krahn DD, et al. (1992) Taste responses and preferences for sweet high-fat foods: evidence for opioid involvement. *Physiology & Behavior 51,* 2:371-9

Drewnowski A, Popkin BM. (1997) The nutrition transition: new trends in the global diet. *Nutrition Reviews, 55*:31—43

Esseltsyn CB. (2008) *Prevent and Reverse Heart Disease: The Revolutionary, Scientifically Proven, Nutrition-Based Cure.* Penguin

Foreyt JP, Goodrick GK. (1992) *Living Without Dieting.* Harrison

Fortuna JL. (2012) The obesity epidemic and food addiction: clinical similarities to drug dependence, Department of Health Science, California State University, *Journal of Psychoactive Drugs. 2012 Jan-Mar;44(1)*:56-63

Foster GD, Wyatt HR, Hill JO, et al. (2003) A randomized trial of a low-carbohydrate diet for obesity. 'The low-carbohydrate diet produced a greater weight loss (absolute difference, approximately 4 percent) than did the conventional diet for the first six months, but the differences were not significant at one year.' *New England Journal of Medicine May 22;348(21)*:2082-90

Gearhardt AN, Yokum S, Orr P, et al. (2011) Neural correlates of food addiction. *Archives of General Psychiatry 68,* 808–816

Giovannucci E, Rimm EB, et al. (1994) Intake of fat, meat, and fiber in relation to risk of colon cancer in men. *Cancer Research, 54*:2390-7. 'Long-term daily intake of meat, particularly red meat, such as beef, pork, or lamb (as is common in Western countries), is associated with approximately a three-fold increased risk of colon cancer.'

Goodrick GK, Foreyt JP. (1991) Why treatments for obesity don't last. *American Dietetic Association, 91, 10*:1243

Groshams M, Sabine L, Falk K. (2011) Implications from addiction research towards the understanding and treatment of obesity. *Addiction Biology*

Herman CP, Polivy J, Lank CN, Heatgerton TF. (1987) Anxiety, hunger, and eating behavior. *Journal of Abnormal Psychology*

Herrera CP, Smith K, Atkinson F, et al. (2011) High-glycaemic index and high-glycaemic load meals increase the availability of tryptophan in healthy volunteers. *British Journal of Nutrition Jun; 105 (11)* :1601-6

Hyman M. (2011) *Food addiction: Could it explain why 70 per cent of America is fat?* Retrieved February 2013 from http://drhyman.com/blog/conditions/food-addiction-could-it-explain-why-70-percent-of-america-is-fat/

Hill AJ, Weaver CFL, Blundell JE. (1991) Food craving, dietary restraint, and mood. *Appetite, 17*:187-97

Joint WHO/FAO Expert Consultation. (2003) Diet, nutrition and the prevention of chronic diseases. *WHO Technical Report Series 916*

Kelemen LE, Kushi LH, Jacobs DR Jr, Cerhan JR. (2005) Associations of dietary protein with disease and mortality in a prospective study of postmenopausal women. *American Journal of Epidemiology, 161*:239–249.18. (This study followed nearly 30,000 women for 15 years. It found that coronary heart disease death was associated with red meat and dairy products intake when substituted for servings of carbohydrates. Coronary heart disease death was significantly reduced when animal protein was replaced with vegetable protein.)

Kennedy ET, Bowman SA, Spence JT, et al. (2003) Popular diets: Correlation to health, nutrition, and obesity. *Journal of American Diet Association, 101*:411-20

Kittagawa T, Owada M, Urakami T, et al. (1998) Increased incidence of non-insulin-dependent diabetes mellitus among Japanese schoolchildren correlates with an increased intake of animal protein and fat. *Clinical Pediatrics, 37*; 111-116

Knowler WC, Barrett-Connor E, Fowler SE, et al. (2002) Reduction in the incidence of Type-2 diabetes with lifestyle intervention or metformin

Kopelman PG, Caterson ID, Dietz WH, (2005) Genes and Obesity, Clinical Obesity in Adults and Children, 3rd Edition

Lagiou P, Sandin S, Lof M. (2012) Low carbohydrate-high protein diet and incidence of cardiovascular diseases in Swedish women: prospective cohort study. *British Medical Journal, 2012;344*:e4026

Lobstein T, Baur L, Uauy R. (2009) Obesity in children and young people: A crisis in public health. *Obestiy Reviews, 5,* 1:4-85

Madhavan TV, and Gopalan C.(1968) The effect of dietary protein on carcinogenesis of aflatoxin. *Archives of Pathology, 85*

Manore MM, Barr SI, Butterfield GE. (2000) Nutrition and athletic performance: Position of the American Dietetic Association, Dietitians of Canada, and the American College of Sports Medicine. *Journal of American Diet Association, 100*:1543-56

NHS, Starchy Foods. (2011) http://www.nhs.uk/livewell /goodfood/pages/starchy-foods.aspx

New York Times, 16 Sept. 2010, Teaching Doctors About Nutrition and Diet

Ogden CL, Carroll MD, et al. (2012) *Prevalence of Obesity in the United States,* 2009–2010, National Health and Nutritional Examination Survey

Ontario Medical Association. (2012) *It's Time to Start Taking Obesity Seriously.* Retrieved February 2013, from https:// www.oma.org/Mediaroom/PressReleases/Pages/ItsTimeToStartTakingObesitySeriouslyOntario'sDoctors.aspx

Ornish D, Brown SE, Scherwitz LW, et al. (1990) Can lifestyle changes reverse coronary heart disease? *Lancet 336*: 129-33

Pelchat ML. (2009) Food addiction in humans. *Journal of Nutrition, 2009 Mar; 139(3)*:620-2

Popkin BM, Doak CM. (1998) The Obesity Epidemic is a Worldwide Phenomenon, *Nutrition Reviews, 56,* 4:106-114

Physician's Committee for Responsible Medicine, Atkins Diet Alert. Retrieved February 2013 from www.atkinsdiet

alert.org/advisory.html

Roth G. (1984) *Breaking Free from Compulsive Eating*. New York: Bobbs-Merill

Sacks FM, Bra GA, Carey, VJ. (2009) Comparison of weight-loss diets with different compositions of fat, protein, and carbohydrates. *New England Journey of Medicine February 2009; 360*:859-873

Shugart HA. (2010) Consuming Citizen: Neo-liberating the obese body, communication. *Culture & Critique, 3, 1*:105-126

St Jeor, ST, Howard, BV, Prewitt, TE, et al. (2001) Dietary protein and weight reduction: a statement for health care professionals from the Nutrition Committee of the Council on Nutrition, Physical Activity, and Metabolism of the American Heart Association. 104:1869-74

Streib L. (2007) *World's Fattest Countries*. Retrieved February 2013 from Forbes

Tarnopolsky M. (2004) Protein requirements for endurance athletes. *Nutrition, 20, 7-8*, 662-668

Thorogood M, Mann J, et al. (1994) Risk of death from cancer and ischaematic heart disease in meat and non-meat eaters. *British Medical Journal*

University of Oxford (2009, 20 March) *Moderate Obesity Takes Years Off Life Expectancy*. Retrieved February 2013 from Science Daily

Trinko R, Sears RM, Guarnieri DJ, DiLeone RJ. (2007) Neural mechanisms underlying obesity and drug addiction. *Physiological Behaviors, 91*:499–505

Rajen AS, Basiotis PP. (1998) Is total fat consumption really decreasing? USDA Center for Nutrition Policy and Promotion (The decrease in percent of calories from fat is a result of increased total caloric intake and not necessarily due to decreased fat consumption. The daily fat intake in grams has, in fact, increased, in many cases reversing the trend of Americans consuming less fat in their diet as was reported earlier.)

UK Food Standards Agency. Retrieved February 2013 from www.eatwell.gov.uk/healthydiet/nutritionessentials/starch food. (Cutting out starchy foods, or any food group, can be bad for your health because you could be missing out on a range of nutrients. Low-carbohydrate diets tend to be high in fat, and eating a diet that is high in fat [especially saturated fat from foods such as meat, cheese, butter and cakes] could increase your chances of developing coronary heart disease... So, rather than avoiding starchy foods, it's better to try and base your meals on them, so they make up about a third of your diet.)

Vander, et al. (1998) *Human Physiology*. McGraw-Hill

Volkow ND, Wang GJ, Fowler JS, Telang F. (2008) Overlapping neuronal circuits in addiction and obesity: Evidence of systems pathology. *Philosophical Transactions of the Royal Society B: Biological Sciences, 363*:3191–200

West KM, Lalbfleisch JM. (1966) Influence of nutritional factors on prevalence of diabetes. *Diabetes 15*; 9-18

Westman EC, Yancy WS, Edman JS, et al., (2002) Effect of 6-month adherence to a very low carbohydrate diet program. *American Journal of Medicine, 113*:30-6

Wang CJ, Volkow ND, Logan J, et al. (2201) Brain dopamine and obesity. *Lancet, 357*:354-7

Wansink B, Chandon P. (2006) Meal size, not body size, explains errors in estimating the calorie content of meals. *Annals of Internal Medicine, 145 (5)*, 326-332

WHO Country Comparison, (2013) BMI Adults % Overweight, Most Recent.

WHO Global and Regional Food Consumption Patterns and Trends. 'There has been a remarkable increase in the intake of dietary fats over the past three decades and this increase has taken place practically everywhere except in Africa.'

Willett WC, Stampfer MJ, Colditz GA, Rosner BA, Speizer FE.

(1990) Relation of meat, fat, and fiber intake to the risk of colon cancer in a prospective study among women. *New England Journal of Medicine, 323*:1664-72. (Tens of thousands of women and men were included in this Harvard study which showed that regular meat consumption increases the risk of colon cancer by about 300%.)

World Cancer Research Fund/American Institute for Cancer Research (1997) *Food, Nutrition, and the Prevention of Cancer: a global perspective.* World Cancer Research Fund/American Institute for Cancer Research, Washington, DC.

Wurtman RJ, Wurtman JJ. (1995) *Brain serotonin, Carbohydrate-Craving, Obesity and Depression*. North American Association for the Study of Obesity.

Young VR, Pellett PI. (1994) Plant proteins in relation to human protein and amino acid nutrition. *American Journal of Clinical Nutrition, 59 (5 suppl):* 1203S-1212S

Chapter Eleven

Baumester RF, Smart LB, Joseph M. (1996) Relation of Threatened Egotism to Violence and Aggression: The dark side of self-esteem. *The Psychological Review, 103*:5-33

Berry R. (2004) *Hitler: Neither Vegetarian nor Animal Lover*. Pythagorean Publishers

Black D. (1998) *The Social Structure of Right And Wrong*. Academic Press

Branden N. (1969) *The Psychology of Self-Esteem*. Bantam

Broman-Fulks JJ, Berman FE, Rabian B, Webster MJ. (2004) Effects of aerobic exercise on anxiety sensitivity. *Behavior Research and Therapy, 42*, 125-136

Campbell J. (2004) *Pathways to Bliss*. New World Library

Chaouloff F. (1997) Effects of acute physical exercise on central serotonergic systems. *Medicine & Science in Sports & Exercise, 29 (1)*, 58-62

Dalai Lama (1998) *The Art of Happiness: A Handbook for Living.*

Hodder & Stoughton

DeSciol P, Kurzban R. (2009) The alliance hypothesis for human friendship. *PLOS ONE 4(6):* e5802. doi:10.1371/journal.pone .0005802

Ellis, A, et al. (1997) *A Guide to Rational Living 3rd rev edition.* Wilshire Book Company

Emerson RW. (1841) *Self-Reliance and Other Essays.* Dover ed.

Galper DI, Trivedi MH, Barlow CE, et al. (2006) Inverse association between physical activity and mental health in men and women. *Medicine & Science in Sports & Exercise, 38 (1),* 173-178

Hassmen P, Koivula N, Uutela A. (2000) Physical exercise and psychological well-being: A population study in Finland. *Preventive Medicine, 30,* 17-25

Jordan CH, Spencer SJ, Zanna MP, Hoshino-Browne, E, Correll J. (2003) Secure and defensive high self-esteem. *Journal of Personality and Social Psychology, 85,*969-978

Mruk CJ, 3rd Edition. (2006) *Self-Esteem, Research, Theory, and Practice: Toward a Positive Psychology of Self-Esteem.* New York: Springer Publishing

Piaget J. (1969) *The Psychology of the Child.* Basic Books

Sedikides C, Gregg AP. (2003) Portraits of the self. In M. A. Hogg & J. Cooper (Eds.), Sage *Handbook of Social Psychology* (pp. 110–138). London: Sage Publications

Shorter Oxford English Dictionary, 5th Edition. (2002) Definition of 'confidence' and 'self-esteem'.

Chapter Twelve

Black D. (1998) *The Social Structure of Right and Wrong.* New York: Academic Press

Campbell J. (2004) *Pathways to Bliss.* New World Library

DSM-V, Diagnostic and Statistical Manual of Mental Disorders (2013) American Psychiatric Association

Emerson RW. (1841) *Self-Reliance and Other Essays.* Dover ed. (1993)

Fabry JB. (1987) *The Pursuit of Meaning*. Berkeley, CA: Institute of Logotherapy Press

Frankl V. (1959) *Man's Search for Meaning*. New York: Pocket Books

Frankl V. (1978) *The Unheard Cry for Meaning*. Simon & Schuster

Helman L. (1973) *Pientimento*. Little, Brown

Jaspers K. (1951) *Way to Wisdom*. Yale University Press

Jung C. (1957) *The Undiscovered Self*. Routledge

Jung C. (1961) *Memories, Dreams, Reflections*. Random House

Lama Surya Das. (1997) *Awakening the Buddha Within*. Broadway Books

May R. (1994) *The Discovery of Being: Writings in Existential Psychology*. New York: Norton

May R. (1953) *Man's Search for Himself*. New York: Dell

Milne AE. (1926) *Winnie the Pooh Complete Collection* (2002). The Book People

Star J. (2001) *Tao Te Ching: Definitive Edition, Translation and Commentary of Lao Tsu*. Tarcher/Penguin Books

Storr A, ed. (1998) *The Essential Jung*. Fontana Press

Teilhard de Chardin P. (1955) Le Phénomène Humain, Editions du Seuil, (Eng. trans. B. Wall, 1959) *The Phenomenon of Man*. Collins

Tilloch P. (2000) *The Courage to Be*. Yale University Press

van Deurzen E, Arnold-Baker C, ed. (2005) *Existential Perspectives on Human Issues*. Palgrave-Macmillan

Yalom I. (1980) *Existential Psychotherapy*. New York: Basic Books

Bring Peter into Your Home

Want to benefit from Peter's wonderful therapeutic gift, but unable to visit him personally?

Now there is a solution.

Peter's unique, state-of-the-art therapeutic hypnosis recordings are available in the form of instant MP3 downloads or CDs, so that those who cannot visit him personally are able to benefit from aspects of his therapy in the comfort of their own home.

No matter where you are in the world or in life, Peter's powerful instant hypnosis downloads and CDs can help bring real change into your life.

Why not begin your journey today?

Visit the website:
www.hypnosiscdmp3downloads.com

About the Author

Peter Field MA CH MBACP FRSH is one of the leading hypnotherapists working in Britain today. With more than thirty years international hypnosis experience, he is an acknowledged Master in the healing art of hypno-psychotherapy. In addition to his busy therapy practice in London and Birmingham, UK, he is a lecturer, hypnotherapy instructor, regular BBC contributor and internationally recognised writer on psychotherapy, hypnosis, and health.

In addition to being a Board Certified Hypnotherapist (CH), he is also a qualified counselor, psychotherapist, and nutritionist.

Peter is the originator of CHI-HypnoTherapy™, an integrated therapeutic approach that works systematically with the person's subconscious mind. The result of thousands of hours of clinical experience, CHI-HypnoTherapy™ is designed to bring about rapid resolution of persistent psychological problems and difficulties.

Peter is a Member of the British Association for Counseling and Psychotherapy, the National Register for Psychotherapists and Counselors, The Association for Professional Hypnosis and Psychotherapy, and is a National Guild of Hypnotists Certified Instructor. The National Guild of Hypnotists (U.S.A.) is the oldest and largest professional hypnosis organization in the world.

In 2006 Peter was elected a Fellow of the Royal Society of Health.

www.peterfieldhypnotherapy.co.uk

Index

PSYCHE
BOOKS

The study of the mind: interactions, behaviours, functions. Developing and learning our understanding of self. Psyche Books cover all aspects of psychology and matters relating to the head.